THE TIGER PROTOCOL

THE TIGER PROTOCOL

AN INTEGRATIVE 5-STEP
PROGRAM TO TREAT AND
HEAL YOUR AUTOIMMUNITY

AKIL PALANISAMY, MD

balance

New York   Boston

Copyright © 2023 by Akil Palanisamy, MD
Foreword © 2023 by Mark Hyman, MD

Cover design by Jim Datz with Alexander Lozano
Cover image © Shutterstock
Cover copyright © 2023 by Hachette Book Group, Inc.

Balance
Hachette Book Group
1290 Avenue of the Americas
New York, NY 10104
GCP-Balance.com
Twitter.com/GCPBalance
Instagram.com/GCPBalance

First edition: May 2023

Balance is an imprint of Grand Central Publishing. The Balance name and logo are trademarks of Hachette Book Group, Inc.

The publisher is not responsible for websites (or their content) that are not owned by the publisher.

The Hachette Speakers Bureau provides a wide range of authors for speaking events. To find out more, go to hachettespeakersbureau.com or email HachetteSpeakers@hbgusa.com.

Balance books may be purchased in bulk for business, educational, or promotional use. For information, please contact your local bookseller or the Hachette Book Group Special Markets Department at special.markets@hbgusa.com.

Library of Congress Cataloging-in-Publication Data
Names: Palanisamy, Akil, author.
Title: The TIGER protocol : an integrative 5-step program to treat and heal your autoimmunity / Akil Palanisamy, MD.
Description: First edition. | New York : Balance, 2023. | Includes bibliographical references and index.
Identifiers: LCCN 2022057856 | ISBN 9781538726068 (hardcover) | ISBN 9781538726082 (ebook)
Subjects: LCSH: Autoimmune diseases—Diet therapy—Popular works. | Autoimmune diseases—Ayurvedic treatment—Popular works.
Classification: LCC RC600 .P35 2023 | DDC 616.97/80654—dc23/eng/20221223
LC record available at https://lccn.loc.gov/2022057856

ISBNs: 9781538726068 (hardcover), 9781538726082 (ebook)

Printed in the United States of America

LSC-C

Printing 1, 2023

To four generations of amazing women in my family, I am grateful for your presence in my life:

To my grandma "Teacher" Aaya, who raised six children while working as a schoolteacher and served as a pillar of her local community—may you rest in peace.

To my mom Padma, who believed in me before I even believed in myself—I wouldn't be here without you.

To my wife Aiswarya, for bringing more love and joy into my life than I could ever have imagined, and for always encouraging me to be the greatest version of myself—you are my sun and my moon.

To my daughter Alisha, for inspiring me with your curiosity, and for never ceasing to amaze me with your precociousness.

Contents

PART THREE
REACH THE NEXT LEVEL OF HEALTH

Foreword

THE HIDDEN PANDEMIC

Autoimmune disease has become a silent epidemic in modern times. Unlike COVID-19, autoimmune disorders have insidiously expanded to huge levels without attracting much attention. In just the past 10 years, some autoimmune diseases have increased by 300 percent. Others have risen up to *5,000 percent* in the past few decades.

One out of every five Americans suffers from some form of autoimmune condition. Hundreds of millions of people worldwide are struggling with autoimmunity. The prevalence and cost of autoimmune disease are greater than heart disease, cancer, and diabetes—combined.

There are more than 100 autoimmune conditions affecting people today, including Hashimoto's disease (also known as Hashimoto's thyroiditis), type 1 diabetes, multiple sclerosis, and rheumatoid arthritis. Sadly, the list continues to grow. Recent research has even shown that irritable bowel syndrome, the most common digestive disorder, is autoimmune in nature.

WHAT'S WRONG WITH THE SYSTEM?

Patients with autoimmune diseases are at a disadvantage in our current medical system. Conventional medicine excels at treating acute illnesses and injuries, but is ill-suited to tackle chronic diseases.

Such patients are often prescribed powerful immunosuppressive drugs that can subdue their symptoms—but this comes at a cost. These drugs can have serious side effects and unintended long-term consequences. More importantly, they only treat the symptoms and do nothing to address the underlying causes of autoimmune illness.

WHAT PATIENTS WANT

From my own three-plus decades of clinical experience, I know people are seeking natural alternatives to help them feel better and regain a healthy immune system. I have seen the frustration and despair that autoimmune patients experience. *The TIGER Protocol* is the comprehensive guidebook they have been waiting for—the solution that can transform their lives.

This book offers a revolutionary approach to healing. It introduces Dr. Akil's innovative five-step TIGER Protocol to reverse autoimmunity by addressing the root causes of disease. The program is broken down into actionable and manageable steps that are easy to follow—providing a detailed road map to health.

A TRIPLE THREAT

My friend Dr. Akil is a unique "triple threat" in the field of integrative medicine. He combines expertise in Functional Medicine with extensive training in Ayurveda and an understanding of the paleo diet and ancestral lifestyles.

On top of that, he has compassion and empathy because he has gone through a serious disease himself. As he detailed in his outstanding first book, *The Paleovedic Diet* (which combines a plant-based Paleo diet with Ayurvedic medicine), he overcame a mysterious illness that forced him to halt his medical training. He emerged with firsthand experience of the power of integrative medicine.

With this background, Dr. Akil is eminently qualified to give you the most accurate and reliable information on autoimmunity. I have the utmost confidence in his approach and the content he has put together.

FUNCTIONAL MEDICINE

Functional Medicine, which seeks to detect and treat diseases by addressing root causes (as opposed to conventional medicine's penchant for managing symptoms), is a movement I have been at the forefront of for decades. I am delighted to see Dr. Akil, one of the world's top experts in Functional Medicine, sharing how this powerful approach can be used to treat autoimmunity.

In addition, Dr. Akil has combined the best of leading-edge research and insights from Functional Medicine with the ancient wisdom of Indian Ayurveda to offer a complete healing plan for patients with autoimmune disorders.

Ayurveda has a great deal to offer in our modern fight against autoimmune ailments. There is a reason why it has survived for over 3,000 years! In this book, Dr. Akil has seamlessly integrated this ancient wisdom with modern science.

A MOUNTAIN OF RESEARCH

Although not widely known, there is an extensive body of research in integrative medicine. (For example, there have been over 50,000 papers published on the microbiome in the past decade alone.) Dr. Akil has read tens of thousands of research papers on these topics and brought together their essential points into a single, user-friendly source (with 800-plus references!).

In other words, Dr. Akil has "climbed the mountain" of autoimmune research so you don't have to.

In addition, he has treated thousands of autoimmune patients over a career spanning more than two decades, so you can trust that the recommendations he makes in this book are clinically proven and tested. You'd be hard-pressed to find another book in which all these medical advances and insights are compiled in a single, accessible place.

TREATING ROOT CAUSES

As a Functional Medicine practitioner, I always believe it's best to treat the root causes of health issues. Dr. Akil will teach you his TIGER Protocol to help you identify and address each of the key root causes of *all* autoimmune conditions: toxins, infections, gut microbiome, eating right, and rest (or lack thereof).

Right off the bat, this is an important insight into autoimmune diseases. Although there are over 100 different varieties of autoimmunity, the root causes are the same and lead to the same basic dysfunction of the immune system. The particular autoimmune condition you end up with depends on what your "weak link" is, based on genetics and lifestyle.

This news is empowering for patients because they can understand what is causing their autoimmunity and learn what they can do about it.

THE BEST DIET FOR EVERYONE

I truly believe this book can revolutionize our approach to all those on the auto-immune spectrum, whether they are suffering from inflammatory symptoms like fatigue, joint pain, rashes, or digestive issues, or even if they are dealing with full-blown autoimmune disease.

In fact, I would argue that the diet plan outlined in this book, with its emphasis on building gut microbiome diversity with prebiotic and fermented foods, offers the healthiest, most well-rounded approach to eating out there—one that all people should follow.

We know that a diverse microbiome—which depends largely on your diet—is one of the most important factors in living a long and healthy life. *The TIGER Protocol* provides you with the most up-to-date understanding of the dietary approach that can best achieve this, including specific foods, recipes, and meal plans to try.

CUTTING-EDGE MICROBIOME RESEARCH

The section on the microbiome is one of the many gems in this book. The insights Dr. Akil offers about the microbiome are among the most advanced and sophisticated I have seen in any book. Yet he has conveyed these complex concepts in ways the average person can easily understand and implement.

One of the hallmarks of autoimmune disorders, and most modern afflictions, is a loss of gut bacteria diversity and an imbalance in the microbiome. The trillions of bacteria living inside of you have been linked to many autoimmune diseases—but also to such disparate conditions as allergies, asthma, diabetes, eczema, obesity, heart disease, fibromyalgia, and migraines.

It is absolutely crucial for those suffering from autoimmune conditions, or any other chronic illness, to restore and boost the diversity of their gut microbiome. I would go one step further and say that this should be a top priority for *all* people because the hallmark of the modern Western microbiome is a significant loss of diversity compared to the robust microbiome of our ancestors.

Dr. Akil gives you a detailed plan on how to achieve this. He explains in depth which foods contain each of the key classes of prebiotics necessary to strengthen your gut microbiome—inulin, resistant starch, polyphenols, oligosaccharides, and more. He teaches you to leverage herbs and spices for maximum benefit. And his tables on the top polyphenol-containing foods are eye-opening! You will find these and many more strategies on how to improve your microbiome in *The TIGER Protocol*.

TOXINS: THE MISSING LINK

Dr. Akil argues that toxins are overlooked in their impact on autoimmune disease; I couldn't agree more. I have seen repeatedly in my own practice how discovering and eliminating toxins can have a profound impact on patients dealing with autoimmunity.

In my own case, I suffered from undiagnosed mercury toxicity. This led to debilitating chronic fatigue syndrome. But by using the principles of Functional Medicine, I was able to clear out the mercury, heal my gut, and recover completely.

Dr. Akil shines the spotlight on toxins as one of the key unrecognized drivers of autoimmunity and helps you begin your healing journey by addressing toxins first in *The TIGER Protocol*.

WHY THIS BOOK STANDS OUT

Other books on this topic have various concerning issues. Some of them are not written by physicians and give you dangerous advice, like telling you to stop your medications abruptly. (Like Dr. Akil, I believe that any tapering of medications should be done gradually under the supervision of your physician.) Other books present diet plans that are too extreme or try to upsell supplements or programs created by the author.

The TIGER Protocol has none of these flaws. It is unbiased and free of commercial interests. The diet plan it offers is moderate and balanced. The program it recommends is a sage middle ground that is effective without being draconian. It is written by a globally renowned doctor who is a widely respected authority in the field of Functional Medicine.

AN UNMATCHED RESOURCE

I believe every patient with autoimmune or inflammatory issues would benefit from reading this book.

Dr. Akil provides readers with a powerful action plan to prevent, treat, and even reverse autoimmune disorders. *The TIGER Protocol* is packed full of evidence-based guidelines, case studies, and practical tools to help you take charge of your health. It is filled with pioneering new ideas and groundbreaking insights. And best of all, it's exceptionally well-written and enjoyable to read.

You don't have to settle for anything less than feeling your best and having the optimal quality of life—regardless of what your diagnosis is. *The TIGER Protocol* is an unrivaled guide that will empower you with information and strategies to take charge of your health and thrive. The knowledge and tools are in your hands now; it's up to you to take advantage and start feeling better!

—Mark Hyman, MD

INTRODUCTION

In the United States, autoimmune disease is the third most common type of illness after heart disease and cancer, affecting 1 in 12 Americans or an estimated 25 million people.[1] An additional 41 million people have high blood levels of proteins known as autoantibodies, which put them at risk of developing autoimmune disease.[2] Autoimmune conditions occur when the body turns against itself—when its immune system attacks healthy tissues and organs. If you are living with an autoimmune condition, you are likely very keenly aware of this.

Worldwide, it is estimated that autoimmune diseases affect around 5 percent of the population, well over 300 million people.[3] Unlike heart disease or diabetes, autoimmune disease is multifaceted—over 100 different autoimmune diseases have been identified.[4]

In my two decades of medical practice, I have worked with many patients who felt confused, hopeless, or uninformed about their diagnosis of autoimmune disease or experience of its symptoms and, despite conventional therapy, they still struggled with poor quality of life. This motivated me to use my training in Western medicine and complementary therapies to create an integrative medicine approach, which I began using to treat my autoimmune patients.

This turned out to be remarkably effective for both patients with full-blown disease and those who had been told they were on the path to autoimmunity. Through this work, I have formulated a simple protocol based on my success in treating autoimmune patients—a protocol that treats and can potentially reverse the consequences of long-term disease and also takes a person off the path of suffering in years to come.

The foundation of my approach is the use of specific healing foods. Diet can be a powerful healing tool, but typical autoimmune diets are restrictive, and this makes them hard to adhere to. In my work with an active panel of autoimmune patients, I have developed a diet that is less draconian but still maintains clinical efficacy. This broader, more inclusive, and palatable diet is easier—and more pleasant—for people to follow for a longer period of time—thus making it more effective. This book presents a simplified protocol which you can do on your own, via easy-to-follow Phase 1 and Phase 2 diets. This will enable you to eliminate the necessary food sensitivities in the short term, then reintroduce foods to achieve a more diverse and balanced diet, which is key to long-term success in autoimmunity and overall health.

AYURVEDIC ROOTS

When developing this protocol, I was influenced by my training in Ayurveda, the traditional medicine of India. According to Ayurveda, all disease occurs as a result of a six-stage process. Only in the fifth stage do symptoms occur. In the first four stages, unrecognized imbalances are occurring that relate to changes in digestion and accumulation of toxins. A skilled Ayurvedic physician seeks to identify disease in the earliest stages and halt its progression before it becomes worse and triggers symptoms, leading to a disease diagnosis. This inspired me to take a proactive approach to all patients, and especially those who are on the autoimmune spectrum. Prevention is preferable to cure (and usually easier, too).

As a Harvard-trained M.D., my approach involves a strong scientific background in biochemistry and Western medicine alongside my training in Ayurveda and alternative therapies. In my integrative medicine practice, I also might utilize functional medicine—a modality that uses specialized lab testing to diagnose and treat imbalances in the function of different organ systems. Over the past two decades, my comprehensive approach has helped thousands of autoimmune patients to achieve remission, minimize their use of medications, and achieve optimal energy and quality of life.

A WORSENING CRISIS

At the time of this writing, autoimmune disease is the fastest growing category of disease, and, unfortunately, research suggests that this might get even worse. A recent study investigated the prevalence of antinuclear antibodies, a common biomarker of autoimmunity, over a 25-year period in the United States.[5]

An antibody is a protein produced by the immune system that binds to substances the body considers foreign and marks them for elimination by the immune system; this could include microbes, toxins, pollen, etc.—and in the case of autoimmunity, normal body proteins that should usually not cause antibody production. Antinuclear antibody (ANA) is one example of such an autoantibody (antibody to one's own tissues) that binds to components in our human cells.

From around 1988 to 2012, the prevalence of ANA increased by 44 percent; this corresponds to an estimated 41 million individuals in the United States in 2012. Most troubling was that the values for adolescents and teenagers increased nearly 300 percent over the study period.

While not all of these persons will go on to develop autoimmune disease, and a positive ANA is not diagnostic of a specific disease, ANAs are commonly seen in patients with several autoimmune conditions. Autoantibodies like ANA may predate clinical disease by years. The striking increase in these autoimmune antibodies is highly concerning. To this we add the COVID-19 pandemic, which may further exacerbate the situation, as the virus has the potential to contribute to autoimmunity (as I will explain in chapter 1).

A LONG JOURNEY

A survey by the American Autoimmune Related Diseases Association (AARDA) found that it takes the average person about three years and seeing four different doctors before getting a correct diagnosis of autoimmune disease. During that time, patients are often told that it's all in their head or that they are complaining excessively or overly concerned about their health.[6]

Subsequently, once patients actually receive the diagnosis, they will typically be referred to a specialist who will be highly trained and skilled in recommending and managing medications, but perhaps less skilled in addressing root causes such as diet, the microbiome, and toxins. Often, my patients tell me that their specialist told them that food has no impact on their condition, and they have been frustrated that connections they have observed between nutrition and their own symptoms have been dismissed. If any of this sounds familiar, or if you have been seeking to understand the root causes of your autoimmune condition, you have come to the right place.

OPPORTUNITIES FOR EARLY INTERVENTION

Autoimmune disease develops slowly over a number of years before finally manifesting. Sometimes, this development spans decades. Consider the autoimmune liver disease, primary biliary cirrhosis. In this case, the diagnostic autoantibody known as anti-mitochondrial antibody can be detected up to 25 years before the clinical manifestation of the disease. In rheumatoid arthritis, for example, rheumatoid factor autoantibodies sometimes appear 12–14 years before the development of symptoms.[7]

The lengthy process of disease development means that there is a substantial window of time during which early detection and holistic treatment can have critically important benefits. One of the key steps in the development of autoimmunity, linked to many autoimmune conditions, is the development of increased intestinal permeability, also known as "leaky gut syndrome"—which may or may not have symptoms, but can be detected by lab tests.[8] Thus, autoimmunity exists in a continuum—what I call "the autoimmune spectrum"—ranging from asymptomatic individuals with positive antibodies to patients with full-blown autoimmune disease and severe symptoms. The earlier we can identify someone on the autoimmune spectrum, the greater the impact we can have.

THE AUTOIMMUNE SPECTRUM

The autoimmune spectrum is based on our understanding that autoimmunity develops gradually over a long period of time, punctuated by key milestones like the occurrence of leaky gut syndrome, increased subclinical inflammation, and the development of autoimmune antibodies. In addition, studies suggest that changes in the microbiome, the trillions of bacteria in our digestive tract, play a key role in the dysregulation of the immune system.

In the earliest stages, antibodies can be detected but there may not be any clinical symptoms. In later stages, there may be indications that something is not quite right such as fatigue, muscle aches, difficulty concentrating, joint pains, mental health issues, digestive symptoms labeled as "irritable bowel syndrome" (a description of symptoms rather than a specific disease), or other nonspecific signs. We now know that through the gut-brain axis even anxiety or depression can be triggered by inflammation in the body and sometimes be linked to imbalances in the gut.[9] The final stage is when tissue damage occurs, and the autoimmune disease is diagnosed.

I have had a number of patients with positive autoantibodies who did not yet meet the criteria for any particular autoimmune disease—they were still early on the autoimmune spectrum, and often had nonspecific symptoms like malaise, poor sleep, brain fog, mysterious rashes, numbness and tingling, or other unexplained symptoms. They were told by doctors that they would eventually develop lupus, rheumatoid arthritis, or multiple sclerosis (and had to wait until then to begin treatment). Through applying this protocol, nearly all of them have been able to prevent the disease from occurring, and progress toward optimal health.

DRIVING THE IMMUNE SYSTEM

Think of your immune system as a car. In autoimmunity, the gas pedal is pressed to the floor, driving the immune system out of control. Conventional medicines like steroids or immunosuppressants are the equivalent of slamming on the brakes. While these will slow the car down, if we ease up on the brakes (e.g., by reducing medication dose) the car will speed up again since the accelerator is engaged. The root causes of autoimmune disease are pushing the gas pedal down. If we can address them and release the gas pedal, then the car is much more likely to slow down and return to a normal speed. Once the gas pedal is released, both holistic and conventional therapies that seek to put the brakes on the immune system can work better.

Although autoimmune disease can be difficult to treat, people can be empowered to know that they can take action and follow specific steps that might improve the course of their disease. Also, they can understand that their disease is not a complete mystery, that we have some ideas about key mechanisms in the development of autoimmune disease.

Root Causes

The development of autoimmunity is a multistep process, with factors like food sensitivities, infections, leaky gut syndrome, toxins, hormone imbalances, and stress driving the progression—tilting the scales until the body's immune system attacks itself. Dysbiosis, in which there's a lack of good bacteria and too many bad ones in the microbiome, is also implicated in many autoimmune diseases.

The earlier these root causes are identified, the easier it is to work on and potentially reverse them. Therefore, if autoimmunity is recognized in its initial stages, people could have the opportunity to implement diet and lifestyle changes and natural healing protocols to potentially prevent them from progressing further, to the development of a full-blown autoimmune disease. Through specialized lab testing, such as an autoimmune reactivity blood test, it's now possible to identify people at these early stages of autoimmunity. Such a test, offered by certain laboratories, can measure a variety of predictive autoantibodies to various tissues and organs, indicating a latent predisposition to develop an autoimmune condition.

Often, patients who are on the autoimmune spectrum but do not meet the criteria for a disease treatable with medication fall through the cracks in conventional medicine. Patients who have positive antibodies but whose symptoms are mild or nonexistent are often told that there is nothing they can do to prevent the progression of their disease. Unfortunately, they are often told by their physicians that they will probably get an autoimmune disease in a few years, and to return when their symptoms get worse so they can be prescribed medication.

Myths and Misinformation

My patients report having encountered a lot of conflicting advice when they began learning and researching about autoimmune diseases. On the one hand, conventional sources focus on medications and new drugs that are being developed to treat autoimmune patients by suppressing the immune system in some way. That contrasts with some alternative practitioners who promise a complete cure to autoimmune conditions with simple dietary changes, assuring patients that they can stop all of their medications.

First, there is an important distinction between remission vs. cure. Second, altering nutrition can be a good starting point, but is rarely able to totally shift the course of the disease, let alone lead to a full remission. Finally, when it comes to weaning patients off medications, I am very cautious and conservative, and work closely with the patient's other physicians and specialists.

My approach is more of a middle ground, utilizing conventional medications when appropriate but focusing attention on the science-based root causes that have been identified as triggers for autoimmunity. There is a growing interest in how natural therapies and integrative medicine can fit into treatment for auto-immune conditions, but there are many myths and misconceptions about these approaches as well. As a result, most patients that I talk to are confused about these topics and have many legitimate questions.

Cure vs. Remission

In cases where a patient is early on the autoimmune spectrum and does not yet have a full-blown disease, there may be a possibility of a cure. While autoimmune disease is usually not curable, it can be put into remission and allow you to have a normal quality of life without disabling symptoms. I think of remission as a time when a person's autoimmune disease becomes quiet and no longer causes symptoms. Often, a remission can even feel like a cure because a person can feel as well as they felt before they developed the condition.

My clinical experience suggests that remission can last indefinitely. But we live in a society that is hard on our immune systems due to issues with food supply, toxins, and stress, all of which make it challenging for patients with autoimmune conditions to maintain their health. Thus, patients with autoimmunity who achieve remission need to be vigilant and pay attention to their diet, lifestyle, and stress in order to stay in balance.

KEY QUESTIONS

"But I don't have a history of autoimmune disease in my family... Why me?"

This is one of the most common questions. My answer is that family history matters a lot less now when it comes to autoimmune conditions. In today's world, a perfect storm of factors has come together to cause an explosion in autoimmune disorders—even in those without a family history. The dramatic increase in environmental toxins and pollutants is taxing our immune systems such that autoimmunity can arise even if one does not carry the genes predisposing to autoimmune disease.

"Can you tell me why this disease happened to me?"

Most patients with autoimmune disorders have been told it's not fully understood why they got their disease—but I want to tell them that that is not what the science says. In fact, studies show that a number of key factors have been shown to contribute to autoimmune diseases, including toxins, infections, gut imbalances, food sensitivities, and stress. Research into the microbiome and increased intestinal permeability has revolutionized our understanding of the early stages of autoimmune disease—studies show that these gut changes can develop even before the autoimmune disease first manifests.

"Is it true that diet doesn't matter and only medications can impact my disease?"

Typically, patients with autoimmune conditions are told that the only thing they can do is take medications—that diet, lifestyle, stress management, and natural treatments are ineffective. However, a growing body of research supports the benefits of nonpharmacologic interventions like stress reduction techniques, improved diet, gut healing, and certain natural treatments in patients with autoimmune disease. There are areas they can look into that are less well-known but implicated to have significant effects on the immune system, such as the health of the oral microbiome, unfamiliar toxins like mold-related mycotoxins, or the impact of a type of trauma known as adverse childhood experiences (ACEs). There are unique interventions that are very promising, such as a compounded medicine called low-dose naltrexone or certain types of acupuncture.[10]

REDUCTIONISM VS. HOLISM

Patients with autoimmune diseases are typically treated by assorted specialists, who approach the treatment of autoimmune disease at the organ and tissue level. An endocrinologist will treat Hashimoto's as a thyroid disease. A rheumatologist will treat rheumatoid arthritis as a joint disease. A neurologist will treat multiple sclerosis as a nervous system disorder, and so on. And yet, it goes unsaid that the same underlying mechanisms of autoimmune disease apply to all these patients, despite their disparate clinical pictures and different end organs that are affected. This fragmentation reflects the siloed approach of conventional medicine to treat diseases based on the particular organ affected—but this is not the best way to approach autoimmune disease.

Instead, a holistic, integrative medicine approach, incorporating both conventional and complementary therapies, can lead to better outcomes and improved quality of life for a person with autoimmune disease. Such an approach seeks to target the root cause of autoimmune disease, the immune system dysfunction, which is present in all autoimmune disorders regardless of which organ is ultimately affected. There is value in targeting these common mechanisms in all people who are on the autoimmune spectrum.

THE TIGER PROTOCOL

It is for these reasons that I developed the TIGER Protocol for autoimmune diseases. My protocol covers the key root causes that should be addressed to prevent or reverse autoimmune conditions:

T—toxins
I—infections
G—gut health
E—eat right
R—rest

The order of the acronym is important as it presents the best order in which to address these factors. I'll explain why this sequence is optimal. The first step is to address toxins, as it is essential to improve liver functioning prior to the potential pathogen "die-off" that might occur in step two, where we focus on killing the pathogens that cause infection. Killing pathogens can sometimes lead to "die off," wherein the toxins released by the dying pathogens need to be cleared by the liver. If the liver is already overloaded from toxins, this process can create some unpleasant symptoms.

Many infections cause a degree of "leaky gut" syndrome or increased intestinal permeability, so trying to heal the gut in step three without first removing the infections in step 2 will not be effective. In step 3, healing and optimizing gut function helps to improve digestion and absorption of nutrients. This ensures that the beneficial foods added during step 4 can have their maximal impact. Adding in therapeutic foods without first optimizing gut function is not ideal because their healing nutrients may not otherwise be absorbed properly.

In step 5, rest incorporates stress reduction and clearing emotional stress from the body. The other factors such as toxins, infections, and gut imbalances are actually a form of stress on the body, which directly impacts the glands and organs and contributes to overall stress load. Once these are taken care of, then clearing emotional stress will have an even more significant impact in improving the way one feels. For reasons such as these, following the optimal sequence is critical, and I provide detailed practical guidance on how to do so.

HOW TO USE THIS BOOK

The TIGER Protocol is divided into three sections, beginning with a basic explanation of the immune system and how it goes awry in autoimmune conditions. part 1 covers key mechanisms like molecular mimicry and the bystander effect, and I explain the different aspects of the TIGER Protocol in detail. I review the scientific and clinical data that connects each of these five root causes to autoimmunity. We discuss the main factors that are responsible for the skyrocketing increase in autoimmune disorders, such as increasing toxin exposure and chronic infections.

I then review the top five most important bacteria in the gut microbiome. Known as keystone species, these little-known bacteria (such as F. prausnitzii and Akkermansia) play an absolutely crucial but unrecognized role in modulating inflammation, autoimmunity, and the overall health of the gut and the entire body. Studies show that decreased levels in these keystone species are one of the key factors in autoimmune conditions. I introduce the Phase 1 Diet, which is an elimination diet meant to jump-start detoxification, reduce inflammation, and promote weight loss to help get things on the right track.

In part 2, you'll learn how to implement the protocol and put all the recommendations into practice. We discuss detoxification, identifying and treating infections, gut-healing protocols, and how to rest properly. I present the Phase 2 Diet in detail, which is a long-term eating plan that reintroduces key foods and serves as the sustainable foundation for long-term well-being and vitality. This includes the top healing foods for the microbiome, which are evidence-based foods with unique prebiotic effects.

In part 3, I talk about treatments that can help "reboot" the immune system to reduce autoimmunity. Once the root causes have been addressed by implementing the TIGER Protocol, then treatments that are intended to modulate the immune system tend to work much better. These include herbs, botanicals, vitamins, compounded medications, and natural therapies that are intended to quell autoimmunity, like fasting or acupuncture.

In part 3, we'll also put everything together to help you to create a customized healing plan, which includes key vitamins and supplements. I discuss a daily routine that will help build health by addressing all the key components of well-being and resilience. This section also provides guidance for troubleshooting, if, after working through the book, you continue to feel unwell. It concludes with a detailed diet and lifestyle program putting together all the concepts from the book. I review next steps in terms of considering other modalities or selecting an integrative medicine practitioner to work with. Appendixes include TIGER Protocol recipes and a complete two-week menu plan.

One of my colleagues defines health as "the ability to live your dreams." This sentiment is consistent with my worldview that a sense of purpose is crucial in life, as is having aspirations that infuse life with a sense of meaning and direction. Having a body that is well enough to enable one to pursue their goals and ambitions is vital. The holistic approach contained in *The TIGER Protocol* will help you to achieve health—to reduce the occurrence of flare-ups, attain remission with a minimum of medications, and feel your best so that you can live life to the fullest.

PART ONE

UNDERSTAND THE TIGER PROTOCOL

CHAPTER 1

Overview—Immune Systems Gone Haywire

A nurse at her local hospital, forty-four-year-old Brenda was diagnosed with Hashimoto's disease, an autoimmune thyroid condition, after experiencing otherwise unexplainable fatigue, weight gain, and hair loss. She had two young children and her symptoms were making it hard for her to manage her family's busy schedule and demanding job. Her thyroid hormone levels were suboptimal but still technically normal, indicating that the attack on her thyroid gland was not yet critical.

She saw her doctor, who told her that because her thyroid hormone levels were not out of the normal range, she did not qualify for a prescription and there was nothing he could do—eventually her immune system would destroy her thyroid and she should return at that time to be prescribed thyroid replacement hormone. An independent thinker, Brenda was used to finding her own solutions to problems and believed that there had to be another approach.

Does this sound familiar to you? Perhaps for years you have been struggling with similar symptoms, but none of the diagnoses you have received feel appropriate, and the medications you have been prescribed do not help, or else they cause unwanted side effects.

We will come back to Brenda's case later in the chapter, to illustrate that there is often a lot you can do even when you have been told that "there is nothing you can do." But first, let me tell you more about how common challenges with autoimmunity are, and teach you about the basics of the immune system.

As discussed, autoimmune disease rates are skyrocketing, making it the fastest growing category of disease. The incidence of type I diabetes has increased fivefold since 1950 in certain countries.[1] Rates of celiac disease, an autoimmune disease exacerbated by exposure to wheat, have also risen about fivefold in the past 50 years.[2] The growth of autoimmune diseases in children is especially worrisome, with some conditions growing tenfold in the past few decades.[3] Almost all varieties of autoimmune conditions, numbering more than 100, are increasing.[4]

But why are autoimmune disease rates rising so steeply? To answer this question, we have to understand the perfect storm of risk factors that have come together to create this raging epidemic. But first, you need to know a bit about the basics of your immune system.

MEET YOUR IMMUNE SYSTEM

We live in a sea of microbes. They are within our body, outnumbering our human cells, and all around us, and your immune system is a sophisticated network of defense systems that protect you from these microbes. When your immune system is underactive, you become at risk for serious infections. When it is overactive, your risk of autoimmune diseases develops.

Your immune system is distributed throughout your entire body, including your thymus (a gland located in the upper chest), lymph nodes, spleen, bone marrow, liver, blood, and cells that sweep through and scrutinize every organ.[5] At a basic level, it can be divided into the innate and adaptive components. The function of the immune system is incredibly complex; what follows is a simplified explanation so we can explore a few key concepts.

Innate vs. Adaptive

While there is often much interaction between them, the innate and adaptive branches can be thought of as the two main components of the immune system. The **innate** immune system is the first responder—it consists of white blood cells and all the proteins and messengers that trigger an immediate reaction when your body decides that it needs to defend itself against an invader. This response is instant and powerful, but nonspecific, and sometimes damages surrounding normal tissues in its haste.

The **adaptive** branch, a hallmark of more evolved animals, is slower but more targeted and precise; although its reaction may take days to weeks, it ensures a more accurate response, and preserves memory so that the immune system can respond more quickly the next time it encounters a specific pathogen.[6] Memory from these immune cells can last for years or decades.

The adaptive response includes B cells and T cells, including a subtype of T cells called T regulatory cells. Considered the master regulators of the immune system, these cells are crucial for "keeping the peace" within the immune system and play a major role in the development of autoimmune disease, as we will see later.

Molecular Mimicry

The first mechanism through which autoimmune disease occurs involves a case of mistaken identity called molecular mimicry, in which a foreign protein—found on a bacteria, virus, or food—resembles a protein found within the human body. Our immune system generally produces antibodies, which, to review, are proteins that bind specifically to foreign proteins and mark them for attack and breakdown by immune cells.

Antibodies are used by the immune system to distinguish foreign invaders from the body's own cells and should never bind to your own cells or tissues. However, the same antibodies produced against a foreign protein could mistakenly bind to a protein on one of your cells if there is a strong similarity between them—thus triggering the immune system to attack and destroy human tissues, while mistakenly thinking that it is attacking invaders. To use a military analogy, it is a case of "friendly fire."

For example, a common virus known as Coxsackie B virus is implicated in type I diabetes. This is a condition in which the body attacks and destroys cells of the pancreas known as beta cells, which produce insulin necessary for regulating blood sugar. The virus contains a protein that strongly resembles an enzyme found in the pancreatic beta cells; when the immune system produces antibodies against the viral protein they may instead bind to the beta cells of the pancreas, triggering an immune system attack that is considered part of the process by which type I diabetes develops.[7]

Another example is Guillain-Barré syndrome, a disease affecting the nerves which causes weakness of the muscles and even paralysis in severe cases. Most of the time, a preceding infection is identified that triggers this condition. The most common offender is a bacteria called Campylobacter, which is the most common cause of bacterial diarrhea in the United States.[8] Proteins in the outer cell wall of Campylobacter have a striking similarity to those found in human nerves, and the cross-reactivity of these antibodies is known to be one of the major causes of Guillain-Barré syndrome.[9]

Many such examples exist. However, it is important to know that the susceptibility of the individual makes a big difference. Not every person who gets Coxsackie B virus or Campylobacter will develop the associated autoimmune conditions. This illustrates the several-step process needed to develop an autoimmune disease, and why it is necessary to intervene with a multi-pronged approach to reduce autoimmunity, as we will be discussing in this book.

Bystander Effect

The second model of autoimmune development involves a case of "collateral damage" known as bystander effect.[10] In this scenario, the immune system works hard to eradicate and destroy a foreign invader that has entered the body. However, in its overzealous efforts to destroy the pathogen, it may damage and destroy some of the surrounding human tissue as well.

If your immune system identifies a group of virus-infected cells, it recruits a strong inflammatory response and brings large white blood cells known as macrophages to the affected area. These cells release toxic compounds that kill the virus-infected cells but also damage the uninfected neighboring cells in the area.

The bystander effect is also thought to be one of the mechanisms by which toxins such as heavy metals trigger inflammation and autoimmunity, as we will discuss in chapter 2.[11]

T Regulatory Cells

This type of immune cell plays a key role in the development of autoimmune disease; instability in these cells has been linked to increased risk of autoimmunity.[12] Conversely, interventions and factors that lead to improving the number and function of these cells are beneficial in autoimmune disease. They are the key regulators of the immune system, and they help to ensure normal activity and prevent autoimmunity.

This is one of the themes that we will be returning to frequently as we discuss strategies and treatments that favorably impact T regulatory cells. Emerging therapies that seek to reprogram T regulatory cells to treat autoimmune conditions are currently in clinical trials, as I will explain in chapter 12.

GENETICS VS. EPIGENETICS

Genetics is still relevant as family history does play a role in predisposing a person to autoimmune disease. But environmental factors are more important than genes—studies of identical twins have found that in most cases, a twin with an autoimmune disease has an unaffected twin, indicating that non-genetic factors are critical.[13]

Suffice it to say, your genes do not determine your destiny. The science of epigenetics describes how non-genetic factors such as your diet, lifestyle, behavior, and environment can change the expression of your genes.[14]

The choices that you make in your day-to-day life may dictate the expression of those genes—whether they are turned on or off—more so than whatever genes you inherited from your parents. Your genes do not establish whether or not you get an autoimmune disease. All the additional factors we'll discuss, such as toxins, infections, gut microbiome, diet, and stress, are epigenetic factors that can either increase or decrease your risk of autoimmunity—and, if you have an autoimmune disease, your likelihood of remission or exacerbation.[15]

Scientists have coined the term "exposome" to capture all of these epigenetic factors, which encompass external influences such as stress, pollutants, and diet, as well as internal non-genetic factors such as the gut microbiome, chronic inflammation, and oxidative stress. The role of the exposome in the development of autoimmune disease is increasingly being studied.[16]

THE GUT IMMUNE SYSTEM

As you learn more about autoimmune disease, you will learn how fundamental the gut is to autoimmunity and, in fact, all chronic diseases. That's why a focus on the gut is foundational to my approach. In terms of the immune system, the majority of it is actually located in what is called the gut-associated lymphatic tissue (GALT). It is estimated that upward of 70 percent of your body's total immune system is present in GALT.[17] This is because our gut, apart from our skin, is our primary source of exposure to the outside world and foreign material and microbes, and thus the highest level of surveillance is necessary there.

The Microbiome

Older estimates put the number of bacteria in humans at 100 trillion versus an estimated 10 trillion human cells, hence the inaccurate but often repeated slogan that we are only 10 percent human and 90 percent bacterial. Newer, more precise estimates are that human beings have around 38 trillion bacteria and about 30 trillion human cells—still, you are more bacteria than human.[18] Anaerobic bacteria (which do not require oxygen for growth) may comprise more than 90 percent of the bacterial species, as we will discuss in detail in chapter 4.

We know that the microbiome (also known as "microbiota"—I will use these terms interchangeably) is complex and may contain hundreds (or even thousands) of different species in the average individual.[19]

A recent global study of people from 32 countries identified nearly 5,000 genetically distinct species that can be present in a human microbiome, with many of these species yet to be named; data from European and North American populations is plentiful, but South American, Asian, and African data is underrepresented and growing slowly (Data from these regions usually leads to the discovery of new species when included).[20] Our understanding of the microbiome is still in its infancy, although it is rapidly developing. There is much that is undiscovered and still unknown.

We know that gut bacteria play a critical role in many processes, including digestion, synthesis of vitamins and nutrients, metabolism, maintaining the health of intestinal cells, enhancing immune function, and protecting against pathogenic organisms. In addition, gut flora imbalance is implicated in various chronic illnesses including obesity, insulin resistance, and cardiovascular disease.

Some of the most exciting microbiota research involves autoimmune diseases. One of the key metrics to determine the health of the microbiome is diversity— tracking the number of different types of species in the ecosystem. Several distinct imbalances have been identified in the microbiome in various autoimmune disorders, but one of the most common findings is loss of diversity.[21]

In fact, studies show that the hallmark of the modern microbiome in almost all people today compared to the microbiome of our ancestors is a loss of diversity. Scientists have studied well-preserved stool samples from >1000 years ago and discovered dozens of bacterial species that are not found in modern microbiomes.[22]

This loss of diversity and important bacteria from our microbiota is thought to be one of the key factors behind the dramatic rise in almost all chronic diseases in modern times.[23] A lack of diversity in the microbiome has been associated not only with autoimmunity but also systemic inflammation, obesity, diabetes, insulin resistance, elevated cholesterol, allergies, and asthma—so it has wide-raging health implications for most modern chronic illnesses.[24] This will be one of the central themes of this book, as I teach you how to improve the health and diversity of your microbiome, and heal your gut in order to address autoimmunity.

Loss of Diversity

Several factors have been shown to contribute to this reduction in diversity. These include reduced breastfeeding rates, the rise of C-sections, low-fiber diets, increased consumption of processed foods, widespread use of antibiotics, emotional stress, and environmental toxins. Over the years, increased use of antibiotics in livestock, overprescribing of antibiotics by physicians, sterilization of our drinking water, reduced exposure to farm animals and microbe-rich environments, increased use of antibacterial soap and cleansers, and improved sanitation of the environment have all led to dramatic decreases in the microbial diversity that we are exposed to while growing up.

This phrase "while growing up" is key because it appears that the exposure to key bacteria in the microbiome during the first few years of life is critical to the normal maturation and development of the immune system. Our gut bacteria play a key role in educating our immune systems during childhood. There is a key window of opportunity during the first year of life, especially during which breastfeeding and exposure to the right microbes can induce lifelong positive changes that reduce the risk of immune-mediated disorders.[25] A lack of this proper training of our immune cells by the microbiota can have long-term negative consequences for our health.

While antibiotics were one of the most important advances in medicine of the twentieth century, it is clear now that antibiotics are being overused and overprescribed throughout the world. One of the inadvertent consequences of this is rising antibiotic resistance (where bacteria become resistant to multiple antibiotics), which is a major threat to public health.[26] As a result of all of these factors, there is strong evidence that the human microbiome has declined significantly in biodiversity and quality over the past century.

Prebiotics vs. Probiotics vs. Postbiotics

We will be discussing these terms extensively, so let's define them. A **prebiotic** can be defined as a non-digestible substance that selectively stimulates the growth or activity of gut bacteria in order to benefit the host.[27] A key quality is that it is selective and often specifically feeds beneficial bacteria rather than harmful bacteria. Typically, it is a fiber component of a plant food. **Probiotics** refer to the actual live bacteria themselves, whereas prebiotics are the food for these bacteria, which they ferment for energy. Probiotics are found in fermented foods, which we will be discussing in depth in chapter 10.

Postbiotics (a relatively newer term) are substances released or produced by the metabolic activity of the bacteria, which benefits the host, either directly or indirectly.[28] Bacteria produce a large number of beneficial postbiotic metabolites, such as short-chain fatty acids, which we will be discussing in depth in chapter 4.

OUR ANCESTRAL MICROBIOME

As I did in my first book, *The Paleovedic Diet*, I'll take an evolutionary perspective, because it helps us understand why things are the way they are today. Analysis of archaeological remains from a North American desert revealed that hunter-gatherer populations from around 10,000 years ago had a total daily fiber intake of up to 225 grams, including around 135 g of prebiotic inulin per day from the starchy roots of desert plants that were specially cooked in rock-lined earth ovens.[29]

Studies of modern hunter-gatherer diets reveal that they typically contain between 100 to 150 g of fiber per day.[30] Compare this with the average American daily intake of 10 to 15 g of fiber per day and the discrepancy is enormous.

Thus, for millennia, our ancestors evolved eating a diet that was much higher in fiber and prebiotics, and that is what our microbiota evolved to expect. This was likely the key factor in the robustness and diversity of the ancestral microbiome. As the intake of fiber has plummeted over the past 200 years, the food that our bacteria relied on has disappeared. The consequences are serious.

First, many bacteria have not survived and have been lost, which is why analysis of preserved stool samples from thousands of years ago has identified numerous species not found in modern microbiota. Second, many of the bacteria have adapted to feed on another readily available energy source—the mucus layer that lines our intestine, composed of proteins made by your intestinal cells called mucins.[31] This is the protective barrier between your gut bacteria and your intestinal cells.

It may be slightly disturbing, but if you do not feed your gut bacteria what they need, they will literally start eating you (or, at least, a part of you).[32]

Good Fences Make Good Neighbors

The mucus layer is the first line of defense in your gastrointestinal (GI) tract against increased intestinal permeability or leaky gut syndrome. As the bacteria begin to consume this mucus layer due to lack of prebiotic foods and fiber, the once robust barrier becomes thin and sparse. The bacteria are now in closer proximity to our intestinal cells, and more likely to cross over into our bloodstream when the opportunity arises.

In fact, one of the hallmarks of the modern Western microbiota is a shift in microbiome bacterial populations from those that consume fiber to those that break down mucus, leading to a thinning of the protective mucin layer—the loss of "good fences."[33] Reversing this pattern is critical to building up and restoring the healthy gut barrier, as well as resolving increased intestinal permeability (leaky gut syndrome), which is what the gut-healing protocol in this book is designed to do.

Of course, you cannot suddenly start eating 200 g of fiber every day. Many people with autoimmune conditions also have gut issues that preclude their ability to tolerate prebiotics. We will talk about the most high-yield prebiotic foods that you can start incorporating to rebuild your microbiome, including which foods are best tolerated by those with gut issues or food intolerances, as part of a detailed discussion on diet in chapter 10.

THE HYGIENE HYPOTHESIS

One of the interesting observations with autoimmune disease is that people who live in urban areas tend to have a higher risk of developing autoimmune conditions than those who live in more rural areas.[34] This has led to a theory known as the hygiene hypothesis, which suggests that as sanitation, toilets, clean drinking water, and other "hygiene" measures became more prevalent, abnormalities of the immune system triggered the rise of autoimmune diseases.

While this was a promising initial hypothesis, it is an oversimplification. One of the original proponents of the hygiene hypothesis, Graham Rook, has reformulated it as the "Old Friends" hypothesis.

Old Friends

The idea is that these "old friends" are a group of organisms—such as parasites, key bacteria in our microbiome, and others such as mycobacteria—that have co-evolved with human beings over millennia; before widespread sanitation and pervasive antibiotic use, these microbes were present in our food, water, and within our bodies throughout our entire lives.[35] Because we were continuously exposed to them, we evolved to co-exist with them.

Did our immune systems evolve expecting these "old friends" to slow them down and dampen them? That is the essence of the "old friends" hypothesis. If our immune systems were hypersensitive and continuously reacting to these organisms that were always present within us and around us, our bodies would have been in a constant state of inflammation, which would have been harmful and maladaptive.

Moreover, it is a survival strategy of "old friends" to depress and put a brake on the immune system to ensure their own survival. By necessity, they had to suppress our immune systems so that they could live in our bodies for long periods without being killed. If they were unable to quiet the immune system, the human host would have eradicated them and prevented them from establishing a long-term home in the body.

Leaning into the Wind

Rook explains this process, saying, "evolution turns the inevitable into a necessity"—which means that if something cannot be avoided, it will be incorporated into daily function and physiology and eventually become something that the body expects to find in the environment and not have to provide intrinsically.[36] The body will start to rely on it to some extent.

One could use the metaphor of a person leaning into the wind. In this case the wind is the vast number of "old friends" that human immune systems have been exposed to over the previous tens of thousands of years. Since the microbial "wind" has been blowing for most of human evolution, human immune systems have evolved in response to lean slightly forward, effectively being just a bit overactive.

The person who is leaning slightly forward but held in balance by the power of the wind is like the immune system that tends to be hyperactive but is restrained by the parasites and other microbes; when the wind is taken away, the person falls down—i.e., the immune system gets out of balance and is no longer held in check, becoming overactive and thus contributing to autoimmune diseases.[37]

INTERNAL IMMUNE SUPPRESSORS

Our resident "ancient organisms," such as parasites, certain bacteria, and even the widely known *H. pylori*, a bacterium that can infect the stomach and cause ulcers, have evolved over eons to suppress our immune system's inflammatory response so that they can ensure their own survival. Specifically, when *H. pylori* is present in the stomach, it attracts to the local tissues a large number of T-regulatory cells, which modify and quell inflammation; T-regulatory cells, as we discussed earlier, are important for keeping a brake on the immune system and reducing overzealous inflammation, and may protect the immune system from reacting to other substances as commonly occurs in asthma, allergies, and autoimmune conditions.[38]

Because *H. pylori* is also associated with stomach ulcers and gastric cancer, it defies easy characterization as good or bad, and has multiple effects that can be potentially harmful or possibly useful, depending on the situation. This is the case with many microbes.

Parasites and Microbiome Diversity

Research on some of these "old friends" has demonstrated an increase in microbiome diversity in people who harbor certain nonpathogenic parasites. For example, Blastocystis is one of the most common parasites worldwide. In many cases, it simply colonizes the GI tract and does not cause symptoms. In some cases, it may be problematic, necessitating treatment—but most of the time it is not the cause of digestive distress.

In fact, studies show that the presence of Blastocystis in the gut is associated with increased richness and diversity of the microbiome.[39] Another example is Dientamoeba fragilis, an extremely common parasite and "old friend." A study in Europe found that children colonized with Dientamoeba had higher levels of microbiota diversity than those children who tested negative for it.[40] Just as with Blastocystis, it does not appear to be a common cause of GI symptoms and is associated with increased diversity in the microbiome. The presence of these two *may* in fact be a sign of a healthy ecosystem in certain individuals.

Now, this doesn't mean it's a good idea for you to seek out these parasites if they are not already within you—consider, other parasites like Giardia or Cryptosporidium can definitely cause GI symptoms and are a major issue worldwide.

For those common, harmless parasites, it appears that exposure to them during childhood is the most important in terms of training the immune system.

Some practitioners automatically try to eradicate Blastocystis if it is discovered on a stool test, using herbal supplements or, in some cases, prescription antibiotics. I often see patients who have not seen their GI symptoms improve after treatment for Blastocystis in the past, whereas the diversity and health of their microbiome has suffered because of the herbal or prescription antibiotics.

Dramatic Deterioration of Infant Microbiota

Much of the education and training of our immune system appears to occur during the first few years of life, meaning the health of the infant microbiota is key. Unfortunately, studies show that the traditional healthy infant microbiome, which should optimally be dominated by the beneficial species known as Bifidobacteria (which you will learn about in chapter 4), is also weakening and declining—it is increasingly being replaced by an unstable infant microbiome with suboptimal biomarkers and overgrowth of potentially bad bacteria.[41] It is unclear if increased use of antibiotics, a rise in cesarean sections, declines in breastfeeding, and/or other factors are responsible for this.

A longitudinal study in 2016 followed gut microbiome development from birth until age three in a cohort of infants in Finland and Russia. There is a high incidence of early autoimmune disease in Finland, and comparatively low incidence in neighboring Russia, despite geographic proximity. The study found huge differences in the microbiota of these two groups of infants.

In Russia, the infant microbiota was robust and dominated by Bifidobacteria, as it should be, and developed a greater degree of diversity by the age of three; in contrast, the Finnish infants had microbiota dominated by the potentially pathogenic bacteria Bacteroides, which produces a higher degree of an inflammatory compound called LPS (more about this in chapter 3).[42] The major difference between the microbiota of the infants in these two countries is thought to be a key factor behind the dramatic divergence in the occurrence of autoimmune disease in Russia and Finland.

Specifically, the abnormally high levels of Bacteroides bacteria in young children in Finland could explain why the country has the highest rates in the world of type I diabetes, an autoimmune disease that often strikes young kids. The microbiota of children worldwide who are at the earliest stage of preclinical type I diabetes (before they develop full-blown autoimmune disease) is known to be dominated by Bacteroides—and displays reduced diversity and deficiency of key beneficial bacteria, as is commonly seen with other autoimmune disorders.[43]

Over the past 100 years, another key metric of microbiome health has been worsening in infants, and that is stool pH, which we will be discussing in detail in chapter 9. Briefly, the lower the stool pH, the more acidic (and healthier) the environment, and the less likely that bad bugs can proliferate.

Unfortunately, stool pH in the infant gut microbiome worldwide has been steadily increasing from 1926 through current times, from an average of 5.0 up to 6.5, likely as a result of decline in beneficial keystone species such as Bifidobacteria.[44] There has been a corresponding rise in dysbiosis seen in the infant microbiome during this time; it is unclear what the long-term ramifications of this change in infant biology over the past century are (but it's probably not good). Dysbiosis in infant microbiota has been linked to long-term health implications such as higher risk of developing autoimmune disorders, chronic inflammation, asthma, and other immune-mediated diseases.[45]

So, we can see how the changes in the human gut microbiome now evident and unmistakable even in infancy are going to have a serious long-term impact. At a population level, the microbiota of our infants is not looking good, and this mirrors the disruption and imbalance that is seen in today's typical adult microbiota.

With all this in mind, one of the most critical interventions we can focus on is to work on rebuilding and restoring the health of the microbiome in both adults and children. Doing so means curtailing the rapid rise in autoimmunity—and all chronic diseases that are the hallmark of modern times.

THE EFFECTS OF COVID-19

Speaking of modern challenges, it is important to understand how the COVID-19 pandemic can potentially impact this more insidious but equally deadly autoimmune epidemic. COVID-19 has the ability to trigger molecular mimicry, and the pandemic could eventually lead to further increases in autoimmune disorders.

COVID-19, like other viruses, can trigger autoimmune reactions by stimulating production of autoantibodies, which were identified in 50 percent of patients hospitalized with the virus in one study.[46] A number of cases of autoimmune disorders developing after COVID-19 infection have been reported including Guillain-Barré syndrome (which can cause temporary paralysis), multisystem inflammatory conditions, autoimmune anemia, and blood-clotting disorders.[47] Molecular mimicry, a key mechanism in autoimmunity as we discussed earlier, appears to be occurring with COVID as it does with other viruses.[48]

Cases of "long COVID," as it's come to be known, with chronic disparate symptoms that persist long after the infection is cleared, are thought to have an autoimmune mechanism as one of the causes of lingering disability.[49] Moreover, antibodies against COVID-19 proteins made by the body appear to have significant cross-reactivity against multiple tissues in different parts of the body, raising a question about whether this pandemic will contribute down the line to increases in autoimmune disorders.[50] Time will tell—but in my opinion, the potential autoimmune-promoting effects of COVID make it even more urgent that we begin to understand and implement the solutions outlined in this book to start tackling the root causes of autoimmunity.

BRENDA BOUNCES BACK

Let's revisit Brenda, who was told her Hashimoto's couldn't be treated until her hormone levels were no longer within the normal range.

Being a proactive person, Brenda was not satisfied with her doctor's advice, who suggested that all she could do for her Hashimoto's was wait for her thyroid to fail and then she'd be prescribed a medication. Moreover, severe fatigue was making it hard for her to continue working. She sought out our integrative medicine clinic and we began working together with an elimination diet, stress reduction, and nutritional supplements including vitamin D and fish oil.

I diagnosed her long-standing irritable bowel syndrome (IBS) as a combination of bacterial dysbiosis and leaky gut syndrome (using a functional medicine stool test) and put her on the TIGER Protocol. Healing her gut using probiotics and prebiotics led to a complete remission of her IBS. We then used ashwa-gandha and other herbs to strengthen her thyroid and adrenal function, with the goal of optimizing her hormones. After four months, her fatigue and hair loss had resolved, and her weight was normalizing. After 12 months, her anti-thyroid antibodies returned to the normal range, confirming a full remission of her Hashimoto's, which she continues to maintain.

CHAPTER 2

Toxins—The Missing Puzzle Piece

Joseph, 44, had experienced severe numbness and tingling for over a year. He had Hashimoto's disease for years, but it was stable with a thyroid prescription. Used to pushing through physical symptoms, he finally sought care when it became difficult for him to walk. He saw a neurologist, who told him he was "on the way" to developing multiple sclerosis but did not meet all the diagnostic criteria yet, and did not offer any treatment.

When I began working with Joseph, we discovered that his levels of mercury were very high, likely based on his sushi addiction (mercury often contributes to neurological symptoms). His lead was also elevated, likely due to dietary exposure from chocolate and many other foods.

Joseph, like almost all my autoimmune patients, was dealing with high levels of toxins. It's important to learn why toxins are the missing link in understanding why autoimmune disease occurs. We address toxins first in the TIGER Protocol because, I believe, they are the primary factor in the rapid rise of autoimmune disease. Additionally, toxins are often overlooked, even by practitioners of integrative medicine. I commonly see patients who have worked with other holistic practitioners and find that not enough attention has been given to the area of toxins.

Join me as we dive into the research on toxins in autoimmunity. After that we will discuss how to reduce and limit your exposure to these chemicals. In chapter 7, I will introduce the detox component of the TIGER Protocol, to help your body eliminate whatever toxins are within.

DEFINING TOXINS

Toxins can be defined as substances, either man-made or naturally occurring, that can cause harm to organisms. Toxins differ from bacteria in that some bacteria are good and some can be bad, but all toxins are unfavorable.

There's no straightforward way to define a normal range. We seek to regulate toxins with the idea that there is a certain threshold or safe level of exposure. But for certain toxins there may be no safe level—in these cases, toxins can cause harm even at levels defined by government agencies as normal. For example, the Centers for Disease Control (CDC) concluded that there is no safe level of lead exposure in children, but recommended using a reference range of below 5 µg/dL as normal (reduced to 3.5 in 2021); yet even "normal" levels of 2 or 3 are associated with cognitive deficits and IQ decline in kids.[1]

Another example is mercury. Blood levels considered normal by conventional medicine were associated with subclinical autoimmunity, as measured by elevated levels of autoimmune antibodies.[2]

Many toxins are not well-studied, partly because of the staggering numbers of chemicals in use. How many chemicals are being used in the United States alone? The Environmental Protection Agency (EPA) identified more than 86,000 compounds eligible for commercial production in their Toxic Substances Control Act and found that, of these, more than 40,000 are currently in use in commerce.[3] Most of these have not been studied for normal ranges or long-term safety. Chronic low-level exposure is the norm for all of us. Research is ongoing to establish normal ranges for some of these toxins, but will be time-consuming.

1+1=3—SYNERGISTIC HARM FROM TOXINS

In this chapter, we'll look at 20 toxins that have each *individually* been linked to increased risk of autoimmune disease. What happens when we start combining toxins? Alarmingly, when one person has high levels of multiple toxins, the effects become synergistic—their combined effect is greater than the effect of one toxin on its own. In other words, it is not just that 1 plus 1 equals 2 in terms of how a toxin affects your body—it might be 1 plus 1 equals 3 or 4.

Research typically seeks to isolate single factors so that they can be studied. But we are starting to see research on the effects of multiple toxins. For example, one study has shown a synergistic interaction between heavy metals and pesticides, which when both present cause a significantly higher level of cell damage than when either is present individually.[4] More studies like this are needed, because that is exactly what is going on with the multitude of toxins that each of us is currently exposed to.

Toxic Levels Within

You might wonder, *How many toxins can one person have anyway? Perhaps it is rare for a person to have high levels of more than one toxin?* The reality is troubling.

Within the sole category of toxins from pesticides, testing by the US Centers for Disease Control (CDC) found that the average person has 13 pesticides at significant levels.[5]

A study performed by two nonprofits that tested blood and urine samples from Americans for 214 substances found an average of >100 toxins elevated per person, and a total of 155 toxins detected in all. Again, these included insecticides, heavy metals, industrial compounds, Polychlorinated Biphenyls (PCBs), and more—and none of the study subjects had any occupational or residential risks for these exposures, they were just average Americans.[6] In this study, they tested for 214 toxins. If they had tested for more, it is likely the number discovered would have been much greater.

The Youngest of Us

Even babies are at risk. Researchers found an average of 200 toxins in blood tests of newborn babies born in US hospitals, including many of the toxins that increase the risk of autoimmunity such as pesticides, heavy metals, flame retardants, perfluorinated chemicals (PFCs), and other industrial toxins.[7] Our children are born with high levels of toxins transmitted to them before birth, a reflection of maternal exposures before and during pregnancy, placing them at increased risk from the very beginning.

Another study identified 59 chemicals (including many of the toxins we will discuss in this chapter) such as PFCs, Polybrominated Diphenyl Ethers (PBDEs), pesticides, mercury, and lead in the blood of newborns at birth—and, significantly, at higher levels than found in their mothers' blood.[8] This study found that babies experience higher exposures to certain chemicals than their mothers through placental transfer before birth.

Once they are born, babies are exposed to toxins from various sources, some of them unexpected. A study testing breast milk found toxic Per- and Polyfluoroalkyl Substances (PFAS) at levels ranging from 50 parts per trillion (ppt) to more than 1,850 ppt; to provide perspective, government agencies recommend <15 ppt of this toxin in children's drinking water.[9]

The study tested 39 different PFAS and found that older compounds phased out by industry (like PFOA from Teflon) are still present, and there is an increase in the newer generation of PFAS that the chemical industry claims do not accumulate in humans. PFAS are tied to hazardous long-term effects in adulthood, including increased risk of autoimmunity, thyroid dysfunction, kidney disease, and metabolic syndrome.[10]

To be clear, breastfeeding is exceedingly beneficial and one of the most powerful practices to build up a healthy infant gut microbiome. My intention in sharing this data is not to discourage breastfeeding, nor to insinuate that breastfeeding parents are doing something wrong. As stated, it is especially challenging to avoid exposure to toxins, even if you do not have higher occupational or residential risks.

EVIDENCE OF HEALING

When toxins are taken seriously and addressed, it often leads to significant improvements in quality of life, symptoms, and health outcomes. This has been documented by case reports in the scientific literature. For example, clearance of heavy metals can often help with neurological symptoms or inflammatory joint issues—in one case, a woman with rheumatoid arthritis saw a complete resolution of symptoms after a year of chelation therapy removed high levels of cadmium from her system.[11]

Another patient with multiple sclerosis, who was unsuccessfully treated for years with conventional medications, was found to have elevated levels of mercury, lead, and aluminum in urine testing; treatment with an oral chelation agent led to gradual improvement of symptoms and clinical remission in his MS, as well as normalization of heavy metal levels in the urine.[12]

THE BASIS OF MY APPROACH

As I reviewed the research on toxins and autoimmunity, I realized I could easily fill up an entire book covering the myriad of toxins and studies documenting their connection with autoimmunity. For our purposes, I decided to focus on major toxins that are the big players in autoimmunity. This is not an exhaustive list, and I have also not included all the research studies—just enough to clarify the key points.

You may find this data and evidence challenging, even depressing. However, it's crucial to begin to understand it. My goal here is to empower you, for this information to serve as a wake-up call to take action around the issue of toxins and begin to heal your autoimmune issues.

Two Important Case Studies

Most research by necessity has to focus on individual toxins and their connection to autoimmune disease. It's challenging to perform studies analyzing the effects of multiple toxins on the risk of illness, even though this would more accurately reflect real-world exposure. However, one such investigation was performed on the workers who participated in cleanup after the World Trade Center attack in 2001.

They were exposed to a toxic combination of airborne silica dust, lead and other heavy metals, asbestos, dioxin, and other chemicals. A study found significantly increased risk of developing eight different autoimmune conditions in these workers over a 12-year follow-up when compared to healthy controls; the most common diseases were rheumatoid arthritis, spondyloarthritis, inflammatory myositis, and lupus.[13]

Another population with high rates of autoimmune disease from exposure to multiple toxins was studied in The Buffalo Lupus Project.[14] A known hazardous waste site exposed nearby residents to lead, polychlorinated biphenols (PCBs), trichloroethylene (TCE), and other toxins; researchers identified a seven times greater risk of developing lupus (and other autoimmune diseases) in people residing in the area who had been inadvertently exposed to the high levels of toxins.[15]

I mention these studies to illustrate that idea of toxin synergy ("1+1=3") that I introduced earlier. When people are exposed to multiple toxins, there is a dramatically increased risk of developing autoimmunity.

Oxidative Stress—How Toxins Harm

Almost all toxins produce harmful compounds in the body called free radicals—unstable, short-lived molecules that react with and impair cellular machinery. They trigger something in the body called oxidative stress, which directly damages tissues. Oxidative stress is defined as the accumulation of destruction caused by free radicals and other detrimental compounds that harm our DNA, proteins, enzymes, and lipids, leading to cell injury and death.[16] This is partly a result of daily metabolic activity within the body, but greatly amplified by exposure to toxins.

Patients with autoimmune disease typically test for high levels of oxidative stress, and correspondingly low levels of antioxidants—this has been clearly shown in rheumatoid arthritis, lupus, type 1 diabetes, multiple sclerosis, and Sjogren's syndrome.[17] The oxidative stress uses up antioxidants, leading to low levels of systemic antioxidants in their bodies.

A study by British researchers followed the diets of 25,000 people over nine years and found that those who developed rheumatoid arthritis consumed around 40 percent fewer dietary antioxidants.[18] Testing for oxidative stress and measuring antioxidant status is uncommon outside of research settings, but I do not think it is necessary because of lack of standardized testing for antioxidants and the universal prevalence of these issues in autoimmune patients. I have measured oxidative stress markers in some autoimmune patients, and they have always been elevated. The bottom line is that oxidative stress is clearly a huge issue in autoimmunity, and one that must be addressed as part of a comprehensive treatment plan.

The solution to oxidative stress, then, is increasing antioxidant levels in the body, and the best way to do that is with diet. For this reason, both the TIGER Protocol Phase 1 and Phase 2 Diets are extremely rich in antioxidants.

Of course, the main way that toxins cause harm that is relevant here is by disrupting the immune system. As we will see, many toxins damage the immune system in multiple ways, thereby increasing the risk of autoimmunity.

AN OBVIOUS TOXIN

Most people can identify cigarette smoke as a toxin, making it a good place to start, because smoking has clear links to autoimmunity.

Smoking can accelerate the development of autoimmune disease even in persons who do not carry any of the genes that predispose them to autoimmunity. Studies show that smoking significantly raises the odds of developing rheumatoid arthritis in women, even those who have not inherited the established genes that predispose to the disease.[19] Smoking is also linked to the development of lupus, multiple sclerosis, ankylosing spondylitis, Hashimoto's thyroiditis, systemic sclerosis, and many other autoimmune disorders.[20]

If you do smoke and have tried to quit, you know smoking cessation is challenging and best approached with a multidisciplinary program.

Incidentally, a review of 24 clinical trials found that acupuncture is helpful for long-term smoking cessation in combination with counseling and educational programs, so if you are having trouble quitting on your own, consider accessing this type of support.[21]

DEADLY ATTRIBUTES OF TOXINS

Before we explore our list of major toxins, there are three main qualities toxins share that stimulate autoimmune disease, making them particularly problematic:

1. Persistence—a tendency to remain in the environment and not degrade. Heavy metals never break down because they are basic elements and cannot be destroyed. Other toxins such as pesticides and endocrine-disrupting chemicals (EDCs) resist degradation and break down very slowly over a time course of decades or centuries—these are often called "forever chemicals." They recirculate between air, water, and soil in a never-ending cycle.

2. Bioaccumulation—an ability to accumulate in individual animals and concentrate as one goes up the food chain. Many toxins are fat-soluble and are gradually deposited into fat, from which they are hard to release; this contributes to bioaccumulation. This is one reason why sweating can help you detoxify, because toxins stored in the subcutaneous fat just under the skin can be excreted in sweat.[22] Some sources question whether toxins can be excreted by sweating; a considerable number of studies support this viewpoint, however. A meta-analysis of twenty-four studies determined that the heavy metal cadmium appears at higher levels in sweat than in the blood, arsenic clearance via sweat in exposed individuals is many times higher than that of healthy controls, and elevated mercury levels could be normalized by regular sauna use.[23] Research has also shown that sweating is a way to eliminate measurable levels of pesticides, flame retardants, phthalates, and PCBs.[24]

3. Slow clearance—poor excretion from the body. Half-life is defined as the length of time for half of the amount in the body to be excreted under normal circumstances. For example, PFCs have a half-life of elimination of between 4 to 8 years.[25] Heavy metals like lead or cadmium have a half-life in humans of up to 30 years.[26] This means that if 1,000 units are

present in the body today, in 30 years that would be reduced to 500 units through normal detox processes.

Now that we know the harm toxins can cause, let's turn our exploration to 20 of the most harmful toxins implicated in autoimmunity.

MERCURY

Heavy metals have unfortunately become a widespread environmental problem. Mercury is present in certain types of dental fillings (usually known as "amalgams"), batteries, bulbs, fish and seafood, and water sources. The Food and Drug Administration (FDA) issued a warning in 2020 about the potential adverse health effects of mercury amalgams in several populations including pregnant women, women planning to become pregnant, children, people with neurological disease, those with impaired kidney function, and others.[27]

Mercury is also released into the air from coal-fired power plants throughout the world. In the United States, the Environmental Protection Agency (EPA) reports that coal-fired power plants are the largest source of mercury released into the air, accounting for 44 percent of all man-made mercury emissions.[28] This airborne mercury then falls to the ground in rain, dust, or simply through the effects of gravity.

The reason why our fish and seafood are high in mercury is that a lot of this airborne mercury has landed in the ocean, contaminating the plants and animals that live there. Mercury, like most heavy metals, goes through bioaccumulation up the food chain. Large predator fish are highest in mercury as a result; smaller fish tend to be relatively low in mercury and other heavy metals.

For unclear reasons, some people do not excrete mercury (and other toxins) as well as others. We are just beginning to understand the genetic and epigenetic differences that may account for this. Mercury is present in high amounts in certain people, and it is possible to test for this with functional medicine. I often find heavy metals such as mercury and lead to be elevated in my patients with autoimmune disease.

How Mercury Harms

There are multiple ways that mercury can cause autoimmune reactions. First, mercury reacts with certain proteins in the body by combining directly with body tissue. The result is a complex hybrid that is heavy metal plus body cell, a sort of half-human, half-metal chimera.[29] Naturally, the immune system recognizes this as a foreign invader, creating antibodies against this partially human tissue, which can cause cross-reactive damage. Mercury can also stimulate certain immune cells called lymphocytes to grow abnormally, losing their ability to tell the difference between self and non-self. Then they might either directly attack or make antibodies to damage your own tissues.

Methylmercury, which is the form of mercury found in seafood, has been linked to subclinical autoimmunity among young women even at low levels that are generally considered safe in conventional medicine.[30] It has been associated with multiple sclerosis, with MS patients having significantly higher levels of mercury in the blood compared to healthy controls.[31] A number of animal studies have shown that mercury exposure can directly cause autoimmune diseases such as lupus and multiple sclerosis by stimulating the production of autoantibodies.[32]

Interestingly, a connection has been found between certain occupational exposures to heavy metals and lupus—one study showed a connection between lupus and mercury exposure from working in a dental office (or using pesticides in agricultural work, as we'll discuss below).[33] Also, patients with systemic sclerosis, an autoimmune disease that causes thickening of skin and connective tissues in the body, had elevated concentrations of mercury in their urine compared to normal patients.[34]

In Brazil, a study of individuals who eat fish found a significant correlation between mercury levels and the autoantibody ANA.[35] In autoimmune thyroid disease, there is strong evidence that mercury accumulates in the thyroid gland and is one of the key causes. Studies have shown that young women with higher blood levels of mercury had a much greater risk for developing antithyroid markers known as thyroglobulin antibodies.[36]

LEAD

Lead is another heavy metal that has toxic effects. In the past, we were exposed to lead from gasoline, lead paint, and plumbing. While it has been phased out of these sources, lead, like other heavy metals, does not break down or disappear from the environment over time. Moreover, automobile exhaust is a persistent source (due to trace amounts of lead still present in "unleaded" gasoline), which in the United States alone accounts for up to 200,000 tons of lead released into the environment each year.[37]

Leaded aviation fuel is still used by over 100,000 planes in the United States, making airplanes the nation's top source of airborne lead; according to the EPA, people who live downwind of airports have significantly higher levels of lead, although these emissions lead to widespread distribution of lead in the air and eventually the soil.[38]

The end result is widespread global contamination of soil and water, therefore most people today are exposed to lead from many different foods and also the water supply; lead that is absorbed by plants cannot be removed by washing or food processing.[39] Testing has identified lead in most fruits and vegetables, which reflects its prevalence in our soils; interestingly, dried fruits and vegetables appear to be the highest in lead.[40]

Foods that are especially high in lead, likely because these plants are efficient in taking up lead from soils, include chocolate, psyllium husk, and certain spices. I will share guidance on choosing safe brands for these products below.

Toxic Effects of Lead

The immune system appears to be exquisitely sensitive to lead in comparison to other toxins; many mechanisms are being studied for how lead could contribute to the initiation and progression of autoimmune diseases.[41]

Specifically, it can dysregulate the hypothalamus-pituitary-adrenal (HPA) axis, which is the primary regulator of energy levels and stress resilience in the body; it also disturbs cell membranes (the protective outer layer of each cell), disrupts enzyme function (which is involved in countless body processes), and causes the formation of free radicals that can directly damage our tissues.[42] As with other heavy metals, the creation of oxidative stress by lead causes breakdown of intrinsic antioxidants, leading to decreases in levels of key antioxidants such as glutathione.[43]

In addition to immune system disruption, lead also impacts the heart and brain. A study found that as blood levels go up (*within the "normal" range*), the risk of heart disease and stroke increases significantly.[44] Extensive research has proven that lead correlates with reduced IQ, learning problems, and behavioral issues in children, which is why pediatricians often order a serum lead screening for children at one year of age.[45]

The Food and Drug Administration (FDA) states that because "lead can accumulate in the body, even low-level chronic exposure can be hazardous over time."[46] Unfortunately, low-level chronic exposure is now the norm for all of us, because lead is so pervasive in all our foods. Lead tends to accumulate in bone over time, and most of the lead body burden resides in the bone; the half-life of lead excretion from bone is about 30 years.[47]

Lead in Cookware

We love our slow cookers and other cookware but, unfortunately, it is possible that the slow cooker may be another source of lead contamination. Some data suggest that certain slow cookers may leach low levels of lead into the food, especially if acid-containing foods such as vinegar, citrus, or tomato products are cooked in them. An investigation in Utah found that 20 percent of slow cookers were releasing measurable amounts of lead into foods; this is thought to be due either to the glaze that lines the vessels or something in the vessels themselves.[48] A slow cooker or electric pressure cooker (like the popular "Instant Pot") which uses a stainless-steel cooking vessel is a better alternative.

ARSENIC

Arsenic is another ubiquitous heavy metal. It can be found in drinking water and certain foods; due to widespread presence in soil, it is present in many fruits, vegetables, and grains, especially rice.

Conventionally grown chicken and turkey are especially high in arsenic because arsenic-based additives were added to poultry feed for many years to prevent parasites and promote weight gain; a study in 3,000 adults found that people who consumed conventional chicken and turkey had elevated levels of arsenic in their bodies based on urine tests.[49] The good news is that these additives are being phased out, as the FDA withdrew approval for them in 2015.

Arsenic Toxicity

Studies show that arsenic has injurious effects on the immune system, including dysregulation of lymphocytes and T regulatory cells, the body's key peacekeepers that maintain immune balance; it also triggers oxidative stress, systemic inflammation, and the production of proinflammatory cytokines, thus contributing to autoimmunity.[50]

Arsenic appears to increase the risk of infections (which play a key role in autoimmune disease) by impairing immune responses; human and animal studies indicate that chronic exposure to arsenic is associated with increased risk of immune-mediated problems (infections, autoimmunity, and cancer) later in life.[51]

A study in children and adolescents found higher levels of arsenic to be associated with higher odds of developing type I diabetes compared to healthy controls.[52] In a Swedish study, children who developed type I diabetes later in life were found to have high levels of arsenic, mercury, and aluminum at birth (likely transferred to the child in utero during pregnancy), when compared to healthy children who did not have increased levels of these metals.[53] Many studies have also found a relationship between arsenic exposure and type II diabetes, indicating multiple effects on impairing blood sugar regulation.[54]

If you have autoimmune disease, arsenic may contribute to exacerbations through multiple harmful effects. A study in patients with multiple sclerosis found that elevated blood levels of arsenic were associated with disease progression and relapse, which correlated with its ability to raise serum markers of oxidative stress.[55]

CADMIUM

Cadmium is another forever chemical that is pervasive in the environment. It causes significant oxidative stress. Due to high levels in soil, it is present in many fruits and vegetables.[56] Unfortunately, chocolate is one of the highest sources of cadmium as well as lead, because of the tendency of the cacao plant to take up heavy metals from the soil.[57] However, I believe the benefits of dark chocolate outweigh the risks, and later we'll discuss how to select brands that are safe for consumption.

Cadmium is thought to play a significant role in the pathogenesis of rheumatoid arthritis.[58] Cadmium levels resulting from typical oral intake of cadmium through the average diet are associated with the production of autoimmune antibodies.[59] In the autoimmune skin conditions psoriasis and vitiligo, patients were found to have elevated levels of cadmium (and lead) when compared to healthy controls.[60]

The cellular and molecular mechanisms by which cadmium disrupts the immune system have been elucidated.[61] Cadmium is also a known human carcinogen, linked to various cancers such as breast, prostate, lung, and kidney.[62]

TRICLOSAN

The National Institute of Environmental Sciences studied toxic exposures that were associated with development of ANA, the most common autoimmune antibody. They found that most prominent among potential risks was exposure to triclosan, an antibacterial and antifungal agent that the US Food and Drug Administration banned from soaps and hand hygiene products in 2017.[63]

It is still present in many products that people may be exposed to, such as toothpaste. Although this was banned from soaps, triclosan is used pervasively and is one of those "forever chemicals" that are distributed extensively around the world. Studies show that triclosan has been widely detected in lakes, rivers, and sea water from many countries, and is incompletely removed by wastewater treatment plants, thus leading to continued persistence in the environment.[64] This serves to further illustrate that banning some of these pollutants does not necessarily reduce our health risk from them.

ENDOCRINE DISRUPTING CHEMICALS

Endocrine disrupting chemicals, or EDCs, are used extensively in agriculture, consumer products, cosmetics, furniture, electronics, and other industrial applications. EDCs are chemicals that are known to disrupt the function of the human endocrine system, which consists of the glands that produce hormones that regulate metabolism, growth and development, tissue function, sexual function, sleep, and mood, among other things. Scientists have estimated the health-care costs associated with the effects of EDCs to be a staggering $175 billion per year in Europe alone; this is one reason why the European Union is considering regulation of EDCs.[65]

EDCs have been studied in type I diabetes and are thought to promote auto-immunity and increase the individual's susceptibility to autoimmune attack.[66] Examples of endocrine disrupting compounds are pesticides, BPA, PFCs, PCBs, phthalates, and flame retardants. We will review several of these EDCs next.

PFCs

We start getting into a bit of alphabet soup as we review the EDCs but let's discuss PFCs or perfluorinated chemicals. Also known as Per- and Polyfluoro-alkyl Substances (PFAS), they are used to create water and stain resistance in carpets and clothing, nonstick surfaces for cookware, and in various industrial applications.

As we learned earlier, PFCs/PFAS were found to be elevated in breast milk. In addition to immune system dysfunction and autoimmunity, they are also associated with cancer, thyroid disease, and fertility issues.[67] A report by the US Department of Health and Human Services found PFCs associated with elevated risk of autoantibodies and several autoimmune diseases.[68] One study in patients with celiac disease found that elevated levels of PFCs dramatically increased the odds (by up to 9-fold) of developing this autoimmune disorder.[69]

PFCs are part of the nonstick coating Teflon, the brand name for polytetra-fluoroethylene (PTFE); perfluorooctanoic acid (PFOA) is a related compound used in the production of Teflon that also has toxic effects. These have been associated with higher incidence of thyroid abnormalities.[70]

PCBs

PCBs, polychlorinated biphenols, are an industrial chemical that was manu-factured from 1929 until it was banned in 1979; despite the ban, due to strong persistence in the environment and ease of spread, they are now widely distrib-uted and found all over the world—the EPA classifies them as "probable human carcinogens."[71]

PCBs (and other EDCs like flame retardants) have been associated with auto-immune thyroid disease.[72] Animal studies have linked PCBs to various autoim-mune disorders, and in humans increased exposure to PCBs is associated with elevated levels of the autoantibodies for autoimmune type I diabetes.[73]

Due to high levels in water, fish tend to take in and concentrate PCBs. PCBs are quite high in farmed salmon, due to PCB contamination in their feed as well.[74] Since PCBs tend to bioaccumulate, they are also present at higher levels in non-organic dairy, beef, and chicken.[75]

Pesticides

Over 1,400 pesticides have been approved for use by the Environmental Protec-tion Agency (EPA). They are used extensively in the environment, with over 1 billion pounds used in the United States alone each year; what is disturbing is that the US Department of Agriculture estimates that over 50 million people in the United States get their drinking water from groundwater potentially con-taminated by pesticides and other agricultural chemicals.[76]

Pesticides have been linked to various autoimmune conditions, multiple types of cancer, and other health problems; the CDC has determined that 93 percent of Americans tested had detectable levels of the insecticide chlorpyrifos and 99 percent had detectable levels of DDT, with the average person carrying about thirteen pesticides.[77] This is concerning because the CDC tests for only a frac-tion of the total number of pesticides to which we are exposed, but still found that a significant number of people tested had potentially harmful body levels of certain pesticides above government safety thresholds.

Children with newly diagnosed type I diabetes were found to have significantly higher blood levels of 8 out of 9 pesticides tested when compared to healthy controls.[78] In adolescents with type I diabetes, higher levels of measured pesticides were associated with worse impairment of pancreatic beta-cell function (the cells that produce insulin) and poorer control of blood sugar.[79] Celiac disease also can be a consequence. One study found that women who had above average levels of pesticide exposure had an 8-fold increased risk of developing celiac disease.[80]

A study of 77,000 women found a significant link between household insecticide use and the development of rheumatoid arthritis and lupus.[81] Women who personally applied insecticide had a three times higher risk of developing either condition compared to women who did not work with pesticides directly. There was a clear "dose-response" for both rheumatoid arthritis and lupus with increasing frequency and duration of exposure—the greater the cumulative exposure, the greater the risk of developing either disease.[82]

This confirms studies done in agricultural workers. An analysis of over 300,000 death certificates in the US over 14 years concluded that farmers who were exposed to pesticides at work were significant more likely to die of an autoimmune disease, including rheumatoid arthritis, lupus, systemic sclerosis, or other autoimmune conditions.[83] A study of male pesticide applicators over an 18-year period found that rheumatoid arthritis was linked to increased use of several different pesticides such as fonofos (70% increased risk), carbaryl (50% increased risk), and chlorimuron ethyl (45% increased risk).[84]

The solution is simple. Wherever possible, avoid household pesticide use and use nonchemical alternatives. If you can manage it, seek out organic foods. Studies have shown that organic produce, as you would expect, is consistently much lower in pesticide residues. Research has also found that, with few exceptions, organic produce is higher in vitamins and minerals than conventional fruits and vegetables.[85]

Organic fruits and vegetables have also been shown to be substantially higher in antioxidants such as phenolic acids, flavanones, stilbenes, and anthocyanins; in addition to protecting against autoimmune disease by reducing levels of oxidative stress, these beneficial compounds also are protective against heart disease and cancer.[86]

Glyphosate

Glyphosate is the world's most heavily used pesticide, owned and produced by Monsanto under the name Roundup. Global glyphosate usage is at a staggering level of 6.5 million tons annually (over 13 billion pounds), and projected to grow steadily in the years ahead.[87] Genetically engineering glyphosate-resistant genes into food crops enables glyphosate to be used at higher doses, leading to higher glyphosate residues on wheat, corn, and other crops.[88] Glyphosate is classified as "probably carcinogenic to humans" by a World Health Organization (WHO) Committee that performed an independent scientific review of over 1,000 studies.[89]

In terms of autoimmune disease, there are two mechanisms through which glyphosate is particularly dangerous. First is its effect on impairing liver detox pathways. Glyphosate inhibits cytochrome P450 liver enzymes, which are critical for breaking down environmental toxins.[90] Second, it has destructive effects on the microbiome by causing a decline in beneficial bacteria—demonstrating antibiotic properties—and predisposing to overgrowth of pathogenic bacteria.[91]

Consequently, glyphosate exposure may play a central role in the pathogenesis of celiac disease.[92] Women who either applied or were exposed to glyphosate had a 40 percent higher risk of developing rheumatoid arthritis compared to non-users.[93]

Although the safety of glyphosate is debated,[94] it is preferable to minimize glyphosate intake. Unfortunately, glyphosate residues cannot be washed off food crops, so it is best to avoid foods that normally contain it, especially conventionally grown soy, corn, and wheat.

GMO Foods

Glyphosate is commonly used on genetically modified foods. Foods made with genetically modified organisms include many potential negative effects; the bottom line is that I recommend avoiding GMO foods because of flaws in industry-sponsored research on safety, and the potential risk of toxicity over time.[95]

There is no requirement that foods containing GMOs must be labeled as such. The most well-established regulation pertaining to GMOs is organic certification–foods that are certified USDA organic are not allowed to have GMO ingredients. The nonprofit Non-GMO Project enables foods to be labeled with a "**Non-GMO Project Verified**" seal, which is something to look for if organic is not available.

BPA

BPA, or bisphenol A, is a hormonally active chemical that is a known EDC; the US Centers for Disease Control and Prevention estimates that 5–6 billion pounds of BPA are produced worldwide each year.[96] Studies show that 93 percent of people in the United States have detectable levels of BPA in their bodies.[97]

In the scientific literature, 11 different autoimmune triggering mechanisms have been identified by which BPA may be a contributing risk factor to autoimmune disease development and progression.[98] BPA causes significant oxidative stress, just like most other toxins.[99] Multiple animal studies indicate that exposure to BPA can promote the development of autoimmune type I diabetes.[100] In terms of human studies, children with type I diabetes have higher levels of urinary BPA than healthy controls.[101] Incidentally, elevated urinary BPA levels are also associated with cardiovascular disease, type II diabetes, and elevated liver enzymes, indicating multiple harmful metabolic effects.[102]

BPA is often found in plastic water bottles, although newer BPA-free plastic may not be so great. In these products, Bisphenol S (BPS) is widely used as a chemical replacement for BPA. Unfortunately, some research suggests that BPS may have toxic effects as well.[103] In animals, exposure to BPS causes irregular heartbeats, the same way that BPA does, by affecting the response of the cells to estrogen. This is not surprising because the chemical structure of BPS is similar to BPA.

BPA is present in thermal paper, which is used to print receipts in most stores, which is concerning because BPA absorbs readily through the skin. Studies have shown that cashiers have much higher levels of BPA in their bodies compared to the average person due to occupational exposure.[104]

Waterborne Toxins

Local municipal drinking water could be high in toxins, some of which are not even regulated by the EPA. For example, the industrial pollutant TCE, or trichloroethylene, is one of the most common groundwater contaminants in the United States. TCE is often utilized in metal cleaning and degreasing agents and used to manufacture various fluids. Both animal and human studies have demonstrated clear autoimmune effects from exposure to TCE, often at low levels typically found in drinking water.[105]

Moreover, the US Department of Agriculture estimates that over 50 million people in the United States get their drinking water from groundwater potentially contaminated by pesticides and other agricultural chemicals.[106] A Harvard study found markedly elevated PFAS in the drinking water supplies of 6 million people.[107]

In addition, an Associated Press investigation revealed that pharmaceuticals including antibiotics, anticonvulsants, hormonal drugs, and psychiatric medicines were present in the drinking water of at least 40 million Americans.[108] When you take medicines, some of them are absorbed but the remainder passes through and makes it eventually into the water system; this is why you shouldn't flush unused drugs down the toilet.

It's for these reasons that I recommend avoiding tap water. I also suggest avoiding bottled water (plastic exposure) and spring water, because widespread environmental contamination has reached even the most pristine springs. I offer recommendations on how to filter your water later in this chapter.

The Environmental Working Group offers a free online Tap Water Database (https://www.ewg.org/tapwater/) where you can check the quality of your local drinking water. When I checked my local water utility, I was concerned to see several toxins at very high levels, including arsenic, chromium, nitrate, and others—with no safe levels established for some of these.

WHAT EXPERTS SAY

Dr. Douglas Kerr, neurologist and autoimmune disease researcher at Johns Hopkins University, writes that there is "almost universal agreement among scientists and physicians that the environmental toxins and chemicals to which we are increasingly exposed are interfering with the immune system's ability to distinguish self from non-self. Most of the risk of autoimmunity comes from environmental exposures rather than from genetic susceptibilities."[109]

Dr. Joseph Pizzorno, one of the world's leading authorities on research in integrative medicine and a doctor with >40 years of experience treating patients, writes "Toxins are now the invisible primary drivers of countless

health problems.... The relationship between toxin exposure and disease
is far more powerful than any other known disease risk factor."[110]

Lisa Jackson, former head of the US Environmental Protection Agency,
said in a Senate hearing on toxins, "A child born in America today will
grow up exposed to more chemicals than any other generation in our
history."[111]

AIR POLLUTION & OTHER TOXINS

Air pollution includes ozone, greenhouse gases, volatile organic compounds
(VOCs), and particulate matter (PM), which refers to microscopic particles that
can carry a variety of toxins. Exposure to PM causes inflammation, playing a
role in the development of and exacerbation of many chronic diseases including
respiratory, cardiovascular, and metabolic conditions.[112]

Emerging evidence suggests that air pollution plays a role in the development
of autoimmune diseases; some of the suspected mechanisms include triggering
production of proinflammatory cytokines, increased oxidative stress and free
radical formation, and airway damage inducing epigenetic changes.[113] Researchers are beginning to look at the role air pollution might play in conditions like
multiple sclerosis, rheumatoid arthritis, lupus, and type I diabetes.[114]

Even in the relative safety of your own home, indoor air pollution may pose
a threat as well. It includes fumes from gas-powered cooking appliances, compounds released from carpets, furnishings, electronics, dust, mold, and other
sources.

In fact, 45 toxic chemicals have been identified in common household dust
that have been linked to a range of health problems including endocrine disruption, respiratory illness, reproductive toxicity, and (pertinent to our discussion)
immune system dysfunction—the list includes phthalates, phenols, flame retardants, and other toxins.[115] You might spend 90 percent of your time indoors
at home, so it is important to address this with the strategies we will discuss
below. In the interest of time, I'm not going to cover other toxins that have been
associated with increased risk of autoimmune disease. These include flame retardant PBDEs (linked to celiac disease),[116] plasticizers known as phthalates (tied to
eczema, asthma, allergies, and immune dysfunction),[117] and industrial "forever
chemicals" known as dioxins.[118]

Microplastics

Microplastics are tiny pieces of plastic—less than 5 mm—that are now found in almost all our food and water due to omnipresent plastic use. The risks to human health are not yet well understood. Patients with autoimmune inflammatory bowel disease were found to have higher levels of microplastics in their stool, although the significance of this is still unclear.[119] Disturbingly, infants appear to have higher levels of microplastics in their stool than adults, indicating greater levels of exposure from their environment.[120]

The recommendations below will help you to minimize exposure to all these additional toxins as well.

I know that reviewing all these toxins might have been overwhelming. Toxins are everywhere, and the goal is not to completely avoid exposure by trying to make your environment completely sterile—which is unrealistic and impractical. Instead, I want to empower you so that you can make the right lifestyle and environmental choices to counterbalance the toxins we are all exposed to.

THE DETOX EQUATION

So, confronted with all these toxins in our environment, in what we eat and drink, what can we do in response? It comes down to a simple equation:

$$\text{Toxins in} - \text{Toxins out} = \text{Toxic Load}$$

Essentially, it is beneficial to try to reduce your exposure to chemicals as much as possible (the intake side of the equation). This is complemented by regular detoxification, in regular intervals as well as periodic intensive cleansing, which comprise the "toxins out" component, which I will discuss in chapter 7. In the meantime, here are some strategies to reduce exposure to household and environmental toxins.

Reducing Exposure to Toxins

1. **Purify your water**
   - Drink water purified by a reverse osmosis water filtration system, which can filter out a wide range of toxins. Units that can be installed

under your sink are available from most retailers and can often be purchased for around $100–$200. I recommend brands such as iSpring, Pure Blue, or Brondell—but other good brands are out there. If you prefer not to install the unit in your home, portable reverse osmosis systems are available.

- More cost-effective but equally good options for countertop water filtration systems include the Zero water filter (which retails for around $40 and has been independently tested to be superior to most other countertop portable filter brands) and ClearlyFiltered, which will provide you third-party testing data that demonstrates their filter's efficacy.

- Because it's possible to absorb significant quantities of chemicals through your daily showers, as they are aerosolized by the hot water, I recommend a shower filter. A good quality shower filter, which you can install yourself, can prevent this. Recommended brands include Aquasana and Berkey.

2. Purify your air

- Automobile exhaust carries a significant number of pollutants, which you might be exposed to while in traffic. Using the recirculate button (which limits the entry of outside air into the car) and keeping your windows raised while driving can help reduce your exposure to airborne toxins while in the car.

- As discussed above, indoor air can pose significant health risks. Getting a high-quality air filter for your home is a good solution. It is also possible to have a professional grade HEPA filter integrated into your HVAC system through Lennox, Nortek, Aprilaire, or your local HVAC company. If you are not able to get one for your entire house, keeping a portable one in your bedroom is still beneficial. Recommended brands that offer individual room purifiers are Air Doctor, Austin, Blueair, and IQAir.

- Keeping household plants is one of the best strategies to help filter your indoor air. NASA conducted extensive research on the best plants to help keep your air clean and identified the most beneficial species as philodendron, peace lily, Ficus, Boston fern, and several varieties of

palm (areca, lady, dwarf date, and bamboo).[121] In addition, they provide a small dose of nature within your home in case you're not able to
get outside every day.

- To help keep household dust to a minimum, clean your floors with a
  HEPA-filter vacuum and/or a wet mop often, and dust surfaces with a
  damp cloth regularly.

- Remove your shoes upon entering the house. This is a custom in
  Indian (and other) cultures, and the science supports this. Dust and
  dirt from outdoors contain toxins and pathogens that have settled
  from the air, which can be carried into your house if you wear your
  shoes indoors. For example, studies of the bottoms of shoes have
  identified lead,[122] pesticides,[123] and multiple harmful bacteria such as
  Clostridium difficile[124] that were shown to be tracked into the house by
  wearing shoes indoors.

- Avoid commercial air fresheners, most of which have been tested
  and found to release phthalates, volatile organic compounds, and/or
  carcinogens like benzene and formaldehyde into your air.[125] A safer
  option is using essential oils with a diffuser.

- If you make use of a wood-burning fireplace, be sure it is in an
  extremely well-ventilated room. Wood smoke contains benzene, formaldehyde, acrolein, and fine particulate matter that can be injurious.[126]
  Electric or gas fireplaces have fewer emissions and are better options if
  available to you.

3. **Minimize exposure to mercury**

- Studies show that heavy metals such as mercury are prevalent in
  water and certain foods, especially larger fish. Choose low-mercury
  fish (wild salmon, mackerel, sardines, anchovy, flounder) and avoid
  high-mercury fish (swordfish, tuna, marlin, shark).

- If you have mercury-containing dental amalgam fillings, consider
  working with a dentist to have them replaced with safer composite
  materials. Work with a functional medicine practitioner to provide
  detox support during this process.

- When taking a fish oil supplement select a product that has been
  third-party tested for heavy metals (e.g., Nordic Naturals, Carlson).

4. Minimize exposure to lead, arsenic, and cadmium

- Ensure that your house is free of lead-based paint. This is more of an issue if your home was built before 1978, when the United States banned the sale of lead-based paint.

- If you live in an older home, make sure there is no lead plumbing. In 1986, government regulations prohibited the use of lead in plumbing, but if you have any pipes or fixtures that were installed before then, it would be prudent to have them checked. Government regulations are slowly catching up with the science. For example, the Safe Drinking Water Act of 1986 restricted plumbing fixtures to a maximum of 8 percent lead (which was considered lead-free at the time); in 2014, a new law reduced the permitted level to less than 0.25 percent.[127]

- Avoid using a slow cooker or any pots with a glazed surface. Safer options for cookware include glass, cast-iron, and stainless steel.

- If you consume canned food, transfer any leftover food to a different (preferably glass) container before storing in the refrigerator—this reduces exposure to lead and tin as well. Lead appears to migrate into the food in a time-dependent manner, so ensure that you are consuming canned food well before the expiration date.[128]

- When cooking rice or other grains, soak them for at least 15 minutes and discard the water. Evidence supports soaking and washing rice before cooking, which significantly reduces levels of lead, arsenic, and cadmium (common in rice).[129]

- Certain spices may be high in lead, especially dried oregano and dried thyme, according to a study from *Consumer Reports*; they tested 126 products and found that about one-third of them had high levels of lead, cadmium, and/or arsenic.[130] The good news is that at least one product of every spice (except oregano and thyme) was found to be safe and without significant amounts of heavy metals. Details about brands are available in the *Consumer Reports* article online (link in the References).

- Psyllium husk can be high in lead levels—choose brands that provide independent testing data indicating they are low in lead, such as Organic India and Yerba Prima.[131]

- Chocolate can contain elevated levels of lead and cadmium. For details on brands that have been tested to be low in heavy metals visit www.doctorakil.com/toxic-chocolate.

- Lipstick can contain high levels of lead, which are present in the raw materials or dyes used to color the product. Several studies have found that the majority of lipsticks and lip glosses contain significant levels of lead (and other heavy metals like aluminum and titanium).[132] Although ingestion of these products is minimal, if they are being applied regularly, it would be prudent to choose a safe option that does not contain lead. For guidance on safe cosmetics, see the section below on "Updating Your Personal Grooming Products."

5. **Reduce exposure to PFCs and PCBs**

- To lessen exposure to PFCs, avoid fabric protectors (e.g. Scotchgard) and clothing that has been treated with compounds to make it waterproof.
- Avoid using Teflon or other pans with nonstick coatings which may contain the PFCs PTFE and PFOA. WearEver Pure Living cookware, which features a nonstick ceramic coating free of lead, cadmium, PTFE, and PFOA, is another good option.
- To reduce exposure to PCBs (and several other toxins) minimize eating farmed fish, especially salmon.[133] Wild salmon is a good alternative. With all fish, trim the fat before cooking because many toxins are stored in fat. Also try to minimize intake of nonorganic dairy, and conventionally grown beef and chicken.

6. **Decrease contact with BPA**

- Plastic water bottles can contain BPA; other BPA-free plastic is not great either. Stainless steel or glass water bottles are safe.
- When purchasing canned food, look for cans that have a "BPA-free" label, indicating a can lining without BPA. Try to avoid purchasing food packaged in plastic as much as possible.
- Limit handling of paper receipts, which contain BPA; opt for electronic receipts if available.

7. **Reduce pesticide exposure**

- Purchase organic fruits and vegetables whenever possible. Every year, the Environmental Working Group releases a list of fruits and vegetables called "The Dirty Dozen" that have the highest pesticide residues even after cleaning and washing at home.[134] Try to always purchase organic versions of these:

- apples, strawberries, grapes, cherries, peaches, pears, spinach, celery, tomatoes, bell peppers, chili peppers, potatoes, cucumbers, nectarines, and green leafy vegetables like kale and collard greens.

- The same group also identified fifteen vegetables called "The Clean Fifteen" that have the lowest pesticide residues. It is acceptable to purchase conventional versions of these if you are not able to get organic for whatever reason:

  - corn, onions, pineapple, avocado, broccoli, cabbage, frozen peas, papaya, asparagus, mango, watermelon, sweet potato, honeydew melon, cantaloupe, and cauliflower.

- As much as possible, avoid using insecticides or pesticides around your home. Take advantage of natural pest control strategies and non-toxic pest repellents.

8. Green your household chemicals

- According to the Environmental Protection Agency, chemicals released into our homes by home care products can make indoor air five times more polluted than the air we breathe outdoors.

- Choose household cleaners that are free of toxins. Many natural brands are available (e.g. Seventh Generation, Dr. Bronner's, and Mrs. Meyer's Clean Day). You can also make your own household cleaners using ingredients like white distilled vinegar and baking soda.

- When painting, select paints with low levels of volatile organic compounds (VOCs).

- When bringing back clothes from the dry cleaner, allow them to air out in a garage or well-ventilated space before putting them in your closet. This will allow the clothes to release chemicals used during dry cleaning, so they do not accumulate in your closet.

9. Update your personal grooming products and practices

- Lipsticks, mascara, eyeshadow, and eye pencils may contain high levels of lead, arsenic, and other heavy metals.[135] To evaluate your cosmetics, visit www.safecosmetics.org or www.ewg.org/skindeep.

- Select antiperspirant that does not contain aluminum, a heavy metal that is difficult to clear from the body.
- When choosing skin-care products, shaving creams, or cosmetics, choose natural products that do not contain parabens, phthalates, toluene, synthetic colors or fragrances, or other artificial ingredients.
- Minimize nail polish, which contains phthalates, formaldehyde, and toluene.
- Avoid fabric softener sheets; they transfer chemicals to your clothes. If you still want to use them, choose products without added fragrance.

10. Reduce exposure to flame retardants such as PBDEs

- Flame retardants are ubiquitous chemicals in couches, cushions, and mattresses that are known disruptors of the endocrine and immune systems.
- Look for organic and "green" building materials, carpeting, baby items, mattresses, and upholstery. Be wary of "greenwashing"; look for certifications like the Greenguard Gold certification, which means the product has been independently tested and complies with the strictest limits for chemical emissions standards.[136] Furniture products filled with cotton, wool, or polyester tend to be safer than chemical-treated polyurethane foam; some products also state that they are "flame-retardant free."

- Clean your home regularly to reduce household dust, which has been shown to contain high levels of flame retardants.
- Research has shown that washing your hands frequently (and especially before meals) reduces body levels of flame retardants, since we often pick up small amounts of these chemicals on our hands through contact with objects at home or at work throughout the day—and transfer them to our mouth inadvertently.[137] Another study found that children who washed their hands at least five times a day had levels of flame retardants on their hands 30 to 50 percent lower than children who washed their hands less frequently.[138] Washing your hands regularly is an easy way to reduce exposure to these chemicals.

STRATEGIES FOR DETOXIFICATION

With the prevalence of chemicals in our environment, it is impossible to avoid exposure completely. Nonetheless, you now have a wealth of information and tools you can use to reduce your exposure to toxins. Additionally, regular detoxification is crucial to help consistently reduce your body burden of these chemicals. In chapter 7, we will talk in detail about the other side of the equation—how to clear toxins from your body.

Let's return to Joseph, who was having trouble walking and had been told he was on his way to multiple sclerosis.

Joseph was surprised to find out that his mercury and lead levels were so elevated. We also found dysbiosis with harmful bacteria and yeast in his gut and increased intestinal permeability. His stress levels were through the roof, but he was skeptical of applying mind-body techniques to combat it.

We began the TIGER Protocol detox, with an elimination diet and supplements such as glutathione to support liver function. Joseph began hourlong biweekly sauna treatments to help detoxify. Follow-up testing revealed that his mercury and lead were normal. I then had him complete an elimination diet and gut-healing protocol with herbs to clear the bad bacteria and yeast from his gut, probiotics to increase his beneficial bacteria, and the amino acid L-glutamine to treat leaky gut.

Eight weeks later, Joseph reported his symptoms were 60 percent improved. I suspected stress was a key factor, but as he was unwilling to attempt meditation, I referred him to a HeartMath practitioner, who trained him to use a biofeedback device that displays visible proof of improvement in stress physiology. Because he was data-driven, this approach was appealing to Joseph, and he practiced it regularly. After six months, he reported full resolution of his numbness and tingling, and improved energy. He never needed to return to the neurologist.

CHAPTER 3

Infections—Disrupting Immune Balance

At just 12 years old, Devi had been diagnosed with Crohn's disease. She had struggled with abdominal pain, bloating, and constipation for over a year. Her symptoms were dismissed as "irritable bowel syndrome" until she finally saw a gastroenterologist, who ordered a stool calprotectin test. Often used to diagnose autoimmune inflammatory bowel disease, a normal level is less than 50. Hers was over 900. A colonoscopy and biopsy confirmed Crohn's disease. Because Crohn's typically causes diarrhea and not constipation, her diagnosis was delayed.

Her father, who was knowledgeable about integrative medicine, immediately put her on a gluten-free, dairy-free diet, which improved her symptoms by about 20 percent. Her gastroenterologist tried various medications on her, but her symptoms did not improve.

This case illustrates a key lesson I learned from a professor in medical school—patients don't read textbooks. There are certain symptoms that are classic for certain diseases, such as diarrhea in inflammatory bowel disease (IBD)—but patients may have unfamiliar manifestations of IBD and other autoimmune conditions. Sometimes it takes a bit of detective work and an open mind to come up with the right diagnosis.

In this chapter, we will review the research on the role of infectious microbes in autoimmunity. Infections with bacteria, viruses, fungi, and/or parasites often play a key role in autoimmune conditions. In my experience, infections and imbalances within the digestive tract are a crucial factor in most patients with autoimmune disease. In certain cases, identification and treatment of infections can help patients with autoimmune disease achieve remission.

In a few cases, patients with chronic systemic infections were actually misdiagnosed as having autoimmunity, and when their infection was fully treated, the autoimmune disease completely resolved.

TERRAIN THEORY VS. GERM THEORY

Before we begin discussing the various microbes that are being studied in auto-immune diseases, let's take a step back to discuss a philosophical difference. In Western medicine, we tend to focus exclusively on the germ, and have a laser-like focus on identifying it (and then the right drug to eliminate it). This can be traced back to Louis Pasteur, who in the nineteenth century advanced his theory that germs cause disease, and that killing or avoiding these organisms is the only way to stay healthy.[1] Don't get me wrong, this has led to wonderful advances in science, such as the development of powerful antibiotics that can be lifesaving in certain situations—so there is real value in this perspective.

However, in integrative medicine we focus on the terrain, which refers to the internal environment of the host. Terrain theory was advanced initially by Antoine Bechamp (a contemporary of Pasteur), who believed that the host environment could be modified to be favorable or unfavorable to microbes.[2] The goal is to make the inner milieu as inhospitable as possible to pathogens. Modern science has confirmed that this is physiologically possible, as we will discuss later (e.g., an acidic large intestine limits the growth of pathogens, while an alkaline colon encourages them).

I believe that both theories have value, but I feel that we have moved a bit too much toward germ theory and do not emphasize terrain enough. Let's take the example of the gut microbiome. We know that it is important to ensure a healthy and balanced ecosystem—which can automatically regulate the levels of bad bugs and keep them in check. My goal is to help you create a robust, diverse, and balanced microbiome—with the richness and resilience of a rainforest. We do not want to have a single-minded focus on eradicating bad bacteria in our gut, because as we will see, sometimes whether a bacteria is good or bad actually depends on multiple factors. My focus is on enhancing the overall vitality and well-being of the entire microbiota community, which will go a long way toward limiting the effects of pathogens.

The emphasis on creating a healthy terrain is a key tenet of Ayurveda as well. Every factor that impacts health influences the terrain, including diet, lifestyle, sleep, exercise, and stress. Of course, I also believe that in some cases one must focus on killing the bad bugs. It is important to understand in-depth the different microbes that can be harmful in autoimmunity, and that is why we are spending an entire chapter on this topic.

ADVANCED TIP

In my own practice, I sometimes follow the functional medicine approach of ordering specialized laboratory tests and I will be describing this approach in chapter 13. However, I always have patients complete the TIGER Protocol first before considering testing for infections. The reason for this is that by clearing toxins, changing their diet, and building up their terrain, patients naturally boost their immune vitality, and this often allows their immune systems to take care of and clear infections on their own.

Therefore, if we test at the very beginning, we may identify multiple chronic infections that would have gone away eventually on their own as part of the TIGER Protocol. By testing (if necessary) after making all the therapeutic changes first, we can see what is left over and deal with a smaller, more manageable set of infections—if any are remaining. Most of the time, testing is not necessary because the TIGER Protocol helps the body remove whatever infections are present.

DYSBIOSIS

The microbiome is known to play a fundamental role in the development of autoimmune disease. Specifically, a condition known as dysbiosis, which can be defined as having too few good bacteria and too many bad microbes (bacteria, yeast, and/or parasites), is being implicated in multiple autoimmune disorders. In fact, it is being studied in most modern chronic illnesses, illustrating the far-reaching impact of the gut microbiome on human health.

Characteristic microbiota "signatures" of bacterial dysbiosis (patterns of imbalance) have been identified in multiple sclerosis, rheumatoid arthritis, lupus, and ankylosing spondylitis.[3] Less common autoimmune conditions such as systemic sclerosis have also been linked to dysbiosis—the typical findings are decreased levels of beneficial bacteria, and abnormally elevated levels of potentially pathogenic bacteria.[4]

You can think of dysbiosis more broadly as a condition of disruption or imbalance in the microbiome that has a negative impact on health. It is the opposite of symbiosis (also called eubiosis), which is a state of mutually beneficial coexistence.[5] In this ideal state, our gut bacteria are supporting every aspect of our health, and we are nourishing and feeding our bacteria optimally. Reversing dysbiosis and achieving symbiosis in the microbiome is one of the most important goals for any patient with autoimmunity—and, in fact, for all people.

Leaky Gut Syndrome

Dysbiosis usually leads to leaky gut syndrome. Normally, intestinal cells are bunched together so that nothing slips by them, like your fingers when you interlace them together. In leaky gut syndrome, the connections between intestinal cells break down and this creates little gaps. These gaps lead to increased intestinal permeability, which is the definition of leaky gut syndrome.

Originally discovered in celiac disease, which leads to severe intestinal permeability, leaky gut has now been established as a key step in the development of many different autoimmune diseases.[6] Once dismissed as a fad by some in the medical community, the condition is now supported by hundreds of research papers.

When the gut exhibits increased permeability, partially digested food particles can slip between the intestinal cells and into the blood. This can be exacerbated if you have low digestive enzymes (something I see commonly in my patients) and are already not breaking down your food properly. The immune system does not recognize these strange-looking, partially digested proteins, and creates antibodies to attack them. This is the first step in the development of food sensitivities, as the immune system begins to react to foods that it did not react to previously.

In addition, opportunistic bacteria and yeast, environmental pollutants, and other toxins can slip through the gut barrier into the blood, spurring the immune system into hyperactivity.

Causes of Leaky Gut

What causes leaky gut syndrome? Changes in the gut microbiome are one of the key contributing factors. These include dysbiosis, declines in the all-important keystone bacteria (which we will discuss in the next chapter), or other infections such as viruses, fungi, or parasites. Also, inflammatory bowel diseases such as ulcerative colitis or Crohn's disease lead to colonic inflammation and leaky gut. Certain food sensitivities (such as gluten sensitivity) can predispose one to the development of leaky gut syndrome, which then leads to worsening food sensitivities in a vicious circle. Excessive alcohol[7] is also a trigger, and stress has a powerful impact by directly weakening barrier function.[8]

Leaky Gut Consequences

Why is leaky gut a problem? As intestinal permeability worsens, the immune system produces a glut of antibodies and sends out inflammatory chemicals and "killer" cells to attack the perceived enemies entering the bloodstream. Certain chemicals known as cytokines are produced in greater quantity, and these can have damaging effects on surrounding tissues. Both the excess antibodies and cytokines can subsequently attack other organs—sometimes depending on where each person has their "weakest link," essentially the most susceptible part of their body. The hyperactive immune system can then mistakenly attack the body's own tissues in this area, starting the individual on the path to autoimmune disease.

Gateway to Autoimmunity

Disruption of gut barrier function is often seen at the very earliest stages of autoimmunity. Even before a patient has a diagnosable autoimmune disease, leaky gut can be present and may often be the first step in the development of the condition. In this state, movement of undigested food, bacteria, and toxins across the overly permeable gut barrier can then lead to abnormal immune responses in distant organs, resulting in inflammation and tissue damage.[9] Basically, things get into the blood that are not supposed to be there, and this agitates the immune system, eventually causing autoimmune reactions and chronic inflammation.

In my experience, almost all patients with autoimmune disease have some degree of increased intestinal permeability. Those who do not still show signs of dysbiosis on stool testing. Without a doubt, intestinal permeability is one of the most important areas to intervene in for all those on the autoimmune spectrum.

We've learned that leaky gut can lead to the immune system going haywire in autoimmunity. However, it is actually possible for immune hyperactivation to occur in autoimmune disease even without the presence of leaky gut. When dysbiosis occurs, it is detected by a specialized type of GI cell called the dendritic cell.

Dendritic cells are part of the immune system and reside close to the gut barrier, just behind our intestinal lining cells. They are constantly sampling the environment of bacteria within the gut, scanning for invaders. They do this by extending cell structures (called pseudo-pods) between the junctions of the cells that line the intestine, all the way into the area where bacteria reside.

Remarkably, they do this while preserving gut barrier integrity and without disrupting intestinal permeability at all.[10] Essentially, they are pushing a periscope up into the GI interior and sampling for pathogens. If they detect bad bacteria, they can trigger an immune response and activate the immune system—even in the absence of increased intestinal permeability.[11] This is why correcting dysbiosis, even if leaky gut is *not* present, is essential in autoimmunity.

DYSBIOSIS SELF-ASSESSMENT

Here's a simple self-assessment to determine whether or not you may be experiencing dysbiosis. Answer yes or no to each of the following questions:

- Do you have more than one food sensitivity or food allergy?
- Did you receive two or more courses of antibiotics in the past year?
- Do you have gas and/or bloating after meals?
- Do you frequently experience either diarrhea or constipation?
- Are you prone to getting stomach upsets or "gut bugs"?
- Do you notice an intolerance to carbohydrates, especially legumes and fiber?
- Do you dislike regularly eating fermented foods?
- Is your diet low in fiber (as defined by less than 40 g of fiber per day)?
- Are you plagued by chronic sinus congestion or recurrent sinus infections?
- Do you experience significant chronic stress?

How Did You Do?

Count the number of "Yes" answers that you have.

Score: 7 to 10. You are at high risk of dysbiosis, based on multiple risk factors. In addition, you experience a number of symptoms that often correlate with abnormalities in the microbiome. You should pay significant attention to improving the overall balance of your bacteria.

Score: 2 to 6. Your microbiome may have been adversely impacted by the presence of negative factors such as antibiotic use or previous GI infections. Your diet may not be the most supportive of your gut bacteria.

As a result, you have a significant risk of dysbiosis, and should start follow-ing the TIGER Protocol Phase I Diet to begin improving your microbiome.

Score: 0 or 1. Congratulations! You probably have a vital and robust microbiome and are unlikely to have significant dysbiosis. You have a lot of positive things in your favor to support the health of your microbiome. You want to continue working to maintain and possibly strengthen your gut bacteria.

LPS—HOW DYSBIOSIS HARMS

To understand the full impact of dysbiosis you need to know about lipopolysac-charide (LPS)—which I learned about while studying microbiology in medical school. It is a combination of lipids and carbohydrates (polysaccharide, specifi-cally) that makes up the outer cell wall of many bacteria found in the gut. LPS protects these bacteria so they are not broken down by bile salts or other enzymes found in the GI tract.

When dysbiosis occurs, there is usually a significant increase in the num-bers of bacteria that have LPS. As bacteria die, their cell walls break down and the LPS is released into the environment. This means the release of LPS is an incidental occurrence and not an intentional action by bacteria trying to cause harm.

Even with an increase in LPS in the gut as a result of dysbiosis, if LPS remains within the interior of the gut, it does not cause a significant problem. It is estimated your gut contains a total of 1 million nanograms (one gram) of endotoxin—but if even just 100 nanograms enter the bloodstream (a tiny fraction of the whole amount)—that's enough to trigger inflammatory activation within the body and brain.[12] So you can see how critically important the integrity of the intestinal bar-rier is, because it functions to keep LPS from entering the circulation.

Toxic Effects of LPS

As we discussed, the gut lining is designed to be an impermeable barrier which keeps LPS and other deleterious compounds found inside the GI tract from get-ting into the circulation. However, when the gut lining becomes compromised and displays increased permeability, as in leaky gut syndrome, LPS begins to enter the bloodstream and triggers a violent inflammatory response.

For this reason, LPS is also called an endotoxin, a toxin that comes from within. Many of the pathogenic bacteria that can trigger serious infections tend to contain LPS, and so its presence in the blood is interpreted by the immune system as a sign of a potentially life-threatening infection such as sepsis, a commonly fatal condition where bacteria enter the bloodstream and spread throughout the body.

Because it is so dangerous, the immune system is primed to detect even low levels of LPS and trigger very strong reactions, because the body believes that it is under serious attack by deadly bacteria. The immune system triggers a strong response by activating hundreds of inflammatory genes, proteins, and immune system signaling compounds called cytokines to try to combat a possibly deadly infection.[13] For example, absorption of LPS triggers the increase of a number of major pro-inflammatory cytokines in the body, such as interleukin-6, interleukin-8, TNF-alpha, and NF-kappa B.[14]

LPS in Autoimmunity

Because autoimmune disease features increased intestinal permeability and systemic inflammation, LPS is commonly elevated in autoimmunity. In fact, in research studies, LPS levels in the blood are used to gauge the severity of both leaky gut syndrome and systemic inflammation in autoimmune and other disorders. For example, in a study of autoimmune hepatitis patients, levels of serum LPS were directly correlated with the severity of increased intestinal permeability, as well as the severity of the underlying autoimmune disease in each patient.[15] LPS testing is only available either in research studies or from a few functional medicine laboratories.

LPS in Other Conditions

In addition to autoimmunity, high levels of LPS are also implicated in obesity, diabetes, heart disease, metabolic syndrome, Alzheimer's disease, chronic inflammation, and fatty liver—making it a quintessential gut-related finding of modern chronic illnesses[16] (just like reduced microbiome diversity as we discussed in chapter 1). The gut-healing program outlined in this book is designed to reduce levels of endotoxin and heal the gut so that LPS does not continue to leak into the bloodstream. For example, high intake of prebiotics such as inulin (which is present in several foods in the Phase 1 and 2 Diets) has been shown in studies to reduce blood levels of LPS.[17]

Incidentally, LPS is thought to also play a major role in depression, which is now understood as an inflammatory condition associated with dysbiosis.[18] Studies show significant increase in antibodies against LPS in patients with depression; LPS also crosses the blood-brain barrier and increases inflammation within the brain.[19]

LPS and Diet

Dysbiosis, and the associated elevated intestinal permeability, is the most common cause of elevated LPS in the blood. In terms of dietary factors, fructose can also cause elevation in LPS, increasing it by up to 40 percent, which is why I strongly recommend avoiding artificial fructose sources such as high fructose corn syrup.[20]

Fat appears to be important as well, with saturated fat possibly being worse for LPS absorption. High levels of saturated fat in a meal appear to transiently increase absorption of LPS into the blood after the meal.[21]

However, I do not believe that saturated fat is harmful in terms of increasing cardiovascular risk. A large meta-analysis reviewing studies including 350,000 people concluded that there is no evidence that consuming saturated fat is associated with increased risk of heart disease or stroke.[22] Another systematic review evaluating studies with over 600,000 people found that there is no evidence to support the recommendation to reduce saturated fat intake and increase polyunsaturated fat consumption in order to prevent cardiovascular disease.[23] And yet, there may be a slight impact in terms of LPS and dysbiosis. With that in mind, I recommend that patients on the autoimmune spectrum focus more on monounsaturated fat, and moderate intake of saturated fat.

ADVANCED TIP

Early on in my practice, I was excited to measure LPS levels in patients with autoimmune disease. I found that almost all of them were elevated—indicating increased intestinal permeability—and the same patients had dysbiosis, small intestinal bacterial growth (SIBO), or other GI infections that were responsible for the elevation in LPS. When these underlying causes were treated and addressed, LPS levels would return to normal.

> I have transitioned to testing and treating the underlying causes of LPS elevation without measuring LPS directly. Since all these tests typically require some out-of-pocket expense, this has been a more cost-effective strategy for patients.

MYCOBACTERIA

Mycobacteria are a subtype of bacteria that are known for their thick cell walls, which allow them to lay dormant for decades and make them resistant to antibiotics; the most famous member is mycobacterium tuberculosis (TB), which is rare in the United States but still a big issue in certain countries.

When it comes to autoimmunity, evidence points to the role of mycobacterium avium subspecies paratuberculosis (MAP) in a few conditions, with the strongest data for type I diabetes. A systematic review identified seven studies that show an association between MAP infection and the development of type I diabetes.[24] A potential mechanism of molecular mimicry has been identified— anti-MAP antibodies produced by the immune system can cross-react with a protein found in the beta cells of the pancreas that secrete insulin, leading to inadvertent destruction of the pancreas by the immune system.[25]

MAP bacteria are often found in cows and cow's milk; due to the hardy nature of mycobacteria, MAP can sometimes survive pasteurization. It is theorized that MAP contamination of milk might explain the correlation between cow's milk exposure and the development of childhood type I diabetes seen in some studies.[26]

In cows, MAP causes a chronic bowel disease called Johne's Disease, which strongly resembles Crohn's disease, an autoimmune bowel disease in humans; this led researchers to explore the possible role of MAP in Crohn's disease.[27] A review of over ten studies found that individuals with Crohn's disease were between 2–7 times more likely to test positive for MAP when compared to healthy controls.[28]

One challenge with mycobacteria is that they are hard to culture in the lab and difficult to detect with usual methods. A 2021 study used a new staining method to look for MAP in intestinal biopsies of patients with Crohn's, and found 18/18 Crohn's disease patients tested positive, whereas MAP was found in 0 out of 15 samples from healthy controls.[29]

MAP bacteria are also being studied for a potential role in multiple sclerosis; further research is needed to clarify the role that MAP infection might play in the development of autoimmune diseases, and the feasible treatments that could be helpful.[30]

THE VIROME

In addition to the bacteria in our body, we harbor a potentially even larger number of viruses, collectively called the virome. A review paper in the prestigious journal *Nature* summarized our current knowledge on this topic.[31] We are just beginning to understand the role of the vast undiscovered world of viruses within us.

As with bacteria, the largest community of viruses in our body appears to reside within our intestines. As with the microbiome, each distinct body location such as the mouth, respiratory tract, and skin has its own distinct viral community. In fact, many of the viruses in our body are likely to be those that infect bacteria (which cause infections) and are called bacteriophages, or phages for short—they play a significant role in regulating the bacterial networks of the microbiome.[32]

The virome appears to be influenced by breastfeeding, diet, medications, age, geography, and health status. Just like the microbiome, viruses colonize the human body soon after birth and assemble gradually over time to create a mature ecosystem.

The Virome and Autoimmunity

Research into the effect of the virome on autoimmune conditions is fascinating. One study identified distinct changes in the virome in young children who developed antibodies associated with type I diabetes; at this earliest stage of the autoimmune condition, a decline of virome diversity and increase in certain viral species was observed.[33] It is interesting that reduced diversity of the virome may be seen in those with autoimmunity compared to healthy people, just as with the microbiome.

The virome is also implicated in celiac disease. In one study, frequent exposure to a virus known as enterovirus (a common, mild virus that affects the GI tract) early in life was associated with higher risk of celiac disease autoimmunity.[34] Interestingly, there appeared to be a synergistic interaction with gluten— in children reporting higher intake of gluten, the risk conferred by exposure to these viruses was significantly greater. This makes sense given that both food sensitivities and infections contribute to autoimmunity.

Another study identified distinct changes in the virome associated with auto-immune inflammatory bowel disease (IBD) in children.[35] Several studies have also shown similar changes in the virome in adults with Crohn's disease[36] and ulcerative colitis.[37] Further research will reveal more about the role of the virome in the pathogenesis of IBD and other autoimmune conditions.

VIRAL INFECTIONS—EPSTEIN-BARR VIRUS

Epstein-Barr virus, or EBV, is one of the viral infections that has been extensively studied regarding its connection to autoimmunity. Epstein-Barr virus infection can activate some of the genes that promote autoimmunity; when EBV infects human cells, it activates several genes associated with the risk for lupus, multiple sclerosis, rheumatoid arthritis, inflammatory bowel disease, type 1 diabetes, and celiac disease.[38]

EBV infection is nearly ubiquitous in people worldwide, with nearly 95 per-cent of humans testing positive.[39] Most people acquire the virus in early child-hood and are asymptomatic. The virus, like chickenpox and many others, remains in the body for life but is usually dormant. If one acquires EBV in later childhood or adult years, it can manifest as infectious mononucleosis or "mono," the syndrome of fever, sore throat, and swollen glands that usually causes severe fatigue and then slowly resolves on its own.

EBV and Autoimmunity

EBV has been connected with a number of different autoimmune disorders. The correlation between EBV and lupus is particularly significant. Many studies have linked EBV to the development of lupus. They have shown that patients with lupus have poor control of EBV infection in their bodies and struggle with limiting reactivation of the virus, as reflected in increased viral loads and ele-vated antibodies directed against EBV.[40]

EBV is also suspected to play a role in the pathogenesis of rheumatoid arthri-tis (RA). Research has shown that RA patients have decreased immune system control of EBV compared to healthy controls; high viral load and elevated EBV antibodies are also commonly seen.[41] Moreover, EBV DNA has been identified in the inflamed cartilage and joints of patients with RA.[42]

EBV has been studied extensively in MS. It is thought to be a "necessary but not sufficient" factor in the development of MS, because MS does not seem to develop in patients who are negative against EBV.[43] EBV-specific antibodies have been found in the cerebrospinal fluid (which bathes the brain) of patients with MS, and EBV-infected cells have been detected in the brains of MS patients.[44]

One of the mechanisms involved with EBV and MS is likely molecular mimicry, because several EBV antigens have been shown to be cross-reactive with proteins affected in multiple sclerosis, such as myelin basic protein in nerve cells.[45] In other words, the immune system makes antibodies against Epstein-Barr virus proteins, but these same antibodies can bind to and then damage the myelin sheath in the nerves because of the strong similarity between these two.

Testing for EBV

Antibody testing can provide clues to the activity of EBV in the body. There are two main types of antibodies directed against infections—IgM and IgG. IgM antibodies are produced during acute, active infection, and IgG antibodies are typically produced at a later stage to provide immunity against future exposure.

Elevations in EBV IgM antibodies in a patient can indicate that they are experiencing either initial EBV infection or reactivation of prior EBV infection. In addition, there is an EBV antibody called Early Antigen (EA) antibody which appears in the acute phase of illness; despite being an IgG antibody it can indicate active infection.[46]

Another EBV test is a DNA polymerase chain reaction (PCR) blood test, which identifies whether there is viral DNA in the blood indicating ongoing, active replication of the virus. Although EBV testing is complex and beyond the scope of this discussion, these are some clues that the virus is active in a person and potentially contributing to their symptoms. Working with a practitioner is the best way to investigate this.

For our purposes, we will focus on creating an inhospitable environment for EBV. Later in the book, we'll explore herbs and natural supplements with antiviral properties that may help ward off EBV.

THE MYCOBIOME

Being aware of the mycobiome, or the fungal organisms within us, has become a critically important piece to our understanding of microbes.[47] Fungi comprise their own kingdom (a major biological category of life), separate from plants and animals. They include yeasts, molds, and mushrooms, and typically reproduce by forming spores. Less numerous than bacteria and viruses, fungi are estimated to comprise 0.1 percent of the total microbes in the gut; the three dominant organisms are Malassezia, Candida, and Saccharomyces, while smaller players include Cryptococcus, Aspergillus, and others.[48] In total, the gastrointestinal tract harbors at least 260 fungal species, some of which also play an active role in the gut-brain axis (the two-way close communication between the gut and the brain).[49]

Fungal infections—Candida

Candida is one of the most common fungi and among the most well-known. While in the past it was controversial whether candida had a significant impact on human health, that is now clear due to mounting research evidence. However, it is important to test for it to identify whether an overgrowth is present.

Functional medicine stool testing, or urine testing with an Organic Acids Test (OAT) can identify elevated levels of candida and its metabolites. It is definitely not possible to infer the presence of excess candida only by symptoms (which are indistinguishable from many other conditions), completing online questionnaires, or doing simple home-based tests.

Candida is the fungal organism most studied in autoimmune conditions; it is being investigated for its role in the pathogenesis of multiple sclerosis and other neurological disorders.[50] One study showed that infection with three different species of candida was independently associated with higher odds of having multiple sclerosis.[51] Another study found that patients with multiple sclerosis had candida species that were significantly more virulent than those in healthy controls, as measured by levels of an enzyme that they use to invade host tissue.[52]

Studies are also investigating the role of the mycobiome in autoimmune GI disorders. A study of Crohn's disease suggests that candida may be one of the initiators of the inflammatory process in this autoimmune condition (along with bacterial dysbiosis).[53] Candida is being examined for its possible role in the pathogenesis of celiac disease, because of possible molecular mimicry between gluten and one of the proteins on the yeast's surface.[54]

Just as with bacterial dysbiosis, fungal dysbiosis appears to play a key role in influencing immune responses and potentially triggering the immune system to be hyperactive.[55]

Biofilms

Crucial to understanding how fungi (and bacteria) operate is the concept of biofilms, which are communities of microbes that aggregate within a matrix of secreted polymers. These microbes gather in biofilms in order to improve survival and increase resistance to antimicrobials and the immune system. Candida is one of the fungal species that is known to produce biofilm, which contributes to its resistance to host defenses and antifungal agents.[56]

Bacteria form biofilms as well. It is important to remember that a biofilm is not a harmful feature of bad bacteria, but rather an essential element of how bacteria organize and grow, to participate in social cooperation, resource harvesting, and defense against antimicrobials.[57] It is part of a normal lifestyle that bacteria often choose.

We want to focus on shifting the biofilm within us from dysbiosis to symbiosis, and not destroying and eliminating the biofilm—again, moving away from germ theory's focus on killing and emphasizing the importance of a balanced terrain.

MIXED SPECIES BIOFILM

Fungi and bacteria appear to have a strong connection within the gut and interact in manifold ways. For example, they can come together in biofilm. Research has documented rapid formation of "mixed-species biofilm" between the potentially pathogenic fungi and bacteria Candida and Citrobacter, as well as Trichospora and Staphylococcus.[58] Such a mixed-species biofilm provides mutual benefit for both fungi and bacteria but unfortunately (from our human perspective) often increases their resistance to antimicrobial treatment.[59]

PARASITES

The role of parasites in autoimmunity is mixed and complex. On one hand, parasites can cause a degree of low-grade immune suppression. They do this partly as a survival strategy to ensure that they can persist in the host without being killed by the immune response. During long-standing chronic infection, they downregulate the host's immune response and also may suppress autoimmune responses by reducing reactivity to bystander pathogens and antigens.[60]

We discussed in chapter 1 how parasites can be some of the "old friends" that our immune systems evolved with over millions of years that help to keep autoimmunity in check. It appears that any beneficial exposure to parasites for this purpose of immune system training has to occur during the first few years of life, and being infected with parasites later on does not carry the same benefit.

At the same time, those who suffer from parasites have a slightly weakened immune system and are more susceptible to colds, flus, and other infections (which can play a role in contributing to autoimmunity). I have seen this time and again in my own patients.

Some of my autoimmune patients have presented with parasites as the cause of various unpleasant GI and even systemic symptoms; stool testing typically reveals gastrointestinal inflammation and increased intestinal permeability. In these cases, treatment of the parasites can improve GI symptoms and the course of the autoimmune condition.

Some parasites can also directly trigger an autoimmune response. In Chagas disease cardiomyopathy, infection by the parasite Trypanosoma cruzi leads to autoimmune tissue destruction in the heart through molecular mimicry and bystander tissue damage.[61]

ARCHAEA

Archaea are a group of single-celled organisms that originally were thought to be bacteria but were later discovered to have enough distinct features to form their own category.[62] Archaea live in the GI tract and are methanogens—they produce methane by breaking down excess hydrogen produced by other bacteria.

Normally, at baseline levels, methanogens in the GI tract are helpful because of their ability to remove excess hydrogen and produce a small amount of methane, which leads to a net reduction in the amount of gas in the intestine—meaning a small amount of methanogens is a good thing. However, if the methanogens become overgrown, as part of a condition called Small Intestinal Bacterial Overgrowth (SIBO) or Intestinal Methanogen Overgrowth (IMO), the excess methane they produce can cause problematic symptoms such as gas, bloating, abdominal pain, and constipation.[63]

SIBO is being studied in various autoimmune conditions, especially those that affect the gastrointestinal system such as inflammatory bowel disease[64] and autoimmune liver disease.[65] We will be discussing SIBO in more detail in chapter 13.

TIGER PROTOCOL APPROACH TO INFECTIONS

An important part of the TIGER Protocol is making the body inhospitable to all types of infections. As we discussed earlier, in integrative medicine we focus on making the "terrain" of your body resilient to bad microbes and building up your natural immunity and resistance to infections. The Phase 2 Diet, which we'll dig into in chapter 9, is designed to build up your keystone species, increase the diversity of your microbiome, and lower your intestinal pH—which makes your GI tract inhospitable to harmful pathogens.

However, we're not going to ignore the bad bugs. Because dysbiosis is so prevalent in patients on the autoimmune spectrum, I am going to put you on a two-week protocol (outlined in chapter 8) to clear out as much as possible any pathogens that might be in your system. In that chapter, we will also talk about how to use specific foods, vitamins, spices, and herbs to boost your innate immune defenses and decrease any dysbiotic bacteria, viruses, fungi, parasites, and archaea in your body.

In the beginning of the chapter, we met Devi, a 12-year-old girl who had just been diagnosed with Crohn's disease.

> Despite a gluten-free, dairy-free diet and taking various immunosuppressants, Devi's symptoms were not improving. I ordered stool testing for her and identified significant dysbiosis with the Cryptosporidium parasite, as well as candida overgrowth.
>
> While a first round of an herbal formula was not effective to eradicate the parasite, a second formula did the trick. To clear the candida, I had her eliminate sugar from her diet, and put her on antifungal herbs including neem. After three months, follow-up testing revealed that her dysbiosis had improved and the parasite and candida were no longer present. At that time, we began using prebiotics to build up her beneficial bacteria.
>
> Gradually, her abdominal pain, bloating and constipation resolved, and she began to have normal daily bowel movements. An avid soccer player, Devi was able to rejoin her school team. After we addressed the infections, the diet she was on and the medication she was taking became much more effective and finally began to work, leading to long-term remission.

CHAPTER 4

Gut—The Foundation of (Immune) Health

Maria presented with poorly controlled psoriasis, an autoimmune skin condition. She had been diagnosed with gestational diabetes after her first pregnancy and had subsequently developed metabolic syndrome characterized by high blood pressure, insulin resistance, and obesity; this was alongside fatty liver, identified by abnormally high liver enzyme blood tests, which was likely related to the insulin resistance. Now, at 40 years old, even daily use of topical steroids did not solve her psoriasis.

Although she did not have any GI symptoms, my first step was to take a look at her microbiome. It was highly disrupted. It showed significant intestinal permeability, high levels of the harmful bacteria pseudomonas, and low levels of Bifidobacteria and lactobacillus. It showed an absence of the beneficial bacteria Akkermansia, which was below the detectable limit of the test. Her butyrate, one of the most important anti-inflammatory short-chain fatty acids in the gut, was quite low.

I suspected that her dysbiosis was a major contributor to her symptoms, although Maria was not convinced of this because she felt fine from a digestive point of view and had no GI symptoms whatsoever.

In almost every branch of integrative medicine, the gut is considered to be the foundation of health—and functional medicine and Ayurveda are no exception. For patients on the autoimmune spectrum, addressing gut health may be one of the most important factors in turning their health around.

You are about to embark on a fascinating journey into the inner workings of an indispensable organ that affects every aspect of your physical and mental life—that's right, scientists consider this to be an organ in its own right and often call it the "forgotten organ"—your microbiome.[1]

In chapter 1, I introduced the concept of the microbiome, which we are going to delve into much more deeply here. First, I'd like to introduce several of the most important players in the microbiome. Known as keystone species, these little-known bacteria play an absolutely pivotal but unrecognized role in modulating inflammation, autoimmunity, and the overall health of the gut and the entire body. For example, the vitally important Faecalibacterium prausnitzii is usually the most abundant bacteria in the entire microbiome and fundamental to health but not widely known.

One reason for this is that certain bacteria are relatively easy to grow and culture in the lab. These are aerobic bacteria that survive in the presence of oxygen in the air. For that reason, they have been well studied and characterized. A good example is *Escherichia coli* (*E. coli*), which was discovered in 1884 by the German pediatrician Theodor Escherich and has been extensively studied since.[2]

Other bacteria, and in fact most of the bacteria in the microbiome, are anaerobic and difficult to culture—they die in the presence of oxygen in the air—and therefore had not been scrutinized until newer, more advanced techniques were recently developed.

It's important to note that there is a great deal of variation from person to person in terms of a healthy microbiome. Two individuals may show only limited (or in some cases no) overlap in microbial species in their microbiota.[3] Still, patterns do appear. In the following sections, we'll take a look at five of the most important keystone bacteria identified so far and review the normal functions and typical ranges of abundance of these bacteria within people.

FAECALIBACTERIUM PRAUSNITZII

I came across this bacterium, commonly known as F. prausnitzii, when I was researching COVID-19 and the microbiome. Faecalibacterium prausnitzii (named after German bacteriologist Otto Prausnitz) is typically the single most abundant bacterium in the entire microbiota of healthy adults, comprising anywhere from 5 to 15 percent of the total bacterial population.[4] In recent years, an increasing number of studies have documented the tremendous importance of this bacteria in a number of inflammatory and immune-mediated conditions. As I began to review the research, I found that there was definitely a connection between COVID and gut health.

The COVID Connection

In patients with COVID-19, there were changes in the composition of the gut microbiome consistent with dysbiosis. Certain beneficial keystone species that are known to modulate the immune system, such as F. prausnitzii, were depleted in a study of 100 patients with COVID-19, and the dysbiosis persisted even after clearance of the virus.[5]

Another study in patients hospitalized with COVID-19 found a drop in beneficial bacteria, and overgrowth of opportunistic pathogens (i.e., dysbiosis); levels of Faecalibacterium prausnitzii were inversely correlated with severity of the disease.[6] This means that the higher the levels of this bacteria, the less serious the case of COVID-19—it appears to be protective against the development of severe COVID disease, although more research is needed to confirm this. I was intrigued by the fact that patients with severe COVID-19 seem to have significantly reduced levels of Faecalibacterium prausnitzii and other beneficial bacteria.

Key Butyrate Producer

As I learned more about this bacterium, I began to understand just how important it is, even though it is not very well-known. Faecalibacterium is an anaerobic bacterium, which means that it dies in the presence of oxygen. Therefore, while it thrives inside the GI tract, it dies quickly when exposed to air in the laboratory and therefore it is difficult to grow and culture.

It is one of the main producers of butyrate, one of a class of important compounds produced by the gut microbiota called short-chain fatty acids or SCFAs. These short-chain fatty acids promote the function of the regulatory T cells that we discussed in chapter 1, which are crucial for regulating the immune system and promoting healthy immune responses rather than autoimmunity.[7]

I think of butyrate as "gut ambrosia" because it has so many benefits. Butyrate serves as the primary fuel for the intestinal cells.[8] It reduces GI inflammation, normalizes intestinal permeability, supports healthy mucus production for the gut lining, and enhances motility of the colon (helping things move through at the proper rate).[9] It also has a variety of systemic benefits including limiting the negative effects of LPS, reducing body-wide inflammation, enhancing insulin sensitivity, supporting healthy mood, and having anti-cancer effects.[10]

Butyrate helps reduce a condition known as visceral hypersensitivity, in which the nerves in the intestine become hypersensitive to normal amounts of gas and movement in the GI tract—this is thought to be one of the key issues in patients with irritable bowel syndrome.[11] It even improves the gut-brain axis and can help to heal "leaky brain," which is an impaired blood-brain barrier commonly associated with impaired intestinal permeability.[12] Thus, butyrate is without a doubt one of the most critical anti-inflammatory compounds in your body—and it must be produced by your keystone bacteria, such as Faecalibacterium.

ADVANCED TIP

Functional medicine stool testing can measure the levels of butyrate and other short-chain fatty acids in the gut. You can take two approaches to help raise butyrate levels in the GI tract—try to increase the levels of your good bacteria that are supposed to produce butyrate, or you can take it as an exogenous supplement. My preference is the former.

Usually, using prebiotics to raise the levels of keystone bacteria is effective and subsequently leads to increased production of short-chain fatty acids including butyrate. Follow-up stool testing can confirm this. If that is not successful, then a butyrate supplement could be considered. While human data is limited, animal studies indicate that exogenous butyrate may help improve intestinal permeability and reduce inflammation.[13] Work with your local practitioner if you wish to try butyrate supplementation.

Connection to Autoimmunity

Reductions in Faecalibacterium have been seen in autoimmune conditions including celiac disease, Crohn's disease, ulcerative colitis, and psoriasis, as well as other chronic illnesses such as type II diabetes, colon cancer, and irritable bowel syndrome.[14]

It appears to be especially important in Crohn's disease. Studies show that lower levels of F. prausnitzii are associated with higher rates of recurrence of exacerbations in Crohn's disease; increasing levels of this bacteria reverses the dysbiosis seen in animal models of colitis.[15] The anti-inflammatory effects of this bacterium are mediated by multiple mechanisms, including raising levels of the beneficial T regulatory cells in the immune system via butyrate and other metabolites, and inducing the production of cytokines that reduce inflammation such as interleukin-10.[16]

Raising Faecalibacterium Levels

There is no probiotic available on the market that contains F. prausnitzii. The best way to raise levels of Faecalibacterium is with a diversity of prebiotic foods, as we will discuss in chapter 10.

AKKERMANSIA MUCINIPHILA

The keystone bacteria Akkermansia muciniphila is another one of the most abundant bacteria in the microbiota, comprising between 1 to 5 percent of total species.[17] It is an anaerobic bacterium, so it thrives in the oxygen-poor environment of the gut but dies in the presence of oxygen.

Mucus Lover

Akkermansia is named after the Dutch microbiologist Antoon Akkermans.[18] "Muciniphila" is Latin for mucus-loving, referring to the fact that Akkermansia feeds on the mucus that lines the intestine (the mucin layer, as we learned in chapter 1). By feeding on mucin, it actually triggers increased production of mucin, which has the net effect of thickening the mucus layer overall, strengthening barrier function in the GI tract, and preventing leaky gut syndrome; one of the ways it does this is by triggering an increase in the number of the cells that produce mucus—called goblet cells—in the gut lining.[19]

Low levels of Akkermansia have been associated with increased intestinal permeability, which is central to autoimmune disease pathogenesis as we discussed earlier.

Akkermansia Improves Gut Health

Studies show that Akkermansia helps reinforce gut barrier function and reduces plasma levels of LPS.[20] As discussed earlier, translocation of LPS into the blood increases systemic inflammation as well as insulin resistance, and can be used as a marker for increased intestinal permeability. Akkermansia induces further beneficial changes by producing acetate and propionate, two of the most powerful anti-inflammatory short-chain fatty acids besides butyrate.[21] Through multiple mechanisms, Akkermansia can have a powerful impact on healing the gut.

Metabolic Powerhouse

Akkermansia appears to have important effects on metabolism. Low levels are seen in cases of obesity and cardiometabolic disorders.[22] It appears that decreased levels of Akkermansia raise the risk of fatty liver disease, the most common liver condition in the modern world.[23]

Higher levels of Akkermansia are associated with the healthiest metabolic status as measured by blood sugar, triglycerides, and waist-to-hip ratio—and appear to increase the effectiveness of weight loss interventions, making it more likely that a low-calorie diet would lead to significant weight loss.[24] In other words, having high levels of this bacteria makes it more likely that you will actually be successful at losing weight on a diet.

Links to Autoimmunity

Studies on Akkermansia in autoimmunity are mixed; in most autoimmune diseases, it appears to be low, but a few studies have found high levels. For example, in psoriasis and type I diabetes,[25] low levels of Akkermansia have been identified. Three studies in ulcerative colitis have shown reduced levels of this keystone species, as well as one study in Crohn's disease.[26]

In contrast, in infants with eczema, one study found high levels of associated Akkermansia[27] while a different study found low levels.[28] In rheumatoid arthritis (RA), one study found that Akkermansia was elevated in the RA group whereas another study reported lower levels associated with RA.[29]

Controversy and Confusion

As we have discussed, in most autoimmune conditions, Akkermansia levels are low (or the research is mixed). The exception seems to be multiple sclerosis, where a couple of studies have found elevated levels of Akkermansia.[30] Some theorize that high Akkermansia may be overconsuming the mucus lining, thus degrading the gut barrier and causing leaky gut syndrome. Therefore, I have heard some patients say that they do not want to increase their Akkermansia levels, for fear of increasing the risk of multiple sclerosis or other autoimmune conditions.

I think this is unlikely because studies show that the net effect of Akkermansia consuming mucus is a remodeling of the gut layer, which leads in fact to strengthening of the gut barrier and *thickening* of the mucus lining in both human and animal studies.[31] We know that a damaged gut barrier produces more mucus as it tries to heal, just like any damaged mucous membrane (this is why your nose produces mucus during a cold).

The purpose of increased mucus production in the gut is to try to reduce inflammation and heal the compromised lining. I suspect that in multiple sclerosis the gut lining is damaged by other causes (e.g. infections, food sensitivities, stress, toxins, etc.), which then causes it to produce more mucus; the increased levels of mucus are happily consumed by Akkermansia, thus raising their numbers. I share the view of researchers who believe that the elevated Akkermansia is a result of a disrupted gut barrier and not a cause of it.[32] More studies are needed to clarify this.

Akkermansia is unique among the keystone bacteria in that it consumes mucus. That is why the research picture is not straightforward as with other beneficial bacteria which are consistently low in autoimmune disease. Thinning of the mucus layer in autoimmune disease may deprive Akkermansia of a key food, thus reducing its levels; conversely, the body's response to try to heal leaky gut by increasing mucus production could raise Akkermansia levels in other patients.

Boosting Akkermansia Levels

It is possible to boost Akkermansia levels with diet or probiotic/prebiotic supplements. Studies show that consuming inulin-based prebiotics can have a beneficial impact on insulin resistance, fatty liver, overall fat mass, and intestinal permeability, likely through the prebiotics' effects on Akkermansia.[33]

Initial studies looking at a probiotic form of Akkermansia have shown favorable outcomes; a randomized double-blind placebo-controlled trial found that taking oral Akkermansia for three months led to improved insulin sensitivity and decreased body weight, fat mass, serum insulin, liver inflammation, and hip circumference in overweight adults.[34] As expected, taking Akkermansia as a probiotic reduced levels of LPS, indicating strengthened barrier function and reduced translocation of LPS from the gut into the bloodstream.[35]

With Akkermansia, consuming certain foods rich in red polyphenols such as pomegranate and cranberry can help raise levels[36] (I will review all these foods in chapter 10). For patients with autoimmune disease, I do not recommend Akkermansia supplements, because of the controversy described above. However, I believe that raising levels of Akkermansia through the diet—which feeds the native keystone strain of Akkermansia already present in each person's gut—is likely to be very beneficial, and does not have a risk of worsening autoimmunity.

Effects of Fat and Fasting

Animal studies indicate that high fat intake may have the effect of reducing levels of Akkermansia. It is possible that saturated fat may have a negative impact on Akkermansia, whereas beneficial omega-3 fats from fish are likely to help, although further studies are needed to confirm this.[37]

Intermittent fasting may also have a beneficial effect. One study showed that intermittent fasting, consisting of around 16–18 hours of fasting per day, led to a significant increase in Akkermansia levels after one month of practice.[38] This is yet another benefit of the intermittent fasting practices that we will discuss in chapter 14.

ADVANCED TIP

Pasteurized (heat-killed) Akkermansia has shown to work just as well as the live version—does this seem puzzling? It becomes clearer when we understand how Akkermansia works. One of the key proteins on its outer surface is vital—Amuc-1100, an outer membrane protein on the cell wall of Akkermansia, has been found to activate intracellular signals that actually enhance the intestinal barrier and optimize intestinal permeability; this same protein has been shown to induce production of anti-inflammatory cytokines such as interleukin-10 (IL-10).[39] Essentially, even if the Akkermansia bacteria is pasteurized (and killed), these proteins on its surface would be able to exert their beneficial effects on immune function and intestinal permeability when introduced into the GI tract via an oral probiotic.

BIFIDOBACTERIUM

Bifidobacterium is well-known because it was discovered a long time ago and is a common ingredient in many probiotics. In 1899, French pediatrician Henry Tissier discovered that children with diarrhea had low levels of an unusual Y-shaped gut bacterium when compared to healthy children. Based on its appearance, he named it Bifidobacterium after the word "bifid," which refers to something divided by a cleft into two parts.[40] Normal levels in the gut are between 1 to 5 percent of the microbiota, and over 250 subtypes of Bifidobacteria have been identified.[41]

Bifidobacteria are one of the first species to colonize the gut. Through vaginal childbirth and the prebiotics contained in breast milk, levels of Bifidobacteria can rise to comprise up to >90 percent of the microbiota in breastfed infants.[42] These levels gradually decline over the first three years of life to approach an adult level closer to 5 percent as the ecosystem shifts to resemble the adult microbiota.[43]

GI Defender

Bifidobacteria help to synthesize B vitamins and antioxidants, educate and train the maturing immune system, support healthy gut barrier function, and protect against pathogens in several ways.[44] Bifidobacteria also produce short-chain fatty acids, but instead of butyrate they produce acetate and lactate, which are beneficial in their own right; they inhibit the growth of bad bacteria such as *E. coli*, reduce inflammation, and protect you from infections.[45] Bifidobacteria can help maintain healthy intestinal permeability and lower inflammatory LPS levels.

Ties to Autoimmunity

Several studies have found decreased levels of these bacteria in conditions such as autoimmune diseases, obesity, diabetes, asthma, autism, and skin disorders. For example, a decline in the relative abundance of Bifidobacteria (and Faecalibacterium prausnitzii), as well as a reduction in overall diversity, was found in the microbiota of patients with autoimmune hepatitis.[46] Patients with celiac disease also exhibit decreased levels of Bifidobacteria and their microbiome when compared to healthy controls.[47]

Therapeutic Uses

Studies show that taking Bifidobacteria as a probiotic (which I will review in chapter 9) can help reduce inflammation in type 1 diabetes, celiac disease, inflammatory bowel disease, multiple sclerosis, and psoriasis.[48] Moreover, they appear to play a key role in the gut-brain axis, which is the close two-way link between the gut and the brain. Studies show that certain strains of Bifidobacteria may have a beneficial impact on depression and anxiety.[49]

As a keystone species, Bifidobacteria's abundance in the microbiome is crucial to help ensure the health of the whole ecosystem. One reason for this is the "cross-feeding" that occurs between Bifidobacteria and other good bacteria in the microbiome. Cross-feeding is where metabolites produced by one species of bacteria have beneficial effects on other species, mediating interactions within the microbiota. Consider, for example, that the lactate Bifidobacteria produce is consumed by beneficial Eubacteria, which in turn produce butyrate.[50]

BACTEROIDES

Bacteroides is the main member of one of the most common categories of bacteria in the microbiota called Bacteroidetes, comprising anywhere from between 10 to 25 percent of the gut microbiota.[51] It is an anaerobic bacterium that cannot survive in the presence of oxygen. Its cell membranes contain LPS.

Bacteroides is what is called a pathobiont, which is an organism that is usually neutral or beneficial but can become harmful under certain circumstances, making this situation more fraught and complicated than that with the three keystone species we discussed earlier.[52] Nonetheless, because Bacteroides makes up such a significant percentage of the microbiota, it is critical to understand it, and learn what you can do to keep its levels in a healthful range and prevent it from causing harm.

The Jekyll and Hyde of Bacteria

Bacteroides can wreak havoc if it escapes from the gut—it is the most common anaerobic bacterial cause of non-GI infections in the body (abscesses, bone or blood infections, etc.). However, it does have some positive effects. It aids in the normal development and maturation of the immune system, provides resistance against pathogens such as Salmonella and *C. difficile*, and breaks down otherwise undigestible food components into compounds that support the growth of beneficial gut bacteria.[53] Bacteroides produces the short-chain fatty acid propionate, which has been shown to help resist infection by Salmonella.[54]

However, if Bacteroides levels start to become too high, they are associated with negative consequences such as reduced microbiome diversity and insulin resistance.[55] Bacteroides also performs an activity called protein putrefaction, where it breaks down protein to form harmful compounds. In this process it can ferment proteins to produce amines, indoles, and ammonia, which have negative effects. Bacteroides can transform our primary bile acids, produced by the liver to aid in digestion, into so-called secondary bile acids, which are potential carcinogens that can cause DNA damage in our colonic cells.

ADVANCED TIP

Although we discussed LPS in chapter 3 as a single entity, there are actually distinct types of LPS on different bacteria that vary in their degree of toxicity. For example, the LPS in Bacteroides is actually much less inflammatory—at least 100 times less—than the LPS in more pathogenic bacteria such as E. coli, Salmonella, Shigella, Klebsiella, Pseudomonas, and Citrobacter (part of a more pro-inflammatory group of bacteria called Proteobacteria).[56]

This is because the LPS in Bacteroides has a slightly different structure from LPS in, for example, E. coli. We are fortunate because Bacteroides is a substantial part of our microbiome, comprising up to 25 percent or higher in some cases, whereas E. coli is a much smaller player that may comprise 0.01 to 0.1 percent of a healthy microbiota. Even though Bacteroides has an LPS that is less inflammatory, it is nonetheless provoking and can have some negative consequences.

Regulates Detox via Beta-Glucuronidase

Bacteroides is one of the main producers of beta-glucuronidase, an enzyme that is the primary mediator of how the microbiome affects detoxification in the body. High levels of this enzyme hinder the clearance of toxins from the body and therefore limit detoxification. The liver packages compounds that it would like to get rid of, such as toxins and excess hormones, together with glucuronide, and secretes that into the GI tract where it should be eliminated via the stool. Beta-glucuronidase breaks off this glucuronide component and allows these toxins or hormones, such as estrogen, to be reabsorbed instead of excreted; so, it is not surprising that increased levels of beta-glucuronidase are implicated in cases of breast cancer[57] and colon cancer.[58]

We can see how dysbiosis in the microbiome can influence detoxification. If you have excessive levels of Bacteroides or other bacteria that produce beta-glucuronidase, that will significantly impair your ability to clear toxins from your body.

Autoimmune Impact

In terms of autoimmunity, high levels of Bacteroides are seen in the microbiota of patients with preclinical type I diabetes, where they have antibodies but have not progressed to develop the disease yet; lack of diversity and deficits in butyrate-producing bacteria are also seen at these stages, indicating dysbiosis.[59]

While Bacteroides does have some beneficial effects, it really does have two sides—therefore it is critical to keep its levels within a healthy range. Strategies that have been shown to reduce growth of Bacteroides include maintaining an optimal acidic pH in the colon, limiting intake of animal fats and dairy products, and incorporating certain prebiotics into the diet, such as FOS, GOS, and polyphenols (to be reviewed in chapter 10).

LACTOBACILLUS

While Lactobacillus species are among the best-known bacteria because of their widespread use in probiotics, they actually comprise only about 0.01 to 1 percent of the gut microbiota. They are famous because of Nobel Prize-winning Russian scientist Elie Metchnikoff (often considered the "father of probiotics"), who isolated *Lactobacillus acidophilus* in the early 1900s in the yogurt of a population of Bulgarian peasants, and attributed their longevity and good health to the benefits of this bacteria.[60] Since they are relatively easy to grow and culture, they have been studied and incorporated into various probiotics supplements over the years.

Lactobacilli derive their name from their ability to ferment carbohydrates into lactic acid, which has led to their use in the production of a variety of fermented foods. Lactobacillus has significant health benefits, including protecting the microbiota against the growth of pathogens, promoting the development of beneficial regulatory T cells in the immune system, producing beneficial short-chain fatty acids, producing certain neurotransmitters such as gamma-aminobutyric acid (GABA), and helping with the transformation of polyphenols so that they can either be absorbed or utilized by the microbiota.[61] They also play a key role in protecting the integrity of the gut barrier and maintaining normal intestinal permeability.[62]

Primary Vaginal Species

More so than in the gut microbiota, Lactobacillus plays a larger role in the vaginal microbiota (in which paradoxically low diversity is the hallmark of a healthy ecosystem, and increased diversity is associated with pathogenic conditions like bacterial vaginosis).[63] Lactobacilli are typically the dominant, most prevalent species in the healthy vaginal microbiota, and therefore one of the first species to colonize the newborn gut microbiome after normal birth.

Influence on Autoimmunity

Children with autoimmune type 1 diabetes have significantly lower levels of lactobacillus than healthy children.[64] Patients with autoimmune hepatitis have been shown to have fewer Lactobacillus in their microbiota than normal people, and these levels progressively decline as their autoimmune condition progresses and worsens.[65] Several studies have shown that taking various Lactobacillus species can help reduce inflammation and pain in patients with rheumatoid arthritis.[66] I review probiotics containing Lactobacillus in chapter 9.

HONORABLE MENTIONS

There are of course hundreds of species of bacteria in the microbiota, and we are just beginning to understand the function of many of them. Although we don't have time to discuss all of them in detail, I would like to include several other bacteria as "Honorable Mentions" because of their contribution to butyrate production and other beneficial effects in the gut. Butyrate, as we discussed earlier, is one of the most essential anti-inflammatory compounds for the whole body.

Other key butyrate producers in the gut include Eubacterium, Ruminococcus, and Roseburia species[67] (each of which may comprise up to 10–15% of the bacteria in some people with a healthy microbiome) and smaller players such as Coprococcus, Subdoligranulum, and Anaerostipes.[68] Many of them work together and participate in cross-feeding in order to create a healthy gut ecosystem. As I mentioned earlier, keep in mind that there is a great deal of individual variability in the microbiota, and percentages may vary significantly between people.

It is ideal to have most of your microbiome comprised of bacteria that produce short-chain fatty acids, especially butyrate. The advantage of having a robust group of multiple different butyrate producers in the gut is that if certain species are greatly reduced, from antibiotics or other interventions, other species can "pick up the slack" and take over to produce the necessary amounts of butyrate to ensure a healthy milieu.

ASSESSING YOUR MICROBIOME

The simplest way to gauge the health of the gut microbiome is by the quality of one's bowel movements. This is consistent with our scientific understanding that stool is about 60 percent bacteria by weight.[69]

Generally, a well-formed stool that is not overly hard or painful to pass is normal. A minimum of one bowel movement a day is ideal, and anything less frequent is not optimal. Surprisingly, there is ambiguity in the medical literature about the definition of constipation, but some sources define constipation as fewer than three bowel movements per week—by this standard, one might think it's normal to have a bowel movement every other day.[70]

From my perspective, while it might be normal and not uncommon, because the prevalence of constipation is so high now, it is suboptimal for autoimmune patients to go without a daily bowel movement. There are a lot of things your body is trying to get rid of through stool, and it is best to assist the body with this through daily elimination.

Your Home Stool Test

Although advanced molecular techniques allow for detailed analysis of the microbiome through stool testing, there is a basic test you can do at home without any equipment—you can test your gut transit time. This is essentially the time it takes for food to pass all the way from your mouth through your GI tract and out of your body—you can think of it as how long it takes food to go from mouth to toilet. This is important because it can make a substantial difference in the health of your digestive tract and microbiota, and is associated with microbiome diversity and cardiometabolic health.[71]

Testing transit time is simple—eat two tablespoons of chia seeds or white sesame seeds, and don't chew them too well. It is best to avoid these foods for a week before the test and eat the food by itself at least an hour away from other foods. Record the time of consumption. When you first start to see the appearance of these foods in your stool, the difference between ingestion and exit time is the gut transit time. This test can also be done with corn on the cob;

a study in Africa with university students found that ingesting whole-kernel corn and monitoring its passage was also an effective way to determine transit time.[72]

This test assesses motility—how quickly something moves through the GI tract—which is a crucial element of digestive function. Although studies indicate "normal" to be up to 30–40 hours, I believe that optimal gut transit time should be between 12 to 24 hours; even though slower transit may be considered normal, it is not ideal to go above 24 hours, because of all the negative consequences of slow transit.[73] When things are not moving through like they are supposed to, many deleterious things can happen.

Bristol Stool Scale

The Bristol stool scale is a well-known metric, developed by a healthcare team from Bristol, England, which rates the consistency of stool on a spectrum from 1 to 7; type 1 is a hard, small stool consistent with constipation, and type 7 is completely watery, indicating diarrhea. Optimal is somewhere in the middle, like type 4—described as soft, smooth, and sausage-shaped.[74]

The Bristol stool scale was once thought to correlate very well with gut transit time. Typically, hard and more constipated stool is associated with slow transit, and loose, watery stool is associated with rapid transit. While in some patients this does hold true, it is not always the case. In addition, frequency of bowel movements does not always correlate with transit time.

I had a patient with soft, Bristol type 4 stool who was happily having daily bowel movements. However, when she tested her gut transit time it turned out to be five days. Although she was having daily bowel movements it was taking an extremely long time for things to pass through her GI tract. Suffice to say, it is important to actually perform this test and not assume that transit time is normal just because one is having daily bowel movements. This test also provides a simple metric that can be used to track the effectiveness of gut treatments. Measuring the gut transit time pre- and postintervention can help to monitor the effects of various therapies.

Negative Effects of Slow Transit Time

Slow transit increases the risk of small intestinal bacterial overgrowth or SIBO, by not allowing bacteria to move through the small bowel at the proper pace.[75] In the large intestine, it can lead to excessive reabsorption of the short-chain fatty acids (SCFAs) produced by the gut bacteria. Those acids are critical to ensure healthy acidic pH in the colon.

Too much uptake of the SCFAs increases the pH of the intestine and leads to neutral or alkaline pH, which enables the proliferation of bad bacteria and harmful yeast like Candida. A process called protein putrefaction can occur due to higher pH and slowed transit, which produces further harmful metabolites. Slow transit time can itself be caused by imbalanced gut bacteria, and through a vicious cycle can predispose to worsening of dysbiosis and pathogenic overgrowth.

There are other detrimental effects of slow transit time. It is more likely to be associated with gas and bloating, because the contents of the bowel are not being cleared appropriately and gas produced by your intestinal bacteria can build up. Through metabolic effects, it is associated with increased visceral fat and higher post-meal blood sugars, both of which are independent risk factors for heart disease.[76]

Just Right

Healthy transit time ensures a balance—it allows enough time for processing and absorption of nutrients and the proliferation of good bacteria, but not so much time that toxins and harmful substances are reabsorbed. The stool also contains LPS and other potentially harmful breakdown products from bacteria that the body wants to get rid of through the bowel movements.

If transit time is too slow, these toxins and damaging substances will gradually be reabsorbed into the bloodstream and will not be eliminated. This is why normal transit time is essential for healthy detoxification.

If transit time is too fast, there is not enough time for nutrients to be absorbed properly. This can be associated with celiac disease, ulcerative colitis, Crohn's disease, or other serious conditions. Very rapid transit time is associated with a reduced microbiota diversity, as it does not allow enough time for growth and establishment of important keystone species.[77] As with most things, there is a healthy middle ground; we don't want things to be moving through too quickly or too slowly.

Improving Transit Time

The most common issue is slow transit time. Because this is usually caused by an imbalance in gut bacteria, completing the gut healing protocol that we'll discuss in chapter 9 can often be helpful.

Other remedies that can be helpful are apple cider vinegar and ginger. Apple cider vinegar (ACV) helps to ensure normal acidic pH in the colon, primarily through its high content of acetic acid (typically 5–6 percent). Maintaining healthy acidic pH in the colon reduces the likelihood of dysbiosis, which can slow down transit time.[78] Additionally, ACV has a direct antimicrobial effect against pathogenic bacteria and candida, further reducing the likelihood of dysbiosis.[79]

Ginger has been shown in studies to improve the emptying of the stomach, which is the necessary first step in normal motility and transit. If digested food does not leave the stomach properly and move through the intestines normally, it can predispose one to pain (indigestion or dyspepsia), reflux of acid (heartburn), and sluggish elimination (constipation).

One double-blind placebo-controlled study used ultrasound imaging to show that ginger was effective at accelerating the emptying of the stomach and gently stimulating stomach contractions, thereby improving gastrointestinal motility.[80] This helps us understand why ginger may be helpful for digestive complaints. One of the most well-established properties of ginger is its ability to reduce nausea and vomiting. Studies have proven that ginger is clearly effective for treating nausea from almost any cause.[81] The effects of ginger on gastric emptying and motility may be part of the explanation for its noteworthy efficacy in treating nausea.

Certain probiotics can be beneficial for improving slow transit time as well. Strains that have been shown helpful to speeding up slow transit are Lactobacillus plantarum[82] (various strains are helpful, and these bacteria are often found in fermented foods) and Lactobacillus reuteri DSM 17938 (also known as Limosilactobacillus reuteri or Lactobacillus reuteri protectis).[83] Multiple brands of probiotics contain these specific beneficial strains.

Now that we've spent extensive time elucidating the gut, let's return to Maria, who was struggling with psoriasis and other issues.

When stool testing identified dysbiosis and low levels of Akkermansia and butyrate, I started Maria on a gut-healing protocol with prebiotic foods and supplements. She took neem capsules to help get rid of the harmful bacteria in her gut. She began consuming red quinoa, red rice, pomegranate, and cranberry, all foods that support Akkermansia. Repeat testing two months later

found that her Pseudomonas overgrowth had resolved, her Akkermansia levels were now above average, and her keystone bacteria, including lactobacillus and Bifidobacteria, were much improved. As a result, her short-chain fatty
acids and butyrate had increased significantly. Her intestinal permeability was
normalizing.

Maria found that weight loss strategies she had tried unsuccessfully before
began to be effective. She started to lose weight and eventually returned to
normal BMI. Her blood sugar and blood pressure improved, and the abnormal
liver enzymes which indicated fatty liver returned to normal levels. Her psoriasis did not completely resolve but started to finally respond to the topical
steroids she was using, and eventually improved.

CHAPTER 5

Eating—Food Sensitivities and the Phase 1 Diet

Sandy was a fifty-four-year-old woman who was diagnosed with Sjogren's syndrome and had severe dry eyes and dry mouth. In addition, the inflammation had caused swelling of both of her parotid glands, located below the cheekbones, creating visible masses on both sides of her face. She had struggled with constipation since college and regularly took laxatives. Despite taking conventional immune suppressants, eyedrops, and a drug to stimulate saliva production, she struggled with persistent symptoms. Her constipation was severe and had caused painful hemorrhoids.

When she came to see me, her quality of life was one of her biggest concerns. Her symptoms hindered her work as a software engineer. In addition, she felt dejected about the unsightly swelling on her face, which was not reducing at all despite maximum drug therapy. She had stopped eating gluten about three months before seeing me, but had not seen any improvement and therefore resumed her regular diet.

Food is fundamental. In this chapter, we will review the different types of food reactions that could potentially play a role in autoimmune conditions, giving particular attention to gluten and dairy—the two most common food sensitivities I find in my autoimmune patients. We will discuss some of the research on the benefits of diet in autoimmune disease. I offer my Phase 1 Diet in detail and teach you how to reintroduce foods after completing it.

ALLERGY VS. SENSITIVITY VS. INTOLERANCE

To begin, let's clarify the difference between food allergy, sensitivity, and intolerance. Understanding the similarities and differences between these three terms is important because we will be referring to them throughout the book.

Food Allergy

This is probably what you think of when you think of an adverse reaction to food. Food allergies are the most severe manifestation, and classically present with difficulty breathing or lip swelling immediately after eating a food one is allergic to. Classic examples are peanuts or shellfish. Allergies can develop at any time in our lives, even in adulthood.

Food allergies can trigger severe, potentially life-threatening infections. For this reason, patients suffering from them are usually advised to carry injectable epinephrine (e.g., the EpiPen) to treat themselves in case of accidental exposure.

Antibodies are proteins synthesized by the immune system to bind to toxins or microbes and mark them for attack by the immune system. In the case of food reactions, antibodies are mistakenly directed against food proteins. There are several different types of antibodies and reactions to food may depend on which antibody is involved—IgG, IgE, or IgA. Food allergies are typically mediated by IgE antibodies, which trigger immediate reactions that occur within a matter of minutes of exposure to the food.

Food allergies generally do not change with time once they are present. Although there are specific desensitization protocols that allergy doctors can put patients through to reduce the risk of dying from anaphylactic reactions, it is unlikely that food allergies can resolve to a significant degree.

Food Sensitivity

Food sensitivities usually cause reactions that are less severe than food allergies, but nonetheless can be very bothersome. These include fatigue, joint pain, rashes, digestive symptoms, cognitive changes, or other nonspecific symptoms. Unlike food allergies, which trigger IgE antibodies, food sensitivities are mediated either by IgA or IgG antibodies.

IgG-mediated food responses are described as delayed hypersensitivity reactions and have been associated in the literature with an array of common clinical conditions, including eczema, migraine, obesity, asthma, irritable bowel syndrome, and—pertinent to our discussion—autoimmune conditions.[1]

Food sensitivities can also develop at any age, but unlike food allergies they may resolve themselves over time. They are affected by the gut microbiota, intestinal permeability, and the overall state of the immune system. Addressing these factors can have a huge impact in the severity of food sensitivities, and in some cases allow patients to resume foods that they were sensitive to in the past.

Food sensitivities are more common in patients with autoimmune conditions. For example, in patients with rheumatoid arthritis, elevated levels of food sensitivity antibodies have been found at higher levels than in normal controls.[2]

Gluten Sensitivity

Gluten is likely the most well-known food sensitivity. Gluten sensitivity actually exists in different degrees of severity; it is part of a spectrum, with celiac disease (the most severe form) on one end and mild gluten sensitivity on the other. Patients with mild gluten sensitivity may test negative using traditional blood tests for celiac disease, but still experience silent inflammation and harmful effects from consuming wheat. In the medical world this is called non-celiac gluten sensitivity (NCGS). Possible symptoms reported in the literature include abdominal pain, rashes, eczema, headache, "foggy mind," fatigue, diarrhea, mood changes, arm or leg numbness, and joint pain.[3] We will be talking much more about gluten later in this chapter.

ADVANCED TIP

The gold standard in gastroenterology is to document celiac disease with a biopsy of the small intestine. However, if the specific affected area of the intestine is missed and not included among the biopsies, then one might falsely conclude that the patient does not have celiac disease. To work around this, I typically begin screening for gluten sensitivity with a celiac blood test. If it is even slightly positive, I stop there and conclude that gluten sensitivity is present. If the blood test is negative, I do further testing to look at stool IgA antibodies against gluten or gliadin (another component of wheat). This is an effective way to identify NCGS. Various labs offer this test, such as Enterolab and Diagnostic Solutions Laboratory.

Food Intolerance

Finally, we have food intolerance, which is distinct from allergy and sensitivity because it does not involve the immune system. Food intolerance is essentially improper processing or breakdown of a food component that can subsequently lead to all the same symptoms that food sensitivities can trigger. However, instead of an immune response mediated by antibodies, food intolerance is usually a result of aberrant or imperfect functional response of the digestive tract to that food component—essentially, your digestive tract does not properly process the food, which then leads to various symptoms.

The most common food intolerance is lactose intolerance, an inability to break down the lactose sugar found in dairy products. As we get older, the majority (about two-thirds) of us lose the necessary intestinal enzyme—lactase—that is necessary to break down lactose; as a result, consuming dairy products with too much lactose can trigger gas, bloating, or diarrhea in many individuals.[4]

FODMAP Intolerance

FODMAP, or Fermentable, Oligo-, Di-, and Mono-saccharides and Polyols are foods containing certain carbohydrates that are poorly absorbed and pass into the large intestine where they are fermented by bacteria. Examples of foods high in FODMAPs are grains such as wheat, barley, and rye, vegetables such as asparagus, onion, garlic, and cauliflower, high-lactose dairy such as milk and cottage cheese, and fruits such as apple, banana, and watermelon.

Often, SIBO is the main cause of FODMAP intolerance, so one of the primary treatments for SIBO is a low-FODMAP diet which eliminates most of these foods. This works by essentially starving the bacteria in the intestines, thereby reducing their levels of overgrowth. However, this is not intended to be a long-term diet.

Once the SIBO is treated and resolved, a person should gradually return to consuming FODMAP-rich foods. This is important because these foods are very high in prebiotics, which are essential in the long run to maintaining the diversity of the microbiome—a crucial factor in health and longevity, as we discussed earlier. We will talk about SIBO more in chapter 12.

ACHIEVING DIVERSITY WITH DIET

Let's shift gears and talk at a high level about diversity before we explore the details of specific foods. Diversity is the key benchmark of microbiome health—the more diversity, the better. It is known that populations that follow a more ancestral, less urbanized lifestyle tend to have a higher diversity. In fact, loss of diversity is one of the hallmarks of the modern disrupted microbiome and is extremely common in patients with autoimmune conditions.[5]

When it comes to diversity, the Hadza, a tribe from Tanzania that still follows a hunter-gatherer lifestyle, are the superstars in this area, with some of the most rich and diverse human microbiomes ever recorded; their diet consists of wild foods including meat, honey, berries, baobab (an African fruit), and tubers that are exceptionally fibrous.[6] While it is not possible to replicate the microbiome of the Hadza, and probably not desirable to do so (because each microbiome is uniquely adapted to the local food and environment of its host), it is possible to boost diversity and thus improve the status of the modern microbiome. Dietary interventions are key.

The Modern Paleo Diet

A recent study looked at urban Italian adults adhering to a modern version of the paleo diet and found striking increases in microbiota diversity in those following such an eating plan. When compared to Italians following a standard Mediterranean diet, those following a paleo diet had unexpectedly high levels of diversity in their gut microbiome, almost approaching the levels seen in traditional populations such as the Hadza and other groups from around the world.[7]

Since this was a cross-sectional study, it is possible that other factors were at play. For example, those following a paleo diet may also be more health conscious and more likely to exercise than other adults, so further study is needed to isolate the effects of diet alone. Nonetheless, it is striking to see that certain adult populations in modern, urban locations are able to achieve highly desirable microbiota diversity close to the lofty levels seen in traditional hunter-gatherer populations.

In this study, the "modern Paleolithic diet" was defined by the consumption of vegetables, fruit, nuts, seeds, eggs, fish, and lean meat, while excluding grains, legumes, dairy products, salt, and refined sugar.[8] The basic template is similar to what I am recommending here.

However, I have a much broader and more expansive definition of the modern paleo diet. I believe that properly prepared legumes, certain gluten-free grains, and fermented foods should be made staples of our modern diets—and these are all elements that can raise microbiome diversity hopefully even higher. By including these specific foods that I recommend in the TIGER Protocol, you can start to increase the diversity of your microbiome hopefully even higher than the desirable levels attained by people eating the "modern Paleolithic diet" from the Italian study.

In chapter 10, I will present my Phase 2 Diet, which is entirely focused on augmenting and enhancing the diversity of your microbiome. The Phase 1 Diet is more restrictive but necessary during the short-term phase of detoxification and gut healing. In the long run, adopting the Phase 2 Diet is the best nutritional strategy you can take to ensure a robust, diverse microbiome—and, thus, a balanced immune system.

HOW FOOD SENSITIVITY AFFECTS YOUR MICROBIOME

A healthy gut microbiota is associated with tolerance to a wide variety of foods; conversely, imbalances in the gut microbiota such as overgrowth of potential pathogens can be associated with, or in some cases even trigger, food sensitivities. For example, the beneficial keystone species Bifidobacteria, which we discussed in the previous chapter, facilitate the breakdown of gluten into compounds that are less inflammatory than intact gluten proteins, thus helping to improve digestion of and tolerance to gluten.[9]

In contrast, the opportunistic pathogen Pseudomonas produces enzymes that interact with gluten to make it more inflammatory and thus increase the likelihood that the immune system will react to it. Intestinal biopsies in patients with celiac disease, the most severe form of gluten sensitivity, demonstrate higher levels of Pseudomonas; this bad bacterium may be playing a role in the development of the gluten sensitivity that characterizes the disease.[10]

Disruption of the microbiome by antibiotics could possibly precipitate the development of celiac disease. A large Swedish study analyzing thousands of people diagnosed with celiac disease found that these individuals were more likely than healthy control subjects to have taken antibiotics within the preceding several months.[11] Interestingly, the risk increased in proportion to the number of courses of antibiotics a person was prescribed; the drug metronidazole, which is a broad-spectrum antibiotic that disrupts flora, had the highest association with celiac disease.[12] It's necessary to note, though, that this is only correlation, and correlation does not imply causation—we cannot say that taking antibiotics caused the person to develop celiac disease.

However, as a physician, it is plausible to me because the antibiotics would have caused reduction in the beneficial species that promote tolerance to gluten, and an increase in the opportunistic pathogens that make gluten more inflammatory. From these studies we see that the balance of bacteria in the microbiota plays a considerable role in determining whether a person develops sensitivity to gluten and/or other foods.

Gluten Sensitivity—It's Everywhere

In the last fifty years, there has been a dramatic increase in gluten sensitivity and celiac disease—studies show an alarming 400 percent increase.[13] Gluten is the most common food sensitivity that I see in my autoimmune patients. The primary reason is likely the disruption in their microbiome, which limits their tolerance to gluten and other foods. A secondary factor in the rise of gluten sensitivity has to do with the wheat itself. Genetic modification and selective breeding to increase crop yields over the years has dramatically changed the genetics and chemical composition of wheat.

The type of wheat that we currently consume is called dwarf wheat, named for its short stature relative to other varietals. Introduced during the Green Revolution in the 1960s, dwarf wheat is highly prolific and produces a lot more grains per acre, which is an outstanding trait for productivity and profitability.[14] However, its nutritional content has declined over the years—ancient grains such as einkorn wheat are 200 to 400 percent higher in vitamin A, vitamin E, and the antioxidant lutein as well as certain minerals when compared to modern wheat.[15] Dwarf wheat is also significantly higher in starch content, especially in a type of starch called amylopectin A that contributes to a higher glycemic index for wheat and has been associated with insulin resistance.[16]

Unfortunately, dwarf wheat is much higher in gluten than older strains of wheat—modern wheat has up to forty times as much gluten as the wheat that your grandparents might have eaten.[17] Moreover, the types of gluten present in the wheat were transformed. Specifically, modern wheat contains high levels of an allergenic gluten protein known as glia-α9, which is notably absent in ancient grains; it's not surprising that most patients with celiac disease react negatively to glia-α9.[18]

The genetic engineering process that creates dwarf wheat also resulted in a plant with extra sets of chromosomes, encoding new proteins with unpredictable effects in humans. Dwarf wheat has forty-two chromosomes, unlike einkorn wheat, possibly the oldest form of cultivated wheat, which has a simple genetic structure of fourteen chromosomes.[19] This is significant because modern wheat has a lot more genes encoding more proteins than any grain that our bodies are used to encountering and processing.

Modern wheat has much more gluten, different types of gluten that people are more sensitive to, far more new genetic material, higher starch content, and lower levels of vitamins, minerals, and antioxidants when compared to ancient wheat. During the last half-century, our DNA has not experienced major changes commensurate with this radical transformation of wheat, and many people's bodies simply may not be capable of processing modern wheat effectively. Add to this the unprecedented alteration of the human microbiota and you have a perfect storm of criteria that have contributed to striking increases in celiac disease and gluten sensitivity.

For all these reasons, I am not a big fan of wheat. I feel that most patients with autoimmune disease would be better off not consuming much of it.

Dairy Sensitivity

Dairy sensitivity is also unfortunately quite widespread, especially among autoimmune patients. For example, people with multiple sclerosis were more likely to have elevated food sensitivity antibodies against dairy proteins than healthy controls.[20] However, if you tolerate it, full-fat dairy can be a healthy part of your diet. There are various functional medicine lab tests for dairy sensitivity. An equally good option is to eliminate dairy products as part of the Phase 1 Diet, and then reintroduce them systematically and monitor for reactions.

Milk consumption is often limited because of lactose intolerance. Other milk products such as butter, ghee, cheese, kefir, and yogurt are low in lactose and better tolerated. Grass-fed butter is rich in vitamin A, vitamin D, conjugated linolenic acid (CLA), omega-3 fatty acids, and vitamin K_2 (an important nutrient for bone health that is found only in dairy products and a few other foods).

If you tolerate dairy and consume it, I recommend full-fat dairy. Full-fat dairy is a whole food and in order to remove part or all of the fat content, it must be processed significantly. Food processing has unpredictable effects that can sometimes be harmful to health.

A Harvard study of 18,000 women found that low-fat dairy products can potentially reduce fertility.[21] Low-fat dairy products were found to be linked with a higher incidence of infertility, while full-fat dairy products were in fact associated with improved fertility. The authors of the study recommend that women trying to conceive substitute full-fat dairy products for low-fat dairy products. My philosophy is that eating whole foods is superior to eating processed foods, and the research confirms this in the area of dairy products.

It's so important to maintain a healthy gut lining and preserve your intestinal permeability that I recommend you avoid additives that have been linked to damaging this barrier. Common emulsifiers such as carboxymethylcellulose and polysorbate 80 have been shown in animal studies to promote increased intestinal permeability.[22] Carboxymethylcellulose may be identified on food labels as cellulose gum, microcrystalline cellulose, or MCC, and is present in a wide variety of foods.

Polysorbate 80 is often used in ice cream, pudding, whipped cream, condiments, and shortening.[23] Data suggests that polysorbate 80 may cause bacterial translocation across the intestinal lining and be especially problematic for patients with Crohn's disease.[24] Although we don't have conclusive human studies, I follow the precautionary principle and suggest avoiding food additives that have the potential to be harmful. If you see one of these on a food label, I recommend avoiding that food.

Research supports the efficacy of dietary interventions in autoimmune disease. A 2019 pilot study in seventeen women with Hashimoto's disease found that six weeks of the Autoimmune Paleo (AIP) diet improved health-related quality of life and symptom burden.[25] While this study did not find changes in thyroid levels, it did document a 29 percent reduction in inflammation as measured by serum C-reactive protein, and modulation of immune function as evinced by reduction in white blood cell counts—which is remarkable proof of the evidence of diet to cause measurable changes within just six weeks.

A 2017 study in fifteen patients with inflammatory bowel disease (IBD) found that an 11-week AIP diet led to significant improvement in pain and symptom scores and reduction in inflammation as seen visually in endoscopy and measured by stool markers (drop in calprotectin from 471 to 112); clinical remission was achieved by week six in >70 percent of the participants, a result which the study authors said, "rivals that of most drug therapies for IBD."[26]

A 2019 follow-up study in the same cohort of patients with IBD looked at the effects of the AIP diet on gene expression.[27] They found that the expression of 324 genes had been altered by diet, with upregulation of DNA repair, beneficial T-regulatory cell, and gut mucosal healing pathways, and down regulation of inflammatory genes—demonstrating the far-reaching epigenetic power of diet to change the way genes are being expressed.

THE PHASE I DIET

Now we begin our journey into using food as medicine. The key difference between the Phase 1 Diet here and the AIP diet is the inclusion of certain foods that are unlikely to be problematic, based on my clinical experience. These include gluten-free grains such as rice, buckwheat, and quinoa, and mung beans (although I recommend avoiding all other legumes). This makes the Phase 1 Diet less restrictive and more tolerable and practical for patients, without compromising the clinical efficacy.

In Phase 1, we focus on eliminating the foods that are most likely to be triggers to inflammation and autoimmunity. It might seem strange to eliminate foods that you feel you have no trouble with, but the reason for this is that sometimes you may be sensitive to foods that don't cause any symptoms—except to trigger inflammation within.

We also simultaneously bring in some of the most powerful therapeutic gut-healing foods to repair and restore your entire digestive system. This will be a 30-day program, after which you will shift to Phase 2. This is very important, because I often see patients who are on very restrictive elimination diets for too long.

The AIP diet can be beneficial for a maximum of two or three months, but after that I strongly recommend patients begin to reintroduce foods. Staying on an overly restrictive diet for too long is harmful because it reduces the diversity of the gut microbiome. It is also probably not necessary because a lot of these foods are not necessarily damaging once one has healed their gut, addressed dysbiosis, and increased intestinal permeability. There is no evidence that all of these foods are universally harmful.

With this in mind, I have included instructions on how to reintroduce foods after 30 days. The Phase 1 Diet will include two stages, each lasting two weeks—Stage 1, where you focus on detoxification with the guidelines outlined in chapter 7, and Stage 2, where you will be addressing infections and dysbiosis with the recommendations in chapter 8.

The goal of the Phase 1 Diet is to avoid the most allergenic foods and simplify your body's digestive processes, to facilitate removal of toxins from your body, clearance of infections, and healing of your gut. Here are the detailed guidelines:

What to Avoid

- All gluten and gluten-containing foods. These include grains like wheat, barley, rye, and spelt, and processed foods that contain these grains such as most breads, bagels, noodles, pasta, foods that contain flour (white or whole wheat), and cereals.

- All dairy products. Examples include milk, yogurt, butter, cheese, ice cream, cottage cheese, or whey protein. In this phase, I also recommend eliminating ghee. Even though it contains only trace amounts of casein (the protein in dairy that some people are sensitive to), some patients with autoimmune disease react to it.
- Soy products. These include tofu, tempeh, soy milk, edamame, soy sauce (which also contains gluten from wheat), and fake meats made from soy.
- Corn. This includes fresh corn and all foods made from cornmeal or corn flour such as polenta, popcorn, corn chips, and corn tacos.
- Eggs. While eggs are among the most nutritious foods, they are unfortunately also a frequent food sensitivity, especially among patients with autoimmune disease. The good news is that reintroduction of eggs after completing the Phase 1 Diet is usually successful.
- All harmful fats. Examples are hydrogenated oils, trans fats, margarine, and vegetable seed oils such as corn oil, soybean oil, and vegetable oil. Also avoid all fried foods.
- Alcohol. While alcohol in moderation may not be harmful, for the purposes of Phase 1 it is optimal to avoid alcohol so that your liver can potentially be engaged in processing other toxins.
- Caffeine. It is ideal to eliminate caffeine completely, but if for whatever reason you cannot completely eliminate this, try to reduce your caffeine intake as much as possible—limit yourself to one cup of coffee or two cups of tea per day.
- All nuts and seeds. This includes almonds, cashews, walnuts, pumpkin seeds, sunflower seeds, pecans, peanuts (technically a legume but commonly thought of as a nut), etc. While I have found sensitivity to these foods to be infrequent in my clinical experience, to be safe I recommend eliminating nuts and seeds as part of Phase 1. This does not include coconut, which is technically a fruit and not a nut.
- All legumes except mung beans (used to make Kitcheri, a healing Ayurvedic dish made with rice and mung beans—you'll find a recipe on page 286). This includes black beans, pinto beans, kidney beans, lentils, etc. and most important, peanuts (highly allergenic).
- Sugar and artificial sweeteners. This includes white sugar, high-fructose corn syrup, candies, sweets, soda, and any product with added sugar such

as sweetened beverages, juices, jams, or spreads with added sugar (processed sugars feed the growth of bad bacteria). Avoid artificial sweeteners such as sucralose (Splenda), aspartame (NutraSweet), and acesulfame potassium because these can disrupt the microbiome and impair glucose tolerance in both animals and humans.[28]

- Conventionally grown meat, poultry, or eggs, or farm-raised fish (if possible, choose organic, grass-fed or wild-caught).
- Nightshade vegetables. During Phase 1, I recommend elimination of nightshades, which include eggplant, tomatoes, bell peppers, chili peppers, white potatoes, and tomatillos.

What to Eat

- All grass-fed, organic, and/or pasture-raised meats and free-range poultry.
- Wild-caught oily fish, especially salmon, sardines, anchovies, and mackerel. These specific fish are the highest in essential omega-3 fatty acids and the lowest in mercury and other toxins. Every day try to have at least one serving of either fish or meat to ensure adequate intake of protein and other key nutrients.
- Non-starchy vegetables (except corn), aiming for at least nine servings per day. Examples include spinach, kale, chard, collard greens, asparagus, and cucumber. One cup of raw vegetables counts as one serving. Measure the vegetables in their raw form to count the nine cups, but then they can be consumed either raw or cooked. Note that if you cook these nine servings of vegetables, they will reduce to less than nine cups of veggies per day in total, which is fine.
- At least one cup daily of lightly cooked cruciferous vegetables to support healthy liver function (broccoli, brussels sprouts, cauliflower, cabbage, bok choy, etc.). I usually recommend lightly cooking or steaming cruciferous vegetables for a few minutes because excess consumption of raw crucifers can dampen the function of your thyroid gland over time.
- All fresh fruits are allowed. Avoid canned, dried, or processed fruits, or fruits with added sugar. You may have up to two servings of fruit per day. Incorporating berries of all types is beneficial because they are rich in polyphenols, which are prebiotics that feed your good bacteria.

- Starchy root vegetables. You may eat starchy root vegetables such as sweet potatoes, beets, carrots, arrowroot, etc., as long as they are not processed—i.e., no french fries or chips of any kind. This can be used as the "starch" component of your plate as we will discuss below.
- Healthy fats. These include extra-virgin olive oil, coconut oil, avocado oil, and avocados. While it is a common misconception that olive oil should not be heated or used for cooking (I review the research on this in chapter 10), extra-virgin olive oil can be used for cooking.
- Prebiotic foods, such as berries of all types, artichoke, asparagus, leeks, jicama, sweet potato, carrot, radish, and mushrooms. (I have a detailed breakdown of all prebiotic foods at the beginning of chapter 10, but I wanted to give you some examples here to choose from.)
- Fermented foods, such as sauerkraut, kimchi, pickled cucumbers, coconut-milk yogurt, kombucha, etc. (complete list in chapter 10 on page 197). Aim for at least a tablespoon of one type of nondairy fermented food each day.
- Bone broth, which is rich in minerals, amino acids such as glycine, and gelatin, is very healing for the gut. Although it has become a fad to consume bone broth, it is genuinely beneficial for helping to heal the gut, which is why I strongly recommend it. Try to have at least one cup of bone broth each day. You can either purchase premade bone broth, or prepare it yourself at home.
- Coconut, as an oil or other forms, can be used without limitation. Coconut milk or coconut-based yogurt are good substitutes for dairy products.
- Spices. Try to consume a variety of spices every day, especially turmeric, ginger, cinnamon, and ajwain. Other options for seasoning include lemon juice, lime juice, apple cider vinegar, or balsamic vinegar (see Advanced Tip on page 103), garlic, onions, and green onions. Since you're avoiding nightshades, skip any tomato-based condiments. A good substitute for soy sauce is coconut-based alternative Coconut Secret Raw Coconut Aminos.
- Broccoli sprouts, at least half a cup daily. Broccoli sprouts are the richest food source of sulforaphane, one of the most beneficial anti-inflammatory plant-based nutrients. They are much better sources than broccoli and other cruciferous vegetables (which are incredibly nutritious and should be included in your diet too). I will discuss the benefits of sulforaphane more in chapter 12.

- Organ meats, especially liver. Organ meats are extremely nutrient-dense. Liver from any animal, ideally organic and/or grass-fed, is acceptable. It is a misconception that the liver stores toxins and is therefore unhealthy to consume. The liver is a processing plant that contains all the key cofactors and nutrients used for detoxification (that we can utilize and benefit from). Consuming liver helps with our own detox processes without adding to our toxic load.

- Cabbage juice. Try to consume at least one 8-ounce glass of cabbage juice twice daily. You can easily make cabbage juice from fresh cabbage with a juicer or blender. Cabbage juice is rich in glutamine, an amino acid that is beneficial for healing impaired gut barrier function. If you prefer not to consume cabbage juice you can take glutamine as a supplement, as described below.

- Mung beans are acceptable but avoid all other legumes. If you are vegetarian, this is an excellent source of protein.

- (Optional) Kitcheri is beneficial for detoxification. You may consume this up to once a day during the detox.

- Gluten-free grains like white or brown rice, quinoa, millet, gluten-free oats, wild rice, amaranth, buckwheat, and teff can be consumed liberally as long as they are cooked in whole-grain form and well-tolerated. Products made from these grains, such as gluten-free bread or pasta, are acceptable for use too.

- Sweetener options. Stevia extract may be used without limitation. You can also use very small amounts (a tablespoon or less) of raw unfiltered honey, unrefined maple syrup, xylitol, erythritol, and fruit-based sweeteners such as monk fruit extract.

- Beverage options besides water include caffeine-free herbal tea and less than eight ounces per day of 100 percent fruit juice (limited because of the concentrated sugar content).

ADVANCED TIP: BENEFITS OF VINEGAR

For those who tolerate it, vinegar may offer added health benefits. Its acetic acid contributes to maintaining an acidic intestinal pH, which is essential to the health of the large intestine, as I explain in chapter 8. Your own beneficial gut bacteria produce acetic acid and other short-chain fatty acids to help maintain this acidic milieu in the intestine, as we discussed in chapter 4.

Vinegar can enhance your metabolic markers. In a randomized trial, two teaspoons of vinegar decreased the blood sugar spike caused by a meal rich in refined carbohydrates.[29] A Swedish study found that adding 1–2 tablespoons of vinegar to a carb-heavy meal lowered post-meal glucose—and increased satiety, the feeling of fullness after a meal.[30] In a randomized, controlled trial of prediabetics (people with slightly elevated blood sugar but not high enough to qualify as diabetics), Arizona researchers found that consuming 2 tablespoons of vinegar daily led to a significant 16-point drop in blood sugar over 12 weeks.[31]

A randomized, placebo-controlled trial in 175 overweight Japanese people found that taking 2 tablespoons of vinegar daily reduced belly fat as measured by CT scans and led to weight loss of about 4 pounds over 3 months—which is modest but notable given participants did not change their diets at all or increase exercise.[32]

To prevent any negative impact on your teeth from the acids in vinegar, either dilute it in water or rinse the mouth with water after consuming. Do not take apple cider vinegar undiluted because it can irritate your throat. If you are taking any medications, especially those that lower blood sugar, please check with your doctor before incorporating vinegar regularly.

How to Make Your Plate

I recommend you eat three complete meals a day during this time in order to fit in all of the healing foods in the Phase 1 Diet. Using the guidelines above, follow these detailed instructions to make your plate for *each meal*:

- Fill half of your plate with a heaping portion of non-starchy vegetables. Aim for three cups of vegetables (measured raw) per meal, which equals three servings, in order to get you the nine servings of vegetables daily over three meals. You can consume them cooked or raw. You may need to add a side of salad or veggies to achieve three servings per meal; be sure to add a generous amount of broccoli sprouts. Include at least one table-spoon of nondairy fermented foods with each meal.

- Fill one quarter of your plate with protein-rich foods, such as wild-caught fish, grass-fed beef, organic poultry, organ meat from any animal, or mung beans. Aim for about four ounces in size, the equivalent of a palm-sized portion or a deck of playing cards.
- Fill one quarter of your plate with a fiber-rich carbohydrate. This could be either starchy root vegetables or gluten-free grains as described above. You can include whole fruits here. Fruit can also be incorporated as a snack, up to two servings per day total.
- Healthy fats, equivalent of 1–2 tablespoons per meal. Be sure to incorporate plenty of healthy fats, such as extra-virgin olive oil and coconut oil, while cooking each meal. If you are having salad, you can combine olive oil with balsamic vinegar and spices to create a tasty dressing. Avocado can be consumed regularly as well.
- For beverages, consider bone broth, cabbage juice, caffeine-free herbal tea, or 100-percent fruit juice (limited to eight ounces per day).

Other Concerns

- If eating this way is a major transition for you, start with incremental changes. This will also allow your body time to get used to the new eating plan. For example, if you have only been eating one serving of vegetables with each meal, increase to two servings per meal for a few days, and then up to the recommended three servings per meal to reach your nine servings daily.
- Hydration is essential. Drink six to eight glasses of purified water daily. Filtered tap water is best.
- Plan to get enough sleep every night so that you wake up feeling well-rested and energized; most people require at least seven to eight hours, and some may need more.
- Aim for thirty minutes of light to moderate aerobic exercise at least four to five times per week. This could include walking, biking, jogging, swimming, or exercise on gym equipment such as a stairmaster or elliptical machine. Avoid extremely vigorous workouts, such as CrossFit or high-intensity training, during this month.

- Practice a mind-body relaxation technique such as diaphragmatic breathing or meditation for at least fifteen minutes daily. This can be broken up into two eight-minute sessions or practiced in a single fifteen-minute session. For instructions and sample techniques, please see chapter 11.
- Try to sweat in a sauna or steam room 30 minutes, three to four times per week. Sweating enhances detoxification through the skin. I will be discussing the benefits of saunas more in chapter 7.

SUPPLEMENTS TO CONSIDER

It is possible to accomplish gut healing mostly with foods, but I want to provide other options in case you prefer to substitute supplements for some of the foods mentioned. These should be taken during the 30 days of the Phase I Diet.

If you are not open to cabbage juice, glutamine can be taken as a supplement. Glutamine powder is widely available and has been shown to normalize elevated intestinal permeability in adults with leaky gut syndrome.[33] I suggest taking a total of 4 g per day, in two divided doses of 2 g each. It is best taken on an empty stomach at least one hour away from food. Studies show that a dosage of up to 20 to 30 g per day of glutamine is safe and well-tolerated for short-term use in adults.[34]

If you cannot or prefer not to eat fish, I suggest taking an omega-3 supplement. The best source of this is fish oil. Aiming for 1,000 mg per day of combined EPA and DHA (the active components of fish oil) would be beneficial. Research indicates that omega-3 fatty acids have a beneficial effect on intestinal permeability and dysbiosis, and favorably impact the gut-brain axis, in addition to anti-inflammatory properties.[35]

For these reasons, I recommend either fish or fish oil during this stage. For vegetarians, algae-based omega-3 supplements are a good alternative.[36]

STAGE 1 AND STAGE 2

The monthlong Phase 1 Diet is split into two stages, each with a different goal. The first 15 days will focus on detoxification (per chapter 7). We will address infections and dysbiosis during the second 15 days, and I will talk about how to do this in chapter 8. For my additional food, lifestyle, and supplement recommendations for each of these stages, please refer to chapter 7 and chapter 8.

HOW TO REINTRODUCE FOODS

After you have completed the Phase 1 Diet for at least 30 days—both stages 1 and 2—it is time to begin reintroducing foods you have eliminated. The best way to do this is gradually, reintroducing one major category of food every three days. To better facilitate this, keep a food journal to track each food you reintroduce, alongside any symptoms you notice over the next three days. Going without a journal makes this onerous, as it it will be hard to remember all the details as time progresses.

I will walk you through an eight-week reintroduction plan next, but let's first review some general principles.

Do not introduce more than one category of foods on the same day, so you can specifically identify the cause of any reactions. Foods from each category should be reintroduced one at a time. If you have reintroduced nuts, then you should bring back almond, walnut, cashew, etc., individually for maximum accuracy.

In terms of the order to reintroduce foods, I suggest leaving gluten and dairy until the very end. We will talk more about how to reintroduce dairy below. It is ideal to continue to avoid gluten, but if you would like to incorporate it occasionally as a special treat you can attempt the reintroduction at the very end to see how you respond.

Signs that you might be sensitive to a food include gas, bloating, constipation or diarrhea, rashes, headaches, sleep changes, sinus congestion, postnasal drip, muscle stiffness, joint pains, or general malaise. If you are not sure whether you have had a reaction to a food category, consume at least two more servings of the suspected foods to see if your reaction worsens.

When you are reintroducing a particular category, eat foods from that category at least two or even three times in that day to maximize the possibility that your body will manifest a reaction to it if you are indeed sensitive to that food. For example, if you are bringing back almonds you may want to have roasted almonds and almond butter at different times on that day; if you are reintroducing corn you could have popcorn, corn tacos, and polenta on the same day.

If you do not notice any symptoms for seventy-two hours after you reintroduce a food, you can add that category of foods to your "OK list" and move on to the next category. If you reintroduce almonds on Monday and feel completely wonderful through Thursday morning, then you can assume that almonds are fine and reintroduce a different category on Thursday. You can continue to eat foods that have been previously reintroduced successfully, so in this example you could still eat almonds on Thursday and then add another food. After this process, I don't recommend eating any food every single day, so it's good to always vary your diet regularly to reduce your risk of developing sensitivities in the future.

Variety, especially in your plant foods, is crucial to building up the diversity of your microbiome. This is where your food journal will come in handy. Your list of well-tolerated foods will be cumulative, so you should have an expanded list as time goes on. As we will discuss in Phase 2, I recommend consuming at least 30 different plant foods per week in the long run.

YOUR EIGHT-WEEK FOOD REINTRODUCTION PLAN

As you work through this plan, remember to keep at least three days between each food you reintroduce so you can tell whether you react to it or not. Essentially, you are introducing two new foods every week, and will reintroduce 16 foods over the eight-week period.

During these eight weeks, you will reintroduce foods that are less likely to be allergenic earlier, such as seeds and legumes, and reintroduce foods that are more probable food sensitivities later on, including eggs, peanut, and nightshades. This is a suggested schedule for reintroduction, but you are welcome to vary it based on your preferences.

Weeks 1 & 2

Start with nuts and seeds. Select those you enjoy consuming and would like to reincorporate regularly. The first week, choose two nuts, such as almond and cashew, and observe how you feel. If there is no reaction, add these foods to your "OK" list. At the beginning of the second week, you can continue to have almonds and cashews, if you didn't react to them, and then start adding some seeds. For example, you might choose two seeds such as chia and flax.

Weeks 3 & 4

Next you may consider reintroducing legumes. Because these are so beneficial for the microbiome and relatively low in allergenic potential, we are bringing them back now. There are not major differences among the legumes in terms of likelihood of sensitivity, so choose some that you would like to eat regularly. An example would be to reintroduce black beans and lentils in week 3, followed by pinto beans and chickpeas in week 4.

Weeks 5 & 6

I recommend reintroducing nightshades around this time. During week 5 you could bring back tomato and bell pepper, and in week 6, eggplant and potato. Bringing back these foods should open up your options at the grocery store and in restaurants. Chili pepper and tomatillo are also nightshades, but I would suggest reintroducing those later, since they are less commonly present in other foods.

Weeks 7 & 8

You have some different options for week 7. These foods may trigger some of the most common allergies and sensitivities, and so we are reserving them for the tail end of the reintroduction. You can reintroduce eggs, if you have not done so already. If you really like peanut, you could bring it back now and observe your reaction. Other possibilities for foods to reintroduce are corn and soy, depending on whether you plan to eat these foods regularly.

During week 8, I recommend reintroducing alcohol and caffeine if you consume either of those. It is best to reintroduce gluten-free drinks to avoid the possibility of a gluten reaction (e.g., wine and not beer). As for caffeine, you could consider either coffee or tea.

After this initial 8-week reintroduction, you can then go on to dairy.

Reintroduction of Dairy

With dairy products, there is a clear hierarchy of what foods to reintroduce. This is because there is a wide variation among dairy products in their content of lactose and casein, both of which can cause issues. We will be reintroducing dairy products in ascending order of lactose and casein, from foods with the lowest content to foods with the highest content.

Always begin with reintroducing ghee, which is the lowest in allergenic potential and contains negligible amounts of lactose and casein. If you happen to react to ghee, which is rare but can occur, you can try fermented ghee (available online) which is the absolute lowest in dairy proteins.

Next, reintroduce butter. Cream can be brought in at this time if you like. After that, bring back cheeses. Goat's milk and sheep's milk cheeses are lower in casein and should be introduced first. If they are well-tolerated, you can move on to cow's milk cheeses.

In the final stages you can reintroduce yogurt, then kefir, which is a liquid fermented milk product that is very high in probiotics. If you have been used to drinking milk before the Phase 1 Diet, you may choose to try incorporating milk again. If you have not been drinking milk due to lactose intolerance or other reasons, it is not necessary to try it.

With dairy products, I recommend full-fat, and avoiding low-fat products due to negative effects on hormones as we discussed earlier. Sticking with the schedule of two food reintroductions per week, it will take you a few weeks to work through the different dairy products.

Reintroduction of Gluten

As previously stated, I think it is probably best for all patients on the autoimmune spectrum to avoid gluten, for all the reasons I described earlier in this chapter. Additionally, because manifestations of gluten sensitivity can vary widely, it can be hard to discern if one is sensitive by monitoring for symptoms after consuming it. The list of symptoms connected to gluten sensitivity is large and increasing.[37]

It is also possible that gluten may contribute to low-grade inflammation in your gut without causing noticeable symptoms. Some data suggests wheat can increase intestinal permeability even in people without gluten sensitivity.[38] However, if you would like to try to reintroduce gluten, I can offer advice on the best way to do so.

Earlier, we spoke about the genetic engineering of modern wheat, and how ancient grains may be a better option. Interestingly, one study showed that unmodified ancient grains such as einkorn wheat may be better tolerated by people with celiac disease (although of course I recommend that patients with celiac disease do not consume any type of wheat).[39]

Sourdough bread presents another option. Wheat that is prepared in a traditional manner (such as in sourdough bread that has undergone a long fermentation) has been found to contain much less gluten than traditional wheat.[40] Moreover, one study that had patients with celiac disease consume properly fermented sourdough bread (which was found to contain <10 parts per million of gluten) for sixty days found that there was no adverse effect on clinical symptoms or intestinal pathology.[41]

Many modern sourdough breads are prepared using fast-acting chemical methods that require only a few hours and do not utilize the extended fermentation of wheat flour by sourdough bacteria. This doesn't allow enough time for the microbes to break down the gluten to low levels, as in traditionally prepared sourdough.

To be explicitly clear, I'm not recommending that patients with celiac disease or gluten sensitivity consume sourdough bread or einkorn wheat—wheat in any form may not be tolerated. However, these are some healthier options for wheat if you do try to reintroduce gluten after completing the Phase 1 Diet.

Let's revisit Sandy's case, as she was struggling with Sjogren's syndrome and a host of other painful issues.

In addition to major facial swelling as a result of her Sjogren's syndrome, Sandy was plagued by chronic constipation, severe dry eyes, and dry mouth. When I saw her, we performed detailed stool testing with a GI Map test, and I was surprised to find only mild dysbiosis but severe intestinal inflammation and increased intestinal permeability. I concluded that her diet might be contributing and ordered food sensitivity testing with stool and blood tests.

We used the results of the food sensitivity testing—which were surprising to Sandy—to guide her on a detailed elimination diet. She tested sensitive to expected triggers like gluten but also to some foods she was eating daily to try to help her constipation, including flaxseed and almond. When she eliminated these foods, in addition to gluten, she noticed a marked improvement in her constipation. That was why eliminating gluten alone had not been helpful—it was necessary but not sufficient.

With her digestion improving, I started her on an intensive regimen of anti-inflammatory supplements, including fish oil, curcumin, and Boswellia. Over time, the swelling on her face finally began to subside, as her salivary glands returned to normal size. After a year, her symptoms finally abated, and she felt like she could be productive at work again without vexing symptoms. She continued on her regular medicines, but reported feeling better than she had ever felt—even before her diagnosis of Sjogren's.

CHAPTER 6

Rest—Understanding Mental and Emotional Rest and Your Nervous System

Five years after receiving a diagnosis of rheumatoid arthritis, 37-year-old Jane found herself in my office, complaining of recurrent flare-ups of joint pain that required periodic treatment with oral steroids—despite being on a weekly maintenance injection of the immune suppressant Enbrel. She also had lifelong anxiety that would periodically trigger panic attacks.

I worked with Jane for over six months to help her detoxify from high levels of environmental toxins, heal her gut from dysbiosis, and eliminate food sensitivities. To my surprise, her symptoms did not budge, and so we began to delve deeper into the role of stress in her life.

Jane was a high-powered management consultant who loved her job; she was married and mother to a 5-year-old daughter. Jane described severe stress from her work, and felt that she was not managing it effectively. When I asked her what she did to relieve stress, she had a one-word answer—"TV."

In this chapter, we turn toward the mind-body connection and discuss stress, rest, and your nervous system. We'll explore the different types of rest and why each of them is important: physical, mental, and emotional rest.

It's important to distinguish between passive mental rest and active mental rest and address a basic need that does not get enough attention—play. We will talk in detail about emotional rest and cognitive approaches that can help you cultivate a better relationship with your thoughts and feelings—including how to better regulate and manage your emotions.

You will also learn about the autonomic nervous system (ANS) and its role in autoimmune disease, particularly a key metric of the ANS known as heart rate variability, and review studies indicating how optimizing heart rate variability can improve autoimmune ailments. Importantly, we'll discuss childhood trauma and the outsized impact it can have in autoimmune disorders.

PHYSICAL REST—SLEEP

In terms of physical rest, sleep is central. Many have written about sleep, so I won't say too much on it—except to review some highlights from the literature.

Sleep is vital for metabolism, learning, memory, immune function, and the balance of multiple hormones; insufficient sleep has been associated with increased risk of heart disease, diabetes, obesity, mood disorders, dementia, immune system impairment, and other conditions.[1] The benefits sleep provides are wide-ranging and often underappreciated.

Sleep is crucial to healing. One randomized trial conducted by the US Army concluded that sleep was even more important than good nutrition in speeding up wound healing.[2] While you sleep, your body is most active at protein synthesis, the process of creating new proteins which is integral to repairing damaged tissues, healing inflammation, and creating healthy new cells.[3]

Studies show that insufficient sleep impacts two major mechanisms that drive autoimmunity—oxidative stress and chronic inflammation.[4] In addition, sleep deprivation deals a blow to the immune system, leading to worsening of several parameters; in contrast, getting sufficient sleep improves immune function and leads to an enhanced ability to fight off infections.[5] Thus, optimizing your sleep is one of the most important things you can do for healing from autoimmune disease.

Most people do not get enough sleep. Individual needs vary, but a good rule of thumb is that you should be waking up in the morning feeling well rested. If you consistently are, then it is likely that you are getting adequate sleep.

MY PERSPECTIVE ON STRESS

When I talk about stress, I often see my patients' eyes glaze over. This could be because they've heard so much about the effects of stress on health, or perhaps they feel guilty that they are not practicing hour-long meditations or doing whatever it is they think they should be doing to manage their stress effectively.

It is important that the approach and attitude we take to stress should not add to our overall stress level as doing so would only make things worse. This is exactly what was shown in a study with a cohort that was already highly stressed—caregivers for Alzheimer's patients—who actually experienced *worsening* anxiety when instructed to practice a daily mind-body technique—likely due to a perceived added burden from an additional daily task.[6]

My approach differs from this by focusing on innovative science and research you might not have heard of, and then sharing practical tools that are not time-consuming but can make a measurable difference.

The Last Straw

Stress is one of the underlying root causes for the initial development of auto-immunity. Countless patients have shared that their autoimmune condition appeared and was diagnosed during a time of high stress in their life. Stress is often the "straw that breaks the camel's back" when it comes to this disease process. The accumulation of toxins, infections, dysbiosis, leaky gut, and food sensitivities can cause progressive immune dysfunction—until a stressful episode tips things over the edge and causes the emergence of autoimmune disease.

Causes of Flare-ups

Studies have also shown that patients with autoimmune disease are more likely to experience a flare-up or worsening of symptoms when they endure emotional stress. For example, in autoimmune hepatitis, psychological stress was a significant factor associated with relapse of the disease, and those patients who achieved long-term remission had coping strategies that allowed them to manage stress effectively.[7]

Antidotes to Stress

In autoimmune hepatitis, mindfulness practice reduced these stress-related flare-ups—this kind of practice is something we'll explore more in chapter 11. It's an important skill; in patients with rheumatoid arthritis, the practice of Mindfulness-Based Stress Reduction (MBSR) over a six-month period led to a 35 percent reduction in psychological distress and depressive symptoms, and improved parameters of well-being.[8]

In chapter 11, I'll discuss a number of general antidotes to stress, such as meditation, gratitude, and forgiveness, as well as several other specific tools. Passive and active mental rest, as well as play, can alleviate stress.

Passive Mental Rest

I want to differentiate between active and passive mental rest, which both have their place. Passive rest entails a quiet, receptive state. You may be passively taking in something, like TV, a book, music, or video content, or you may be relaxing quietly without doing anything in particular. Human beings are hardwired to need such unfocused time. Passive rest allows your body and mind to unwind and allows space for recharging your physical and mental batteries. This downtime is not a luxury—it is a requirement. It is also crucial for productivity because proper rest allows you to be more focused and efficient when you do return to work.

However, passive rest is not sufficient. For optimal stress reduction, active mental rest is essential as well, using mind-body techniques such as meditation or mindfulness practice.

NEUROPLASTICITY

One of the key advances of modern neuroscience is our understanding of neuroplasticity, which is how many mind-body techniques work. We used to believe that it was only possible to change our brains in childhood. The new science of neuroplasticity has showed us how we can rewire our brains at any age, to help improve our overall health.[9]

The brain's ability to recover after stroke is one example of neuroplasticity in action.[10] Practices that take advantage of neuroplasticity can assist in reducing pain, healing past trauma, improving depression or anxiety, and sharpening memory and focus.

Many of the practices you'll learn, such as mindfulness and meditation, are tools that help with this brain rewiring. I find that in my patients with autoimmune disease, using these tools for neuroplastic healing can sometimes be the missing link in helping them turn their condition around.

Understanding Your Mind

Your mind, which expresses itself through your brain, is constantly generating thoughts. This is a continuous, nonstop process. A study that used functional MRI imaging to track brain activity estimated that the average person has over 6,000 thoughts each day.[11]

Patients who are starting to meditate often tell me that they cannot keep their mind still and notice that it is creating thoughts constantly. They tell me that this must mean they can't meditate, but what's actually happening is that they received insight into the exact nature of the mind—that is just what the mind does.

If this has ever happened to you when you've attempted meditation, know that it is perfectly normal, and not an indication that you can't meditate. This also raises the question of how you define meditation, which we will explore in detail later.

As I mentioned above, every thought is associated with an emotion or feeling. That feeling, if strong enough, can also translate to physical sensations in the body. The important takeaway is that your mind is constantly generating thoughts, and that each thought is paired with a specific emotion.

ADVANCED TIP: INSIGHTS FROM NEUROSCIENCE

The many advances that have been made in neuroscience are relevant practically. A few key insights:[12] Thoughts and emotions go hand in hand and are inextricably linked in your neurobiology—each thought is linked with an emotion. This is a key point that we will come back to later.

Emotions occur when your brain makes sense of sensory input and the environment around you (your inner and outer world) using knowledge and prior experiences. We used to believe that each emotion was located in a specific part of the brain (e.g., fear in the amygdala). We now know that many different areas and networks in the brain can create the same emotion. Emotions also underlie memory formation, which is why powerful emotional experiences are often "etched" deeply in memory.

COGNITIVE TOOLS

Over the years, I have assembled a diverse toolbox of cognitive strategies which I'll share in detail once we've been through the other parts of the TIGER Protocol. These tools are meant to help you develop skills for managing and regulating your thoughts and emotions. They include approaches I will teach you later, such as upleveling, reframing, and choosing better-feeling thoughts. We will delve into these in chapter 11; for now, we'll talk generally about some issues that can affect your journey to heal from autoimmunity.

Beyond Pop Psychology

If you're unfamiliar with these principles, they may feel uncomfortable. Accessing treatments thought to be "alternative"—like meditation and mindfulness—can seem strange, especially when your struggles are rooted in the physical. But there is a real link between feelings and thoughts; thoughts can be associated with either positive or negative feelings, to varying degrees, and study bears this out.

You can better grasp the nature of your thoughts by digging into how you feel, and this is important because what you think helps determine your experience of life. Your thoughts have a huge impact on your body too (the science of placebos, which I discuss in chapter 11, sheds light on this). With cognitive methods, like changing the nature of your thoughts to be more positive, you can help your body to heal.

My focus is on helping you manage and improve your response to things that occur, whatever those events might be. Ignoring difficulties or real challenges in your life, or glossing over them with positivity, can also be detrimental. What's important is how you respond to these challenges, and how you move forward.

Pain vs. Suffering

To explore this further, let's look at the distinction between pain and suffering. Physical pain does not always equate to suffering. Mindfulness-Based Stress Reduction (MBSR) was originally developed to treat patients with chronic pain, and studies show that it can reduce one's perception of pain.[13] Women who have given birth and found the experience meaningful may not classify it as "suffering" despite the excruciating pain.

A Buddhist friend shared a teaching from his tradition about this. It talks about a man who is walking in the forest when he is suddenly hit with an arrow and feels great pain. A few moments later, he gets hit with a second arrow in the exact same spot, greatly aggravating the discomfort. The first arrow represents the actual physical pain, and the second arrow symbolizes how the mind may react—e.g., resisting, judging, or catastrophizing—and exacerbate the pain significantly, thereby increasing suffering. Paying attention to this aspect, what the mind does in response, can make a meaningful difference. We have no control over the first arrow but may be able to elude the second.

I want to acknowledge that it is not easy to implement this when you are in the midst of severe pain. We have all experienced how pain can be all-consuming and intense. And yet, encounters with pain—either physical or emotional—are unavoidable as a part of life. Being human guarantees that something unwanted, such as pain, will appear at times. So, when that pain arrives, the question is, how are you going to respond?

Pain itself is not an objective phenomenon. It is a subjective experience that is created in the brain and can be strongly influenced by multiple factors such as attention, body image, visualization, and other practices we'll learn later in the book. It is also usually not a static sensation; even chronic pain can change a great deal from moment to moment—in intensity, pattern, and quality—if we can tune in to it. Mindfulness can offer guidance here to help you manage your response in a way that enables you to suffer a little bit less. If you are interested in learning more, various mindfulness training courses such as the MBSR Program are available (I have completed this twice and highly recommend it).

Choosing and controlling your reactions to whatever occurs—in your body or in your life situation—is profoundly empowering. To be clear, I don't suggest suppressing your sensations, thoughts, or feelings. What I am talking about is self-regulation—being in the present moment and having the freedom to choose how you would like to be in the here and now. We will also talk later about how to handle your negative thoughts more effectively.

Inner Awareness

A popular bumper sticker says, "Don't believe everything you think." This captures another key point, to create a slight sense of separation between yourself and your thoughts and feelings. You are not your thoughts or feelings. Thoughts and feelings come and go but there is an awareness within you that does not change—I call it "inner awareness."

This perspective allows you to create a little bit of distance from uncomfortable thoughts and sensations, and that can be empowering. For example, if you say, "I am anxious," that itself might possibly increase your anxiety. But if you say, "I am noticing some anxious thoughts and feelings," that gives you a bit of space where you can manage those feelings better and choose your response with some flexibility.

Avoiding Identification

When you completely identify with a thought and feeling, you are fully caught up in it. Continuing with anxiety as an example, if you are constantly worrying about something that *might* happen, this anticipatory anxiety projects you into an imagined future and takes you away from the present moment.

However, if you can focus on your breathing or use another grounding tool to anchor yourself in the present moment, you gain a small degree of separation that enables you to begin to detach from and observe those anxious thoughts. Perhaps you can catch yourself before the worry and anxiety begin to spiral out of control.

Your thoughts and feelings are messengers, and your job is to think about what message they are trying to send you and find ways to process and come to terms with them in an organized way. It is not about suppressing your feelings. Rather, you can feel them, honor them, and then think about the message and meaning that they are bringing to you—which allows you to process them and move through them more quickly.

TRADITIONAL CHINESE MEDICINE

One of my early teachers in Integrative Medicine, who taught me about neuroscience, was also trained in Traditional Chinese Medicine (TCM). The research in neuroscience is consistent with TCM principles, which state that every thought is associated with an emotion, and that emotions cause subtle changes in the body. TCM maintains that emotion is an energy that travels through the meridians, the energy channels that course through the entire body. Each emotion is associated with a different meridian. For example, the lung meridian is associated with grief and the liver meridian is associated with anger.

While this principle has not been researched, we have all noticed how our thoughts and feelings can lead to physical sensations. I have often observed how if I am worrying or thinking about something stressful, I may feel "butterflies in my stomach" or subconsciously tense my shoulder and neck muscles. As soon as I become aware of the worries and fears, and the corresponding physical tension, I can work on consciously letting go of both.

This interaction can work both ways. The simple practice of smiling for no particular reason can lead to a slight upliftment in your perspective and feeling.[14] In one study, participants who held a pen between their teeth to force a smile were more likely to see the world around them in a positive way.[15] People who received cosmetic Botox injections (which limited their ability to frown) reported significantly more positive mood than those who could frown normally.[16] Laughter yoga, where you practice laughing (for no particular reason), can help boost your mood and well-being.

THE AUTONOMIC NERVOUS SYSTEM

The autonomic nervous system (ANS) is the primary mediator of the connection between the mind and body. Optimizing your autonomic nervous system is crucial for all those on the autoimmune spectrum. First, we'll discuss why this matters, and then talk about strategies to actually improve autonomic function.

The ANS is divided into two components: the sympathetic and parasympathetic nervous system. The sympathetic nervous system is responsible for activating the "fight-or-flight" response in our bodies, whereas the parasympathetic triggers the "rest-and-digest" pathways of recovery and rebalancing.

The Sympathetic Nervous System. The fight-or-flight response is primal; it's the part of our nervous system that evolved to keep us alive as early humans. It is adaptive in the short term but counterproductive in the long run. In the short term, the sympathetic system increases blood pressure, heart rate, and blood sugar so that we can either run or fight an animal that is chasing us. The problem is that the stress of modern life leads to people being in this state most of the time.

Activation of your sympathetic nervous system on a long-term basis raises your blood sugar, blood pressure, and inflammation levels, and disrupts your immune system and digestive function.[17] This is significant because we know that chronic inflammation can contribute to worsening autoimmunity, and disruption of gut and immune function can have direct impact on autoimmune disorders.

The Parasympathetic Nervous System. Your body in its wisdom has a counterbalance. The antidote is your parasympathetic nervous system, which enables your body to recharge, recover, and regenerate itself. It counteracts all the effects of the sympathetic. All mind-body practices have the effect of activating the parasympathetic, which helps lower blood pressure, slow the heart rate, boost immune function, and restore digestion.

Your Body Can't Tell the Difference

I always like to take an evolutionary perspective, and the purpose of the autonomic nervous system is to help you survive. To this end, we are wired with a hair-trigger sympathetic nervous system that is attuned to threats in our environment and can initiate rapid responses to boost our chances of survival.

Modern life doesn't present the same type of life-threatening circumstances our early ancestors faced. Now, a car cutting you off in traffic, or your boss yelling at you, or an argument with your spouse, all trigger the same fight-or-flight physiology. Moreover—and this is a crucial point—even your thoughts about those situations and incidents can trigger the same reaction.

Your body reacts the same way, whether it is an actual stressful event or merely your thought about a stressful event. We might have stressful experiences that occur in our daily lives, but we also have memories of past stressors that we often replay and re-live in our minds—and both of these can trigger that sympathetic branch of the ANS.

That is why it is so crucial to identify and become mindfully aware of what is going on in our minds. Doing so can help gradually reframe our perspective on those charged memories and experiences—which can go a long way toward reducing our fight-or-flight physiology. Moreover, we can also use various techniques to activate the parasympathetic nervous system (and its main nerve, the vagus nerve), as we will be discussing in chapter 11.

HEART RATE VARIABILITY (HRV)

HRV is an excellent metric to track the balance of sympathetic and parasympathetic in your body, to gauge the health of your autonomic nervous system. Your heart rate is a measure of how many times your heart beats in a minute. HRV is a measure of the variation in time between your heartbeats.

A low variation in heart rate is associated with activation of our sympathetic nervous system, and chronic fight-or-flight activation. A higher heart rate variability is associated with activation of our parasympathetic nervous system.

Studies show that people with a variety of autoimmune conditions such as rheumatoid arthritis, lupus, and systemic sclerosis demonstrate reduced HRV when compared to healthy controls.[18] In patients with rheumatoid arthritis, lower HRV and the corresponding elevated sympathetic nervous system effects on the heart are thought to contribute to the increased risk of arrythmia and sudden death seen with the condition.[19]

Other Effects of HRV

HRV was initially developed as a tool to help athletes optimize their performance, and it is still used by elite athletes.[20] It was subsequently shown that reduced HRV was associated with the development of diabetes, chronic inflammation, obesity, and psychiatric disorders such as depression.[21]

Studies also show that a lower HRV is associated with hypertension and an elevated risk of heart disease, the number one killer of people worldwide.[22] Therefore, improving your HRV should help not just your autoimmune condition but also reduce your risk of a variety of modern chronic inflammatory conditions.

Measuring and Increasing HRV

A growing number of gadgets make it easy to keep track of your HRV. They include watches like the Fitbit and Apple Watch, devices that use chest straps such as Polar and Garmin, and wearable rings like the Oura. If accessible to you, you can use these devices and the apps associated with them to help you to monitor your HRV and track changes over time.

Dietary factors can have an impact on HRV. The most studied intervention is supplementation with omega-3 fatty acids such as in fish oil. A meta-analysis of 15 studies concluded that supplementation with omega-3s increased HRV (I will be discussing omega-3 supplements in chapter 14).[23]

Simple deep breathing was shown in one study to increase HRV in patients with rheumatoid arthritis or lupus.[24] HRV biofeedback is another tool that can help. Programs like HeartMath utilize this approach, as we will discuss later.

STRESS AND THE GUT

Stress has major harmful effects on the gut, which is pertinent in autoimmune disease. Psychological stress has been shown to directly cause increased intestinal permeability, which we know is a key risk factor for autoimmune conditions.[25]

In addition, we know that stress leads to reduced levels of stomach acid, which is critical for digestion. The secretion of stomach acid depends on parasympathetic signaling through the vagus nerve; recall that the parasympathetic turns on "rest-and-digest" pathways and stomach acid production is part of this.[26] If you are in chronic sympathetic stimulation (fight-or-flight), these signals to the stomach will be turned off. This is important because stomach acid is crucial for digesting your food so you can break it down properly and then absorb all its nutrients. The lack of stomach acid can reduce your absorption of key vitamins and minerals, which is why chronic use of acid-blocking Proton Pump Inhibitors (PPIs) has been associated with several nutrient deficiencies.[27]

The pancreas, which also produces several digestive enzymes, is connected to both sympathetic and parasympathetic nerves, which play a big role in regulating its overall function and secretion of enzymes.[28]

This makes sense from an evolutionary perspective. If your body believes you are running from danger, it will activate the sympathetic nervous system and direct all its energy and attention to the muscles so you can flee—it would make sense to shut down digestion, which is a very energy-intensive process.

Endorphins

Endorphins are feel-good chemicals that help to reduce inflammation and modulate the immune system. The term "endorphin" comes from *endogenous*, which means internal, and *morphine*, the opiate pain reliever. These peptides, when produced by your body, help to relieve pain and increase feelings of pleasure and well-being.

Activating production of endorphins is beneficial. Strategies to help raise your endorphin levels include exercise, massage, laughter, meditation, sex, dance, aromatherapy, dark chocolate, saunas, acupuncture, and taking a warm bath.

One of the therapies we will discuss in chapter 12 to modulate the immune system, low-dose-naltrexone, works by increasing the body's production of endorphins (and reducing inflammation). Placebos can also cause your brain to increase the production and release of endorphins to relieve pain.

EFFECTS OF CHILDHOOD TRAUMA

This is a book about autoimmunity, so it may seem strange to address this topic. It's important to consider childhood trauma because there is an unexpectedly strong link between trauma early in life and autoimmune diseases years or even decades later.

The impact of adverse childhood experiences (ACEs), which include abuse (physical, emotional, or sexual), neglect (physical or emotional), and household dysfunction (e.g., domestic violence, substance abuse, mental illness, divorce), is becoming better understood. Early childhood stress dramatically increases the likelihood of hospitalization with a diagnosis of autoimmune disease later in adulthood.[29]

It is thought that epigenetics, a term that describes how changes in behavior and environment can affect the expression of our genes, is one key mechanism by which ACEs have long-term effects. Stress affects the way that our genes are expressed, which has fundamental impacts on our physiology. Traumatic events affect specific genes that regulate the production of stress hormone receptors in the brain; this impedes the brain's ability to properly respond to stress and tips the brain into a state of constant hyperarousal, which can persist through adulthood.[30]

When children with a high ACE score reach adulthood their stress hormones and fight-or-flight physiology have been upregulated for decades. The result is chronic inflammation, which is at the root of most modern chronic diseases. It appears that early life stress has the long-term effect of creating patterns of inflammation that persist all the way through adulthood, increasing the risk of developing autoimmune disease and other inflammatory disorders.

Medical Effects of ACEs

ACEs impair the normal development of the hippocampus, the part of the brain that regulates memories and helps to process emotions, leading to significantly reduced adult hippocampal size, which causes a vicious cycle that compounds the issue and further reduces resilience and stress tolerance.[31] Interestingly, there is evidence that meditation can actually increase the size of the hippocampus.

Adverse childhood experiences are associated with many poor health outcomes in adulthood, and autoimmune disease is one of those consequences. Compared to people with no ACEs, someone with two ACEs in childhood has twice the risk of being hospitalized with an autoimmune disease decades later as an adult, and a 70 percent higher risk of being hospitalized with a variety of other autoimmune disorders.[32]

This is relevant because ACEs are surprisingly common in the United States population—more than 60 percent of people have experienced at least one significant adverse childhood experience; in fact, 40 percent of people have experienced at least two, indicating that childhood trauma is extremely common in the population.

There are a few alternative approaches to addressing ACEs. You may be familiar with some—Five Elements acupuncture, and Eye Movement Desensitization and Reprocessing (EMDR). The right psychotherapist can also play an instrumental role, especially one who has expertise in addressing trauma.

Importance of Play

We have talked about the crucial importance of activating the parasympathetic, and there are various tools and techniques to help with this. But there's one other fundamental need for all people that is often not appreciated—the need for play. The vital importance of play for the health and development of children—in physical, mental, social, and cognitive aspects—has been well-established.[33] Pediatric research has shown that positive emotions experienced during play help to regulate the body's stress response.[34] Animal research has identified play as an instinctual drive that is crucial to the well-being of animals throughout their lives, with psychological and social benefits.[35]

While research on adults is limited, play can have huge benefits regardless of age, and it is especially important for those with autoimmune disease or other chronic illness. It can aid in relieving stress, boost your creativity and imagination, augment brain function, and strengthen your connections with others.[36]

I resonate with a quote from George Bernard Shaw: "We don't stop playing because we grow old; we grow old because we stop playing."[37]

If you are not sure how to start, here are some ideas on how to incorporate play with a friend or family member:

- play a board game
- do a jigsaw puzzle
- color in an "adult coloring book" (yes, that's a thing)
- throw around a frisbee
- participate in a sport that requires at least one other person to play
- play fetch with a dog or use catnip toys with your cat
- have a pillow fight
- build a snowman or make snow angels
- tell a joke
- sing your favorite song in the shower or with karaoke

- go bowling, go-kart racing, or miniature golfing
- dance at home to a song that you like
- join your kids in their play (dress-up, building something; the choices are endless)

And a few options that require screens:

- make a game out of your exercise. For example, if you are a runner, there are apps that make it seem like you are being chased by zombies
- watch cartoons or funny movies
- spend five minutes playing a game on your phone

Let's get back to Jane, the overwhelmed management consultant trying to manage rheumatoid arthritis, amidst frequent flare-ups.

Despite weekly injections of Enbrel, an immunosuppressant, Jane still required oral steroids. We identified stress as a key factor in her illness. I explained that her main outlet of watching TV provided passive mental rest, but that active mental rest was critical to her healing. I taught her about various stress reduction practices. She began practicing yoga once a week. She used the free mindfulness app Smiling Mind (which I recommend a lot) to practice ten minutes of meditation daily. We also spoke about incorporating play, and she started to watch cartoons with her daughter.

Gradually, her flare-ups began to lessen. She saw a therapist regularly who helped her anxiety with cognitive-behavioral therapy. After a lot of soulsearching, Jane realized that she needed a major change at work. She took a job with a nonprofit that was more meaningful to her but meant accepting a significant reduction in pay. However, she had a huge drop in work stress and had a lot more time to spend with her family and devote to activities that were fulfilling to her. She told me how her new job made her realize just how much unrecognized stress and anxiety her previous position had been causing her.

She finally attained remission, and now has not needed oral steroids for flareups in over three years. Eventually, to the surprise of her rheumatologist, she was able to reduce her Enbrel injections from once weekly to every two weeks without having any increase in symptoms.

PART TWO

IMPLEMENT THE TIGER PROTOCOL

CHAPTER 7

Toxins—Detoxify and Improve Liver Function

Connie was a 51-year-old Haitian-American stay-at-home mom who had successfully raised four children. When her youngest child started high school, she began to experience joint pain, stiffness, and swelling. A few months later she was diagnosed with rheumatoid arthritis.

She saw a rheumatologist and was prescribed methotrexate, which unfortunately did not have any impact on her symptoms, so, another medication, known as Xeljanz, was added. After getting limited relief and becoming concerned about the possible long-term side effects of these medicines, Connie came to see me.

After a detailed history, I found out that she had many mercury-containing dental fillings from her childhood in Haiti. After running blood and urine samples, we determined that her mercury was extremely elevated. In addition, lead levels were very high, likely due to her love of chocolate. Connie asked me, "How am I going to get rid of all these toxins?"

We begin the TIGER Protocol with the all-important first step, addressing toxins. First, we'll review the importance of optimal digestive function and daily elimination for clearance of toxins. Then, I'll teach you about the basic detox pathways in the body including the liver, skin, and lymphatics.

During the first two weeks of the Phase 1 Diet, I recommend you follow the guidelines in this chapter to accomplish optimal detoxification. The healthy diet itself will enable your body to attain a degree of cleansing, and the additional recommendations in this chapter will help to enhance that. We will discuss foods, spices, herbs, and additional supplements that can upgrade your capacity to detox.

IMPACT OF DETOX ON AUTOIMMUNITY

In my own practice, I see how detoxification positively impacts autoimmune diseases. For example, clearance of mercury can often help with neurological symptoms or inflammatory joint issues. Scientific literature bears this out; a particular documented case showed resolution of rheumatoid arthritis in a woman with high levels of cadmium, lead, and aluminum after one year of chelation therapy to remove these metals.[1] Another patient with multiple sclerosis (MS), who was unsuccessfully treated for years with conventional medications, was found to have elevated levels of mercury, lead, and aluminum in urine testing; treatment with an oral chelation agent led to gradual improvement of symptoms and clinical remission in his MS, as well as normalization of heavy metal levels in the urine.[2] Although these are two brief examples, they are representative of many more that show that this aspect of the protocol is critical.

Importance of Elimination

Proper elimination is essential during detoxification because so many toxins are cleared through the stool. The way that your liver, your principal detox organ, clears most toxins is by packaging them into bile (a digestive fluid produced by the liver) and releasing them into the GI tract, so they can be disposed of through the stool. The body tries to get rid of a lot of toxic compounds with each bowel movement.

Ensure that you have at least one stool daily. This is part of what I consider "pre-tox," to prepare the body for effective detox. If you are not having a daily bowel movement, there is a possibility that toxins can be reabsorbed into the body while they are waiting in your intestinal tract.

Fiber Is Crucial

As you are following my Phase 1 Diet, you will already be eating a significant amount of fiber. In this case, I am not recommending fiber to help with bowel movements; rather, the fiber powders I am recommending have unique properties—they bind to toxins in your GI tract and hold on to them as they exit your body via stool. They help prevent the reabsorption of toxins into your bloodstream from your intestines. To that end, I am recommending them during the first two weeks you are on the Phase 1 Diet.

I also recommend that you continue taking either of these fiber powders during the second two weeks of the Phase 1 Diet—the "I" stage of the TIGER Protocol—when we will focus on getting rid of bad bacteria and pathogens in your gut (as we'll review in the next chapter). As bad bacteria, yeast, and other harmful microbes are dying off, they also release certain toxins. These fiber supplements help to bind the toxins from these harmful microbes as they die. In addition, they both have beneficial prebiotic properties to assist the buildup of helpful keystone bacteria in your microbiome. They also help with establishing optimal pH in the intestine, which limits the growth of pathogens—we'll get to that in chapter 8.

There are two good options for getting additional fiber. Regardless of whether you have constipation, normal bowel movements, or diarrhea, you can consider either option. Try one option first, and if you do not react well to it for any reason, then go ahead to the other choice. Research has shown benefit for both these fibers in cases of constipation and loose stools:

Psyllium husk. Psyllium is an excellent prebiotic and great source of fiber that is beneficial in a wide variety of people. It is derived from the shell of the psyllium seed, which comes from the Plantago ovata plant native to India and China. Both the intact psyllium seed and husk are available as powders, but I recommend going with the psyllium husk because it is easier on the stomach and more widely available. Surprisingly, psyllium husk can help in cases of constipation as well as diarrhea by providing additional bulk to the stool.

Psyllium has been shown to help raise the levels of three groups of beneficial bacteria known to produce butyrate—Lachnospira, Roseburia, and Faecalibacterium—especially in patients with constipation.[3] Recall that butyrate is the powerful anti-inflammatory metabolite we discussed in chapter 4. Of note, psyllium has major systemic benefits, including reducing cholesterol, reducing blood pressure, increasing satiety and thus supporting weight loss, and alleviating IBS symptoms.[4]

To add it to your diet, I recommend starting with half a teaspoon per day and building up gradually to 1 tablespoon per day, or whatever dosage is sufficient to ensure daily bowel movements. It is crucial to increase your water intake and ensure that you are drinking at least 2 L of water per day. With all prebiotics, there might be gas, bloating, or cramps as your stomach bacteria shift, but typically the symptoms subside within a week. As you increase the dose, if at any point you begin to see GI symptoms (that do not resolve within a week), decrease back down to the dose where you were not having any noticeable symptoms—and stay at that dose.

PHGG or Partially Hydrolyzed Guar Gum. Thriving in a hot, arid climate, the guar bean is native to India but has been cultivated worldwide now for over a century. Made by grinding and drying the guar bean, PHGG has unique and potent properties as a prebiotic. In addition to being a great source of fiber and helping elimination, partially hydrolyzed guar gum has been shown in studies to help balance your microbiome, reduce small intestinal bacterial overgrowth (SIBO), alleviate IBS symptoms, and selectively feed some beneficial bacteria.[5] It can be helpful in constipation or diarrhea.

It increases levels of keystone species such as Faecalibacterium, Bifidobacteria, and Bacteroides and boosts the production of short-chain fatty acids such as butyrate and acetate.[6] PHGG has shown additional systemic benefits such as regulating blood sugars by slowing the uptake of glucose from the intestine, promoting satiety, and lowering cholesterol levels.[7] My preferred form of PHGG is a patented product called SunFiber®, and there are various brands that contain this product, such as Tomorrow's Nutrition and Perfect Pass.

Start with 1/4 scoop daily for one week, then increase to 1 scoop daily with or without food. Mix into 8–12 oz of water or any other liquid. PHGG dissolves more easily than psyllium husk and is completely tasteless. It is normal to have some increase in gas for a few days as your gut bacteria are shifting. If it is too much, then reduce the dosage to 1/8 scoop or even lower (like 1/4 teaspoon per day) and build up more gradually to the lowest dosage that does not cause any uncomfortable symptoms for you.

It is very important to start low and go slow with the dosage. If you are sensitive to supplements, begin with 1/4 teaspoon per day. As tolerated, you can eventually build up to the one scoop daily or whatever dose is sufficient to ensure normal, healthy daily bowel movements. Every person is different, and you need to figure out the best dosage for you.

Supplements for Constipation

Hopefully, with the fiber inherent in the Phase I Diet and either psyllium husk or PHGG, you will start to have normal daily bowel movements. That is a precondition for effective detoxification.

Some people, especially those with a previous history of constipation, may need additional support for optimal elimination. If you are still not eliminating daily despite the additional fiber, you may take one of the following supplements to assist with this during the detox:

- Triphala—which means "three fruits" in Sanskrit—is a well-known Ayurvedic formula that features equal parts of three dried fruits (haritaki, bibhitaki, and amalaki). It usually comes in 500 mg tablets. Start with one tablet at bedtime with a glass of water. Increase the dosage by one tablet every night to a maximum of three tablets until you are having at least one soft bowel movement daily. The brands Organic India or Banyan Botanicals are certified organic, but other good brands are available. Triphala has impressive detoxification properties and can be an excellent adjunct during the cleanse even if you don't need it to stimulate bowel movements.

- An alternative is magnesium, which is available in various forms such as magnesium citrate, magnesium oxide, or magnesium gycinate. Any form is acceptable for this purpose, although there is variability in absorption of different forms (as I will cover in chapter 14). Most people find that magnesium at a dose of 400 to 600 mg per day is helpful to soften the stool and promote regular bowel movements. Too much magnesium can cause loose stools or diarrhea. In addition, magnesium has many systemic benefits, which we will discuss in chapter 14.

HOW YOUR LIVER FITS IN

Now that we have optimized your digestive elimination, let's talk about the crucial function of your liver in this process. The liver is your principal detox organ—responsible for filtering the blood and removing toxins—although technically it is more of a processing plant and not a filter, because it does not hold on to toxins. Many toxins are fat-soluble, and are stored in body fat and cell membranes, which are primarily consumed of lipids. This makes it hard for the body to eliminate such toxins. The liver must convert such fat-soluble toxins into water-soluble forms that can be excreted from the body.

It does this through a two-step process called Phase 1 and Phase 2 detoxification. Phase 1 is carried out by cytochrome P450, a diverse group of around 30 enzymes.[8] This system efficiently processes toxins into intermediate metabolites—but these can be highly reactive or even harmful unless they are broken down by Phase 2 pathways. Phase 2 requires combining the secondary compounds with other molecules to create water-soluble by-products. In Phase 2, the intermediate compounds are joined to one of six different molecules to be prepared for elimination, e.g., methyl groups (via a process known as methylation), sulfate (sulfation), or glutathione.

These end-products are removed from the body either by the kidneys through urine or by the intestines via bile and stool. Interestingly, the microbiome also plays an important role in the process of detoxification (through the enzyme beta-glucuronidase), as we discussed in chapter 4.

Balancing Phase 1 and Phase 2

Phase 1 and Phase 2 have to be optimally balanced—if the reactive metabolites produced by Phase 1 are not quickly broken down, they can build up and cause cellular damage or uncomfortable symptoms such as headaches, fatigue, dizziness, stomach upset, aches and pains, or nausea. Therefore, it is crucial to support both Phase 1 and Phase 2 during detoxification. What I commonly see in patients is relative overactivity of the Phase 1 pathway and underactivity of Phase 2. This can sometimes produce symptoms such as fatigue, malaise, or excessive reactivity to chemicals.

The food and supplements I recommend during this process support both Phase 1 and Phase 2.

Clues to Poor Liver Function

Before we talk about optimizing liver function, let's discuss how to assess its performance in the first place. It can actually be hard to detect suboptimal liver function. Traditional blood work, consisting of liver enzymes such as AST and ALT, is designed to be a screening tool for hepatitis, a condition of severe liver inflammation which may be caused by viruses, alcohol, or other major insults to the liver.

If you have normal liver enzymes, it means you (thankfully) do not have hepatitis or other serious liver inflammation. However, that does not mean that this key organ is functioning optimally. In fact, your liver could be under duress but that might not show up on traditional blood work which picks up only the most severe dysfunction. Unfortunately, we do not have functional medicine testing to detect subtle imbalances in liver function.

However, there are several clues that could indicate that your liver is not working optimally—which may be due to a high body burden of toxins. Because traditional blood work only detects severe liver dysfunction, we need to look for other indirect signals that indicate that the liver needs support. The following conditions may all be caused by other factors but it's possible that reduced liver function could be one of them:

Poor thyroid hormone conversion. There are two basic thyroid hormones in the body, T3 and T4. T3 is the active form which is used by your cells, and T4 is the inactive precursor. Your thyroid mostly produces T4, and your body must convert it to T3. The majority of that conversion happens in the liver.[9] Having a normal T4 thyroid hormone but a low T3 level may indicate suboptimal liver performance.

It is important to look at where in the reference range thyroid hormone falls—e.g., the upper half of the normal range vs. the lower half of the normal range. T4 and T3 should generally correlate if the liver is working well—for example, they might both be in the upper or lower normal ranges. If T3 is low (or in the lower half of the normal range) while T4 is within the middle or upper half of the normal range, then one can conclude that some of that conversion of T4 to T3 is happening poorly in the liver. This indicates that the liver is not performing one of its key functions properly and could benefit from nutritional support.

Difficulty staying asleep. According to Traditional Chinese Medicine (TCM) the time window from 1 a.m. to 3 a.m. is associated with the liver. In TCM, every two-hour window of the day is associated with a different organ or gland. During a specific window of time, one particular organ is the most active. This is in line with new research showing that different organs such as your heart, liver, and kidney have intrinsic clocks that regulate their activity during the day.[10] Your mitochondria, the energy producers within each cell, are also affected by your daily circadian rhythm.[11]

Even your microbiome is no exception, as it is regulated by an innate circadian clock as well as your overall circadian rhythm.[12] Your bacteria may be more active during the night, which is why I recommend taking probiotics with dinner, so they can interact with your microbiome overnight.[13] These specific nighttime hours are when the liver is most active and if it is overloaded it can struggle and cause you to wake up during that time. If you fall asleep fine but are consistently waking up between 1 a.m. and 3 a.m. every night, this could indicate that your liver is struggling and needs support. Many of my patients used to wake up during those hours but their sleep issues resolved once we worked on naturally supporting their liver.

Severe Premenstrual Syndrome. If you have a period, experiencing severe PMS before your cycle begins may be a clue that the liver is struggling to handle the flux of hormones that typically occurs during that time. The liver has a significantly increased workload in the days before the menstrual cycle begins because of the major changes in female hormones, which need to be metabolized by the liver. If it is not able to process them effectively, the hormone levels can rise beyond optimal, triggering a variety of hormone-related symptoms that are associated with premenstrual syndrome, such as mood swings, breast tenderness, or irritability.

Hemorrhoids. Hemorrhoids are swellings formed by the dilation of veins around the rectum. This condition can be related to the liver due to the way blood circulation works in the body. The rectal veins surrounding the area where hemorrhoids usually form drain directly into the portal vein of the liver. This is a well-known connection in physiology that I learned in medical school. If the portal vein is affected by some sluggishness in the liver, then the backward pressure can cause slight distention of the veins in the rectal area and this can predispose to hemorrhoids. If they do manifest, they may be either internal (not visible) or external hemorrhoids.

Itching. Even in conventional medicine, it's well established that recurrent itching can be a sign of impaired liver function. It may be localized to the same body part, or it may be present throughout the body. Generally, itching from liver issues does not cause rashes, but excessive scratching in response to the itching can cause skin changes. Continuous or severe itching may be a sign of other issues and is a symptom for which you should consult your doctor.

Blood Sugar Issues. The liver plays an important but underappreciated role in blood sugar regulation. While the pancreas plays the largest role in regulating glucose, the liver (and also the adrenal gland) matter too. If someone experiences drops in blood sugar where they become suddenly hungry during the day despite having eaten normally, that indicates an issue with blood sugar regulation. While this could be due to other factors, sometimes it is caused by an underfunctioning liver. If this happens at night, it could impact sleep. If your blood sugar drops at night, then your cortisol may spike upward to raise your blood sugar. This will arouse you and wake you up from sleep. Often, a person in this situation may not know why they have woken up, because their blood sugar has already returned to normal by the time they awaken.

If you're not experiencing any of these signs and symptoms, you might wonder if it's still necessary to undergo the detox process. The answer is yes. We are chronically exposed to a myriad of toxins these days. So many of them impact the immune system, as we reviewed in chapter 2. In my clinical experience, addressing toxins is a very important step to tackle one of the key drivers of autoimmunity. Now, let us continue to another organ that can be important for detox—your skin.

TESTING FOR TOXINS

It is possible to test for toxins using specialized functional medicine tests, which can assess heavy metals and other categories of toxins. However, even these tests only detect around 20 to 30 different toxins. As we discussed in chapter 2, there are over 40,000 chemicals currently in use, and it is simply not possible to test for most of them. For this reason, I think it is better to focus on enhancing the function of your own detox pathways and helping them do their job better in order to eliminate whatever toxins are present. To this end, I will teach you how to optimize the function of your key detox pathways—the liver, the digestive tract, the lymphatic system, and the skin.

SWEATING HELPS DETOXIFY

The skin is your largest organ. The skin tends to absorb a fair amount of anything applied topically, which is why it is important to use natural skin-care products, as we discussed in chapter 2. In addition, the skin can be used for detoxification. Many toxins are fat-soluble and deposited in fat stores within the body, which make them inaccessible to blood or lymphatic circulation that can carry water-soluble toxins to the liver for detoxification.

Here are a few tips on how to optimally detoxify through sweating:

- Sweating must be done in a specific way to release toxins stored in the subcutaneous fat layer just underneath our skin. To do this, sweating must result from the body being gradually heated from an external source, so sweating from exercise does not accomplish as much in terms of detoxification, although exercise has many extraordinary benefits.
- Sweating in a sauna or steam room is effective at stimulating toxin release through the skin. At least fifteen to twenty minutes is necessary to

achieve this objective. I recommend starting with one or two sessions per week.

- If you do not tolerate the heat from a traditional sauna, infrared saunas are a good alternative. These achieve the same benefits in terms of detoxification but do not heat the air around the body. People who are intolerant of traditional saunas often do well with infrared saunas. I discuss saunas in more detail below.

- If you do not have access to any of these, it is also possible to use a bathtub at home. Fill the bathtub with hot water and immerse your body in it for at least fifteen minutes until you feel some sweat on your forehead. You may put a quarter cup of bentonite clay into the water to prevent your skin from absorbing any existing chemicals in the water.

- If you are intolerant to heat or do not have a bathtub, you can sit outside on a warm, sunny day until you break a sweat.

Sauna Therapy

A sauna may be one of the most cost-effective investments a person with autoimmune disease can make, due to multiple beneficial effects. Studies show that sweating in a sauna is an effective way to excrete lead, mercury, arsenic, and cadmium.[14] Research has also found that sweating leads to high levels of other environmental toxins in the sweat—often at higher levels than found in blood and urine, suggesting that sweat may be an effective vehicle of detoxification; examples of toxins that behave in this manner are pesticides, flame retardants (PBDEs), BPA, phthalates, and PCBs (a study even compared sweating from a sauna to sweating induced by exercise and found that sauna use led to higher levels of excretion in the sweat for several toxins).[15] You will recall that these four heavy metals and five environmental pollutants are all toxins that are associated with increased risk of autoimmune disorders, as I outlined earlier.

Saunas stimulate the production of heat shock proteins (HSPs) in the body. HSPs enhance the function of the immune system, clear toxic metabolites from the circulation, and help cellular repair functions.[16] Sauna use raises the levels of beta-endorphins, the body's intrinsic opioid compounds that help with feeling good and reducing pain; this likely contributes to uplifting mood as well.[17] Additionally, saunas activate hormesis, in which a moderate stress on the body triggers activation of a variety of health-promoting mechanisms. Basically, you stress the body a little and then it comes back stronger. Sauna use causes upregulation of certain hormones such as norepinephrine and prolactin and reduction in the stress hormone cortisol; it also leads to increased levels of growth hormone and improved insulin sensitivity.[18]

Research shows that using a sauna four to seven times per week led to a 40 percent reduction in death from all causes over a 21-year time period (using it two to three times per week was associated with a respectable 24 percent decrease).[19] This includes reduced risk of cardiovascular disease and sudden cardiac death.

Contraindications and Cautions

Sauna use should be avoided in pregnancy and heart failure. If you are on medications, check with your doctor before use. If you are intolerant to heat, or prone to orthostatic hypotension (where your blood pressure drops when you stand up), you should use caution.

Always start with the lowest temperature setting. You may want to start with just a few minutes and build up slowly to 20 minutes daily. Hydration is crucial—ensure that you drink lots of water before and after use of the sauna. Some people find additional electrolytes (NUUN, LMNT, or similar products) helpful, especially if they sweat a lot. If you experience dizziness or discomfort of any kind, immediately discontinue use.

Getting the Benefits

You might think that in order to use a sauna, you need to spend money on a gym membership or luxury spa visit. However, portable saunas do not take up much space. They consist of a chair inside a small folding tent that you sit in and then zip yourself up from the inside. Your head typically stays outside the tent. The sauna heats the interior of the tent either with infrared light or a heating element. When you are done, it will fold down and can be put away. Good models are available online starting around $100. Newer products such as sauna "blankets" are available as well, although we need more research to assess if they are as effective as regular saunas.

There are two main types of saunas, traditional and infrared. Traditional saunas use conventional electric heating to heat the air in the sauna to high temperatures (which then heats the body), while infrared saunas use infrared light to heat the body directly, allowing them to have the same effects at lower temperatures. Therefore, they are often easier to tolerate for those who are sensitive to heat. Infrared saunas have another benefit from the infrared light they use—photobiomodulation (PBM), which has been shown to have other health-promoting effects, as I will discuss in chapter 12.

OPTIMIZE YOUR LYMPHATIC SYSTEM

The lymphatic system is part of the circulatory system, comprising a network of channels called lymphatic vessels that carry a clear fluid called lymph around the body. Unlike blood, the lymph fluid is not pumped by the heart, but instead relies on muscular contraction and body movement to move the fluid appropriately.

Keeping a healthy lymphatic system is important for the immune system. Research shows that the lymphatic system plays a key role in immune regulation by helping to transport immune cells to and from lymph nodes, carrying pathogens for removal, and directing the movement of various immune cells.[20] The lymphatic system also helps with the removal of toxins from the body.

Here are some tips for keeping your lymphatic system healthy:

- Regular aerobic exercise is beneficial for lymphatic drainage.
- More gentle activities such as yoga or tai chi are also effective.
- Dry brushing is an Ayurvedic practice in which you use a soft-bristled brush to brush the skin across your entire body before a shower. It can be a helpful way to exfoliate dead skin, improve circulation, and move the lymph fluid throughout the body.
- Use of a sauna also supports healthy lymphatic flow.

SUPERFOODS FOR DAILY DETOXIFICATION

In terms of diet during this detox, your foundation will be the Phase 1 Diet. Here are a few additional foods to give particular attention:

- Beets and especially beet greens are the richest food source of betaine, a natural phytochemical that supports phase 2 liver pathways. They also support methylation, which is a key function for detox and other processes in the body. Incorporate beet greens into soup, salads, or smoothies.

- Regularly consume cruciferous vegetables, which support Phase 2 liver pathways. These include bok choy, broccoli, brussels sprouts, cabbage, cauliflower, collards, kale, and turnips. Making sure they are lightly cooked will ensure that there is no negative impact on your thyroid; extremely high intake of raw cruciferous vegetables may dampen the functioning of your thyroid if consumed for a long time.[21] This is more likely to be true if you have an iodine deficiency, which is why I recommend using iodized salt and eating seafood which tends to be rich in iodine.
- Sulfate addition (or sulfation) is one of the key Phase 2 liver detox pathways—nutritional support for this comes from sulfur-rich foods such as onions, shallots, and leeks.
- Garlic has a variety of health benefits and aids detox by also supporting the pathway of sulfation. Eggs are beneficial too, but you will be avoiding them temporarily as part of the Phase 1 Diet.
- Chlorella is a type of algae that has been traditionally used for clearance of heavy metals. While human studies are limited, one animal study did find reduced brain accumulation of mercury in rats fed chlorella powder while also ingesting mercury.[22] Chlorella is rich in other nutrients including amino acids, vitamins, and minerals and is well-tolerated. Add one to two teaspoons of chlorella powder to a smoothie. Please note that this may turn your stool a green color because of the deep green color of chlorella.

HYDRATION

Before exploring supplements, let's review hydration. This is something basic that we often take for granted but it is indispensable, especially when your body is clearing toxins. I recommend drinking at least two liters of water daily. This is vital during detoxification because the liver processes water-soluble toxins for excretion by the kidney. The best way to support your kidneys' detox capacity is by ensuring adequate hydration. If you are adding regular sauna and exercise to the regimen, which I highly recommend, you may need even more water. A simple rule of thumb is that your urine should be mostly clear during the daytime. If it is yellow it could indicate that your urine is concentrated because you are not getting enough water.

SUPPLEMENTS

It is best to take supplements under the supervision of a licensed practitioner. The recommendations listed here are general guidelines and need to be individualized for each person. If you experience any type of adverse reaction while you are taking a supplement, stop it immediately and consult with your practitioner. Some general guidelines: I always recommend only starting one new supplement at a time. In this case, for example, I would recommend first beginning with glutathione, and then adding in AdvaClear or UltraClear Plus pH after a few days. It is a good idea to start with a low dose and increase slowly.

Glutathione

I consider glutathione to be a core supplement during the detox phase of the TIGER Protocol. Glutathione is considered the "master antioxidant," the most important antioxidant in the body. It is made in the body by the liver using a few amino acids. It is crucial for phase 2 liver detox, as discussed above. Glutathione also is one of the most effective compounds to counter oxidative stress.

Several studies show that autoimmune conditions are associated with increased oxidative stress and impaired antioxidant function, often reflected in low glutathione levels.[23] This leads to more damage from free radicals, and permits toxins to build up to higher levels, leading to a vicious cycle of inflammation and autoimmunity.

Therefore, it is likely that people suffering from autoimmunity are already low in glutathione, and thus expected to benefit from supplementation. It is possible to measure your level of glutathione with a blood test through a standard laboratory. However, if you are not able to have this done, it is still safe to take it as a supplement to support detoxification.

Glutathione appears to be safe and well-tolerated at standard dosages. In terms of contraindications, there is not enough safety data to support use during pregnancy or breastfeeding, so I recommend avoiding it in both of those situations.

There are two main forms of oral glutathione: liposomal and reduced. The liposomal form is packaged inside a lipid sphere called a liposome, which boosts the absorption. Studies show that taking liposomal glutathione is effective at increasing body stores of glutathione and favorably impacting markers of oxidative stress.[24] In terms of dosage, I recommend starting with 100 mg once a day and then building up gradually to 100 mg twice a day with food, not exceeding a max of 500 mg per day.

Reduced glutathione, also known as L-glutathione, has also been shown to be effective at elevating serum levels of glutathione in the body; one randomized placebo-controlled trial found that daily intake of reduced glutathione raised body stores of glutathione and reduced markers of oxidative stress.[25]

Various companies have patented forms of reduced glutathione that have good absorption. Setria® is one form; another, Optitac, was found to reduce fatty infiltration of the liver in nonalcoholic fatty liver disease (thought to affect roughly 20–30 percent of Americans).[26] With reduced glutathione a slightly higher dosage is needed. I suggest beginning with 250–500 mg once a day and building up to 250–500 mg twice a day after meals.

Both liposomal and reduced glutathione have data showing efficacy, and you can choose either one of them as they are equally good.

Additional Supplements

In addition to glutathione, I also recommend choosing one supplement that supports detoxification specifically, just for the two weeks of Stage 1. There are various options to choose from. Again, choose *only one* supplement from the following list of options:

- Metagenics AdvaClear contains vitamins, minerals, and botanicals that support healthy detox pathways in a tablet form. The suggested dose is two tablets twice a day with food. Start with just one tablet once a day and add a tablet every few days, building up slowly to the final dosage.
- Metagenics UltraClear Plus pH is a good option for those who prefer a powder instead of taking a tablet. It contains a base of rice protein combined with vitamins, minerals, and other nutrients that support detox pathways. The recommended final dose to build up to is two scoops twice a day. As with all liver support, it's important to build up to the final dose gradually. Start with half a scoop or, if you are sensitive, a quarter of a scoop twice a day. Increase the dosage by half a scoop per day every three days until you achieve the final dose of two scoops twice a day. If at any point you get uncomfortable symptoms of any kind, reduce the dose to the level that does not cause any symptoms for you. This can also serve as a meal replacement (more like a snack) or a base for a smoothie.

- Standard Process offers a variety of supplements that can be used to support detoxification. The typical supplement I recommend for this purpose is Standard Process Livaplex, a blend of vitamins, minerals, and grass-fed beef liver extract. The dose should be individualized, but with all supplements I recommend the "start low and go slow" approach. If tolerated, work up gradually to a dosage of one capsule three times a day with meals.

- If you prefer not to take a supplement, herbal teas are another option. These are less potent but usually well-tolerated, especially if you are sensitive to supplements. Herbal teas that contain dandelion, milk thistle, or artichoke are good options. Good options are Yogi Tea DeTox or Traditional Medicinals EveryDay Detox.

QUESTIONS AND ANSWERS ABOUT THE PROTOCOL

I'd like to address some common questions you might have before beginning this detox. In my experience, these are some of the typical questions patients have.

How will I feel?

In surveying my patients, there's a wide variety of response to this part of the protocol. Some feel better than they have ever felt in their lives before, describing a profound increase in energy and vitality. Some people do not feel any noticeable difference. Others feel some side effects or unpleasant symptoms as their body begins to release toxins that it has been holding on to for years or even decades. Possible symptoms include headaches, fatigue, aches and pains, upset stomach, rashes, sinus congestion, postnasal drip, and/or general malaise. If this is the case with you, my main advice to you is: Be patient. Usually these symptoms gradually get better as the detox continues. Remember that this is a sign that your body is expelling toxins and this is going to be very beneficial for you in the long run. If the symptoms become too much, stop taking whichever supplement you are taking. Wait two days and resume at a lower dose; increase to the highest dose that you can tolerate that does not cause adverse reactions. Every person is unique, and you have to determine what works for you.

What happens if I "cheat"?

I want to reassure you that it's okay if you are not perfect in following the diet and other recommendations. The effects of the detox are cumulative, and eating something that is not part of the meal plan occasionally is okay if there are no other options. With that said, maximal benefit will likely result from adhering to the program as strictly as possible. Do your best and if for whatever reason you are not able to stick to the diet for a meal or two, it will not throw off the entire detox and invalidate any benefits.

How do I come off the detox and reintroduce foods?

Please refer to my detailed instructions at the end of chapter 5 about how to reintroduce foods that you have eliminated during the Phase 1 Diet.

Now that we've walked through our detoxifcation protocol, let's revisit Connie.

Connie was struggling with rheumatoid arthritis despite being on the powerful medications methotrexate and Xeljanz. Our testing revealed very high levels of mercury and lead. Connie was highly motivated to take action to address the root causes of her condition.

I referred her to a holistic dentist, who worked with her over about six months to remove all her mercury dental amalgams and replace them with composite materials. After that, we completed a four-month heavy metal detox using herbal formulas such as chlorella, cilantro, and modified citrus pectin. Connie also purchased a home sauna and used it regularly. She eliminated chocolate and other sources of lead in her diet.

Follow-up testing after the detox revealed that her mercury and lead levels had come down to normal. We completed the rest of the TIGER Protocol, with a focus on improving her diet, sleep, and physical activity. Soon afterward, she noticed significant reduction in her pain and swelling. Her energy levels improved as well.

Eventually, she was able to discontinue the Xeljanz and remain in remission on just the methotrexate.

CHAPTER 8

Infections—Identify and Eliminate Infections

At 28 years old, Sabrina had been living with lupus for a few years. She had been taking hydroxychloroquinine, the typical first-line medication, for three years when she developed some visual changes. Tests indicated early retinal damage, a possible side effect of the drug.

Frightened, she discontinued the medication on the advice of her doctor. She was reluctant to start a new medicine and began experimenting with diet. After watching a documentary about plant-based eating, she became a strict vegan and cut out animal products, oils, and salt from her diet.

Unfortunately, the diet did not work to improve her symptoms. Instead, she experienced weight loss, fatigue, dry skin, and insomnia. She came across my first book, The Paleovedic Diet, *and learned how Ayurveda recommends different diets for each person based on their body type. She determined that she was an Ayurvedic* vata *body type (which correlates with "wind" and has light and dry qualities), for whom a vegan diet is not recommended.*

Sabrina switched to a Mediterranean template, eating fish and poultry, plenty of olive oil, and lots of ghee after learning its benefits according to Ayurveda. She also started taking fish oil and vitamin D. Her symptoms reduced by about 50 percent, and she was finally able to see me in my office. She asked me what else we could do to control her lupus. The topic of infections was something she had not investigated previously, so we decided to explore that area.

After toxins, we move on to infections, the "I" in the protocol. In this second step, we'll focus the next two weeks on clearing infections. In this chapter, we will discuss how to resolve the most common infections implicated in autoimmune disease. From the food perspective, you will be continuing the Phase 1 Diet. We'll talk about a few additional dietary strategies that are helpful, and have a detailed discussion about nutritional supplements, spices, and herbs.

OPTIMIZING YOUR TERRAIN

As we discussed in chapter 3, our goal is to make the inner "terrain" of your body as inhospitable as possible to pathogens. By making your inner environment unfriendly to harmful microbes, we increase the chances that your immune system will be able to take care of whatever bad bugs are present. A key part of this strategy is optimizing the pH of your digestive tract and making your large intestine slightly acidic. This will go a long way toward optimizing the vitally important terrain of your intestinal microbiome.

Maintaining Optimal pH: Indispensable for Health

What you need to know about pH (which stands for "power of hydrogen" and is measured on a scale from 0 to 14) is that neutral is 7.0—anything below 7 is considered acidic, and anything above 7 is considered alkaline. A healthy pH for the colon is between 5.0 to 6.5, which is considered acidic since it is below the neutral pH of 7.0. At this acidic pH, the growth of pathogens is inhibited. Potentially problematic species such as *E. coli*, Bacteroides, and Desulfovibrio and yeast species such as Candida begin to proliferate when the pH starts to rise above 7.0.

How quickly can stool pH change? Studies show that increasing levels of fiber in the diet can rapidly decrease the pH within just a couple of weeks; in one study, people who doubled their fiber intake from 17 g to 34 g per day experienced a progressive drop in stool pH over a mere two weeks.[1]

Studies also show that higher stool pH is associated with increased risk of colon cancer, likely due to the production of carcinogenic compounds, whereas an acidic colon environment contains more nutrients that are protective against colon cancer.[2] Two different mechanisms are suspected. A process called protein putrefaction, where bacteria break down protein to form harmful compounds, occurs much more at alkaline pH. At higher pH, pathobiont bacteria (bacteria that can be either harmless or harmful at certain times) such as Bacteroides, *E. coli* (yes, it's not always bad!), and Clostridia ferment proteins to produce amines, indoles, and ammonia, which have negative effects on gut permeability and motility.[3]

Additionally, our primary bile acids, produced by the liver to aid in digestion, can be fermented by pathobionts into so-called secondary bile acids, which are potential carcinogens because they can cause DNA damage in our colonic cells and inflammation—a process that only occurs at neutral or alkaline pH. The growth of pathobionts such as Bacteroides, and their ability to produce all these potentially harmful compounds, depends heavily on colon pH.

Improving Mineral Absorption

An acidic pH is critical for absorbing certain minerals such as calcium and iron. Their absorption declines when pH starts getting into the alkaline range. Maintaining this acidic pH is crucial to maintaining healthy absorption and optimal digestive function, preventing dysbiosis, and preventing colon cancer.

Strategies to Maintain Healthy Stool pH

One of the biggest contributors to healthy pH are short-chain fatty acids, which are produced by our healthy bacteria. The most important and well-known of these SCFAs is butyrate, which has a number of beneficial properties. As we discussed in chapter 4, butyrate is the primary fuel for the intestinal cells, and it reduces inflammation, promotes normal intestinal permeability, has anti-cancer effects, and improves the gut-brain axis by even healing "leaky brain," an impaired blood-brain barrier.

The best way to increase production of short-chain fatty acids is the Phase 1 Diet—a high-fiber diet with plenty of plant fiber, which will be used by the good bacteria to produce SCFAs. Thus, the Phase 1 Diet is one of the best eating plans to maintain acidic intestinal pH.

Fermented Foods and Fiber

Fermented foods contain organic acids, such as lactic acid and acetic acid, that contribute to maintaining healthy acidity in the colon. Vinegar is defined by its content of acetic acid; consuming fermented foods that contain vinegar delivers the acetic acid to the intestine, where it helps keep pH at a healthy low level. We'll learn more about the effects and benefits of fermented foods in the next chapter.

In the previous chapter, I suggested taking either psyllium husk or partially hydrolyzed guar gum as an additional fiber source. Both fibers have the effect of increasing the production of short-chain fatty acids, and thereby acidifying the intestine and lowering its pH.

Prebiotic Foods

Your bacteria use the fibers in these prebiotic foods to produce short-chain fatty acids. For example, galactooligosaccharides (GOS) are diverse short chains of galactose molecules that are beneficial prebiotics. Some of the richest food sources of GOS include (in descending order) Jerusalem artichoke, lentils, lima beans, and chickpeas; most other beans are decent sources of this prebiotic.[4]

It is important to note that increasing the consumption of prebiotics may cause more gas and distention. As the bacteria are shifting, and starting to ferment the prebiotic fibers, they will begin to produce more gas (as well as the highly beneficial short-chain fatty acids). This will likely resolve over time as your system gets used to increased intake of these foods.

If it's uncomfortable or problematic, reduce the intake of these foods until symptoms are not bothersome. A good strategy is to start slowly with very small quantities of these prebiotic foods and build up gradually to allow your digestive tract to get used to them. We will spend more time on prebiotic foods in chapter 10.

SPICES

Now that we have discussed dietary factors to curb the growth of microbes, we will move on to spices. These spices come from Ayurveda, the 3,000-year-old traditional medicine of India, which I've studied for many years. It is one of my favorite modalities to incorporate with patients.

In Ayurveda, spices are considered a class of medicines in their own right. In particular, there are four main spices I strongly recommend you utilize during this phase to help improve your balance of microbes. These are ajwain, ginger, garlic, and black cumin. Incorporating these spices will go a long way toward reducing levels of pathogenic bacteria, yeast, and parasites. In addition to providing you with supporting research, I offer you practical tips on how to work them into your daily diet. In the Recipes section, I've included recipes that incorporate these spices. An easy way to achieve the recommended daily intake is to incorporate some of the spices into a smoothie each day.

Ajwain (Trachyspermum ammi, Carum copticum)

Ajwain, also known as ajowan or carom, is a spice that is not well-known in the West but is used extensively in India, both in cooking and in Ayurveda. Ajwain contains a number of beneficial phytochemicals including glucosides, saponins, carvacrol, thymol, and beta-pinene; it is also nutrient-dense and an excellent source of fiber, vitamin B_3 (niacin), and minerals including calcium, phosphorus, and iron.[5] The high concentration of the aromatic compound thymol in ajwain often reminds people of thyme, which is also rich in thymol.

Ajwain is traditionally used in Ayurveda to combat viral and bacterial infections and parasitic diseases. Its antibacterial activity was confirmed in a study examining potentially pathogenic bacteria and fungi—ajwain was effective in *selectively* inhibiting the growth of dysbiotic gut microbes (such as clostridium bacteria and the yeast candida), without having a negative impact on beneficial bacteria.[6]

For these reasons, ajwain can be especially beneficial to address dysbiosis and improve microbial balance in autoimmune patients. It does not harm your beneficial keystone species, while it inhibits the growth of pathogenic bacteria and yeast.

A number of animal studies have demonstrated digestive benefits of ajwain, including treatment of peptic ulcer, improved activity of digestive enzymes, and reduction in stomach discomfort and pain.[7] I like ajwain because of these digestive benefits, and that is why I recommend continuing to incorporate ajwain while cooking even after you finish this protocol.

Ajwain has an excellent safety profile and adverse reactions have not been reported in the literature. It can be consumed in either whole seed or powder form. It can be found commonly in Indian grocery stores and is available online. To improve their flavor, you can cook the seeds first by either dry roasting or cooking them in oil. Ajwain makes a good addition to meat, vegetable, and lentil dishes as well as curries.

I recommend aiming to incorporate one teaspoon of ajwain seeds or half a teaspoon of ajwain powder over the course of a day, distributed between your various meals.

Ginger (Zingiber officinale)

Ginger is the rhizome (technically the underground stem) of the ginger plant. It is used extensively in Ayurveda for its digestive benefits, anti-inflammatory properties, and energizing and stimulating effects. Like most spices, it is an outstanding source of antioxidants; its key phytochemicals include gingerols, paradols, shogaols, and gingerones.[8]

Ginger is often used in Ayurveda to tackle infections and is especially helpful against viruses and bacteria. One study showed that fresh ginger is active against a virus known as respiratory syncytial virus (RSV), a common cause of lung infections, especially in children.[9] Another study demonstrated the potent antibacterial activity of ginger, revealing that ginger was able to inhibit the growth of multidrug-resistant bacteria, which are bacteria that have become resistant to several antibiotics.[10]

Ginger has a powerful capacity to reduce inflammation and pain, providing further benefits for autoimmune patients. A randomized controlled trial found that ginger powder was as effective as the prescription anti-inflammatory diclofenac at reducing pain and improving symptoms in patients with knee osteoarthritis over a twelve-week period.[11] Another randomized double-blind placebo-controlled trial found that ginger extract was better than placebo at reducing pain in patients with osteoarthritis of the knee.[12]

Ginger has an excellent safety profile. The most common mild side effect is gastrointestinal irritation. Because it is quite pungent, high doses of the spice may cause heartburn, diarrhea, or stomach upset.

Ginger as a spice is safe, but there are a few contraindications for use of the supplement. Patients on blood-thinning medications such as warfarin (Coumadin) or clopidogrel (Plavix) should avoid ginger because of possible herb-drug interactions.

As with all supplements, ginger extract should be stopped at least two weeks before any surgery because of possible interactions with anesthesia medications.[13] Ginger is often recommended as a treatment for symptoms experienced during pregnancy such as nausea, although I recommend that pregnant women consult with their physicians before taking any dietary supplement.

There are many ways to consume ginger, and in this case, the more, the better (within the range that does not cause you any gastric distress). It can be used to add an aromatic note to any dish and can also be taken as a tea or an extract. Pickled ginger provides the additional benefits of a fermented food.

If you opt to use ginger powder, I recommend trying to incorporate a total of one teaspoon per day. If you use fresh ginger, I suggest aiming for about a half inch piece distributed throughout the day.

Garlic (Allium sativum)

Garlic has powerful antimicrobial effects. It has antibacterial, antiviral, and anti-cancer properties.[14] In addition to its anti-infective properties, garlic also has been shown to enhance the functioning of the immune system by stimulating beneficial immune cells, modulating the production of immune signaling compounds called cytokines, and reducing inflammation.[15]

The main active ingredient in garlic, allicin, is made when two compounds that are stored in separate compartments of garlic are mixed. It takes about ten minutes for this process to occur.

To maximize the therapeutic benefit, scientists devised a special process.[16] Crush, mash, or mince the garlic and then wait. After ten minutes, the allicin will be synthesized and is heat stable. You may then either consume the garlic raw or cook with the garlic without destroying the beneficial compounds.

I often crush garlic at the beginning of cooking so that it is ready to use later after I have completed other steps. If you heat it right after crushing, you will not be getting many of the therapeutic effects of garlic.

In my practice, we often use garlic extracts as part of treatment for SIBO, small intestinal bacterial overgrowth. In this case, we are using whole garlic as part of a regimen with many other antimicrobial components, so extracts or supplements are not needed. Aim to use approximately one clove of garlic per day.

Black Cumin (Nigella sativa)

While black cumin (no relationship to cumin) is not easy to find, it is a spice that has tremendous healing potential, especially when it comes to autoimmunity. Black cumin is a small, black seed that is somewhat shiny. It is revered as a "hidden gem" in Ayurveda. Also known as *Nigella sativa*, it is a gold mine of medicinal properties—research shows potential health benefits in many conditions including heart disease, cancer, and autoimmune disease. There are more than 100 different compounds in black cumin, including amino acids, essential fatty acids, and thymoquinone, the chief anti-inflammatory phytochemical in black cumin which is not found in any other food.[17]

In clinical studies, black cumin has shown anti-inflammatory, anticancer, pain-relieving, immune-boosting, and fever-reducing properties.[18]

In Ayurveda, black cumin is traditionally used for its antimicrobial activity. These properties, including antiparasitic and antifungal effects, have been documented in multiple studies,[19] which makes it a perfect addition to the protocol.

Black cumin has been shown to be not only rich in antioxidants but also able to strengthen the body's own antioxidant defense systems by modulating enzymes relating to glutathione, the master antioxidant in the body.[20] As we discussed, increasing glutathione levels helps to support phase two liver detoxification, which is very beneficial for those with autoimmune conditions to help keep toxin levels low. Patients with autoimmunity have high levels of oxidative stress and are likely to benefit from increasing antioxidants in their diet.

Black cumin's ability to reduce inflammation and modulate the immune system was examined in a study with rheumatoid arthritis patients. Five-hundred-milligram capsules taken twice daily were able to effectively reduce pain, swelling, and morning stiffness when compared to a placebo after daily use for one month.[21]

Black cumin is a safe compound; the only adverse reactions reported in the literature are two cases of skin irritation from using *Nigella sativa* oil topically.[22] The whole seed is safe to consume as a spice during pregnancy, but the supplement form should be avoided in pregnancy because animal studies suggest that *Nigella sativa* may inhibit uterine contractions.[23]

To find black cumin you have to venture to specialty stores or Indian markets where it is often sold under the name *Nigella sativa* or *kolonji*. It is also available online, and I recommend brands that have organic versions such as Mary Ruth's and NOW Foods. The seeds can be used whole and do not have to be ground into powder. They have a mild peppery taste and add an aromatic flavor to recipes; they can be liberally added to meat, vegetable, and bean dishes and can be used in sauces and soups.

If you are using whole black cumin seed, I recommend trying to incorporate at least one teaspoon per day in total. You can place it in a pepper mill and grind it onto your dishes or cook with it. With black cumin seed powder or oil, I suggest a half teaspoon daily.

SUPPLEMENTS

In addition to regular use of ajwain, ginger, garlic, and black cumin, there are two additional supplements I recommend taking during this time—neem and turmeric. In designing this protocol, I have chosen elements that are likely to be beneficial in multiple ways for autoimmune patients; this is the case with neem and turmeric (and the four spices above). Neem and turmeric not only have powerful antimicrobial effects, but also have anti-inflammatory, antioxidant, and metabolic benefits.

Neem (Azadirachta indica)

One of the most powerful antimicrobials in Ayurveda, neem is revered for its broad-spectrum activity against a variety of pathogens. Studies on neem show that it has antiviral, antibacterial, antifungal, and antiparasitic properties.[24]

Neem also has favorable metabolic effects. A randomized, placebo-controlled trial found that neem extract had a beneficial effect on blood glucose and insulin resistance; pertinent to autoimmune conditions, it was also able to reduce markers of inflammation and oxidative stress.[25] Multiple parts of the plant have been used, but in this case neem leaf is what I recommend.

I recommend taking a 500-mg neem leaf capsule twice a day with food (daily dose of 1,000 mg) for a total of two weeks. Various brands are available, but I would suggest using organic neem. Organic India and Banyan Botanicals are two solid sources for neem. Please note, it is contraindicated in pregnant or breastfeeding women. With men, there is a theoretical risk of impacting fertility if taken long-term because of possible spermicidal effects but taking it for two weeks is safe.[26]

Turmeric (Curcuma longa)

While turmeric is best known for its anti-inflammatory effects, it is a surprisingly potent antimicrobial. Studies show that it has significant antibacterial, antiviral, and antifungal effects.[27] I am including it here because of these powerful effects at helping to clear harmful microorganisms, albeit in a gradual and gentle manner.

Curcumin, the most famous key ingredient in turmeric, reduces inflammation through multiple mechanisms at the cellular level. Because chronic inflammation is the hallmark of autoimmunity, curcumin is especially valuable because of its powerful anti-inflammatory effect. Curcumin is effective at blocking NF-kB, a transcription factor that turns on the expression of genes related to inflammation and has been associated with various autoimmune diseases.

Several animal and human studies have compared the efficacy of curcumin to prescription anti-inflammatories and found it to be equally effective, with fewer side effects. One RCT that compared turmeric against ibuprofen in patients with osteoarthritis of the knee found that 1,500 mg of a turmeric extract per day was as effective as 1,200 mg of ibuprofen in alleviating knee pain and stiffness and improving knee function, with fewer side effects such as abdominal discomfort.[28]

A study involving patients with rheumatoid arthritis (RA) found that curcumin was as effective as the prescription anti-inflammatory diclofenac at reducing pain and disease activity in RA.[29] Another RCT evaluated the use of curcumin to treat chronic anterior uveitis, an autoimmune inflammatory disease of the eye, and found that curcumin was comparable in efficacy to conventional drug therapy.[30]

One of turmeric's key strengths is its antioxidant potential. Its molecular structure enables it to function as an antioxidant and block free radicals directly. However, it also can stimulate the body's own production of antioxidants, which can potentially be even more powerful.

Turmeric has been shown to stimulate production of superoxide dismutase, an enzyme present in all cells that breaks down damaging free radicals; it also drives synthesis of glutathione reductase and glutathione-s-transferase, enzymes that are critical for the body's production of intrinsic antioxidants such as glutathione.[31] Turmeric provides support for phase 2 liver detoxification pathways and can be used to help treat disorders of the liver and gallbladder.

Try to consume as much turmeric as you can, in a variety of different forms. I recommend getting turmeric into your diet every day. Whenever possible, add some black pepper to accompany the turmeric, because this greatly increases the bioavailability and absorption of the turmeric—by 2,000 percent, or 20 times in one study.[32]

I suggest cooking with turmeric powder but also taking it as a supplement, especially during this phase of clearing infections. When turmeric is processed into an extract, the absorption and bioavailability are increased and body tissues will be penetrated better for therapeutic effects—to get it into your whole body, the supplement form is necessary.

One of the most cost-effective brands of turmeric is Root2 Turmeric Extract Curcumin C3 Complex®, available online. If using this product or other "straight" curcumin supplements, you want to work up to 1,000 mg of curcumin daily. Taking it after meals can minimize GI side effects.

Turmeric has also been formulated using other technologies to boost absorption. While typically at a higher price point, these forms do achieve some of the best absorption available for supplemental curcumin. One form is Theracurmin, which uses colloidal nanoparticles to achieve 27x the absorption of traditional curcumin.[33] Longvida is a form that uses fat-containing particles known as liposomes to achieve up to 65x the absorption of curcumin and also cross the blood-brain barrier, to enhance the neuroprotective effects of curcumin.[34] CurcuWin (molecular dispersion technology) and NovaSol (unique micelle structure) are also highly bioavailable forms that both achieve up to 100X the absorption of regular curcumin.[35]

All four of these are patented forms of curcumin that are sold under different brand names by multiple companies—none of which I have any commercial relationship with. Examples of brands that incorporate these forms include Natural Factors and Integrative Therapeutics (Theracurmin), NOW Foods and ProHealth (Longvida), GreenIVe and Natrol (CurcuWin), and Delta Nutrition and Solgar (NovaSol).

You can choose any one of these options. Because dosing recommendations vary based on the formulation, I recommend following the dosage prescribed on the bottle. I suggest taking it for a minimum of two weeks during this phase of the protocol, but then continuing on with it after that for the anti-inflammatory benefits.

Turmeric has a good safety profile. Turmeric is about 2 percent curcumin by weight. Doses of up to 8,000 mg of curcumin (equivalent to 160 tablespoons of turmeric powder) per day have been shown to be safe for daily consumption for at least two months based on clinical trial data.[36] Thus, the powdered spice is extremely safe.

There are some cautions for the use of turmeric supplements. Because of turmeric's blood-thinning properties, patients who are on blood-thinning medications such as warfarin (Coumadin) or high-dose nonsteroidal anti-inflammatory drugs (NSAIDs) should avoid turmeric supplements; for the same reason, it is recommended to discontinue turmeric supplements at least two weeks before any type of surgery. Patients with active liver disease or gallstones should use caution with curcumin because of its potential to stimulate gallbladder contraction.[37] Pregnant and breastfeeding women should not take turmeric supplements because of lack of safety data but can safely use the spice in cooking.

Now that we know how to clear our infections, let's check back in with Sabrina.

When I saw Sabrina in my office, she reported a long history of recurrent vaginal yeast infections and UTIs for which she had taken antibiotics. On physical exam, I noticed that she had a thick white coating on her tongue, which can be a clue to excess yeast in the body. I suspected Candida overgrowth, and both a urine organic acids test and stool microbiome test confirmed high levels.

She also had significant leaky gut and dysbiosis with too many Klebsiella bacteria. I started her on a gut-healing protocol with a focus on clearing out Candida and bad bacteria. I had her fully eliminate added sugar from her diet (which she found surprisingly challenging) and follow the TIGER Protocol Phase I Diet.

Her symptoms improved significantly but did not fully resolve. Since she was understandably reluctant to resume conventional medicines, I prescribed her compounded low dose naltrexone (which I discuss in chapter 12). She achieved remission of her lupus and was able to stay symptom-free on a combination of healthy diet, vitamins, supplements, and the naltrexone.

CHAPTER 9

Gut—Healing Your Gut (and Oral) Microbiome

Karina was a 65-year-old Russian woman who was brought to me by her daughter for evaluation of a rare autoimmune condition known as polymyositis. Her immune system was attacking her muscles, causing pain and inflammation. She was starting to experience weakness and reduced strength in some of her muscles as well.

Although Karina did not speak English, her daughter Sofia was very engaged and motivated. She had taken her mother to the Mayo Clinic and other doctors around the country to try to determine the cause of this uncommon condition, without success.

When she came to see me, Karina's blood level of creatine kinase (CK), a measure of muscle inflammation, was over 2,000 (normal is <200). She had been on the oral steroid prednisone for a long time, without reduction in her CK level. Sofia was interested in uncovering the root causes of her mother's rare disease. She asked me where we should start, and, as is my wont, I suggested we begin with the gut.

We now move on to the "G" part of the TIGER Protocol—improving gut health and reversing leaky gut syndrome—an essential step to successfully treating autoimmune conditions. I suggest following this part of the protocol for four weeks. You have completed two weeks of detoxification in the first step followed by two weeks of clearing infections in the second step. Because gut healing is so important, I strongly recommend you commit to this third step for a month.

As in other chapters, we'll review an evidence-based gut-healing method that patients with autoimmune disease can use to heal their gut. This will improve your microbiome, heal the leaky gut, and help restore normal regulation of the immune system by the gut microbiome.

As part of this protocol, we will discuss foods, spices, and nutritional supplements that can be beneficial. I will also cover the lesser-known oral microbiome and its connection with autoimmune disorders, as well as strategies to improve and optimize it.

DETERMINING INTESTINAL PERMEABILITY

Elevated intestinal permeability may not have any symptoms. I often see patients with no GI symptoms whatsoever, but significantly impaired gut barrier integrity. So how do we test for it? The most commonly used tests are zonulin, the lactulose/mannitol ratio, and serum lipopolysaccharide.

Zonulin

A good biomarker to assess intestinal permeability is zonulin, which can be measured either in stool or blood. It is a protein that causes disassembling of the tight junctions, which are the structures that hold together the intestinal cells and maintain gut wall integrity.[1] Therefore, if these levels are elevated, it reflects higher breakdown of the tight junctions, which is tied to impaired barrier function.

Lactulose/Mannitol Ratio

Another common way to assess gut permeability utilizes differential absorption of the sugars lactulose and mannitol, in a test that has been used since the 1970s.[2] Lactulose is a large molecule that is minimally absorbed in a healthy gut. When permeability is abnormally high, lactulose is absorbed and then excreted in the urine. Mannitol is a sugar alcohol that is absorbed readily by healthy intestinal cells and also excreted via urine.

Both sugars are excreted unchanged in urine in proportion to the qualities absorbed. Therefore, an elevated lactulose/mannitol ratio in the urine, after oral intake, indicates increased gut permeability.

Lipopolysaccharide

As discussed in chapter 3, lipopolysaccharide or LPS is a compound produced from gram-negative bacteria that is typically found within the intestine and not absorbed. In cases of impaired barrier function, LPS can pass through and enter the bloodstream. Elevated serum levels of LPS and a related molecule, LPS binding protein, are biomarkers for intestinal permeability.[3]

All these markers are commonly used in research studies on gut permeability, which I will be reviewing in this chapter.

Dysbiosis

We know that dysbiosis is one of the main causes of increased intestinal permeability in patients with autoimmune disease.[4] With the protocol you completed in chapter 8, you have taken steps to treat and reverse dysbiosis, and improve the balance of your microbiome. Now, we can go on to use diet and supplements to help strengthen gut permeability, because one of the principal causes of its breakdown has been addressed.

ADVANCED TIP: SECRETORY IgA

Another way that I diagnose leaky gut—albeit indirectly—is by abnormal levels of secretory immunoglobulin A (IgA), a marker that is often found in functional medicine stool tests of the microbiome. Humans secrete an estimated 3 g of secretory IgA into the gut lumen each day to modulate both beneficial and pathogenic bacteria, and increased production can signify an upregulated immune response in the gut.[5] This protein is the first line of defense in protecting the gut epithelium against microbes, and levels may increase in response to pathogens of any type (that are neutralized by direct binding of IgA),[6] or as a result of increased intestinal permeability or in some cases allergic responses to food or environmental antigens.[7]

DIETARY FACTORS

First, we will focus on all the foods that can be helpful in normalizing gut barrier function. The Phase 1 Diet has already started the process of gut healing. Now, you can gradually expand on the Phase 1 Diet and begin to reintroduce foods as we discussed at the end of chapter 5.

Below, we'll review the research behind the foods that I'm talking about using to help heal your gut completely.

Fiber Intake

Increasing dietary fiber with plant foods improves intestinal permeability. A study looking at patients with fatty liver, who often have increased intestinal permeability, found that increasing the intake of plant fibers led to reduction in serum levels of zonulin.[8] During this intervention, fiber consumption from plant foods increased from 19 g/day to about 29 g/day.

Incorporating the nine servings of vegetables and two servings of fruits per day that I recommend on the Phase 1 Diet will easily achieve this goal, to support the goal of healing leaky gut. By the way, this is also the optimal intake of fruits and vegetables to achieve maximum risk reduction for cardiovascular disease and early death, according to a review of 95 studies examining the relationship between fruit and vegetable intake and health outcomes.[9]

The Inulin Effect

In terms of specific plant fibers, prebiotic fibers such as inulin appear to be especially beneficial. A randomized, double-blind trial found that food enriched with inulin was able to significantly reduce intestinal permeability in healthy adults over a five-week period.[10]

That is why in both the Phase 1 and Phase 2 Diets I include numerous foods containing prebiotics such as inulin. In the next chapter, I'll teach you about ten different foods that are good sources of inulin. I will also include many foods that contain a variety of other prebiotics, because of their beneficial effects on the microbiome and the gut lining.

Bone Broth and Collagen

Bone broth is rich in gelatin, collagen, and amino acids, which can help in healing the gut. In an animal model of ulcerative colitis, beef bone broth reduced intestinal tissue damage and inflammatory cytokines and biomarkers such as interleukin-6 and TNF-alpha.[11] An animal study evaluating the anti-inflammatory effect of chicken bone broth found that it helped relieve jaw inflammation.[12]

The collagen is likely a key element. It helps enhance tight junctions and improve barrier function in intestinal lining cells.[13] If you prefer not to take bone broth, a good alternative is taking grass-fed collagen powder, which is likely to provide more consistent dosages of collagen than bone broth.[14] An animal study showed that collagen supplements heal tissue damage and help regenerate gut mucosa in ulcerative colitis.[15]

Additionally, collagen may aid in reducing joint pain in adults, making it an attractive option with anti-inflammatory benefits beyond gut healing.[16]

Omega-3 Fats

Essential omega-3 fatty acids, found in fish, flax, and other foods, have also proven beneficial in healing the gut. Studies show taking fish oil helps to address dysbiosis, increases the production of short-chain fatty acids, and supports gut barrier function.[17] This is why I recommend frequent consumption of fish and shellfish as part of a good nutrition plan. If you are not open to eating fish, you can take a fish oil supplement with 1,000 mg of combined EPA and DHA per day.

Vegetarians can take an omega-3 supplement that is sourced from algae, which works equally well. This is preferable to consuming flax oil, which has short-chain omega-3s that need to be converted to the most beneficial long-chain omega-3s—and most people are not very efficient at this conversion. Studies have shown that, on average, only 10 percent of short-chain omega-3s may get converted to long-chain forms, with significant variability based on genetic factors.[18]

The Benefits of Zinc

Zinc is helpful in normalizing increased intestinal permeability. A randomized, double-blind study found that 3 mg of additional zinc can help improve intestinal barrier integrity over just five days (this study was done in children so I would double the dose to 6 mg for adults).[19] This amount of zinc is found in one cup of cooked beans, or 1 oz of pumpkin seeds. For this reason, a zinc supplement isn't necessary, but incorporating these zinc-containing foods is very beneficial for healing leaky gut.

Fermented Foods

Fermented foods deserve special mention. Not only are they full of beneficial bacteria and organic acids, which heal the gut and support the microbiome, but they have an anti-inflammatory effect on the body as well.

One study in children found that a fermented porridge was more effective than conventional porridge in resolving increased intestinal permeability as measured by lactulose/mannitol ratio.[20] Fermented foods that have been shown to be beneficial for GI health in randomized controlled trials include sauerkraut, natto (a fermented soybean dish), and kefir.[21] Increased intake of fermented foods was also linked to reduced social anxiety, illustrating the power of the gut-brain axis.[22]

Boosting Microbiome Diversity

In a fascinating study, six weeks of fermented foods significantly reduced inflammation and markers of immune system dysregulation while raising microbiome diversity.[23]

What was interesting was that the bacteria from the foods themselves was a very small subset of the new bacteria that emerged in stool samples—there were many new bacteria showing up that were not present in the fermented foods. Somehow the bacteria in fermented foods was creating an environment that was favorable to the microbiome, allowing new species to flourish.

The beneficial organic acids found in many fermented foods, such as lactic acid and acetic acid, help to acidify the colon. As we discussed earlier, an acidic intestinal environment helps our good bacteria to thrive and limits the growth of harmful microbes—in some cases, this environment can even help the body to get rid of bad bacteria.[24] Through this mechanism, fermented foods improve the balance of bacteria in your microbiome.

Fermenting food has been one of the strategies used by many cultures from around the world for preservation. It is likely that we have co-evolved with the bacteria found in fermented foods. In our modern era, our food—for lack of a better term—is too sanitized, and we desperately need to introduce new bacteria into our systems. Adding in fermented foods is one safe and effective way to accomplish this.

This study also evaluated multiple markers of the immune system, allowing an in-depth analysis of how the immune system was doing. When you visit your regular general practitioner and ask for a measure of inflammation or a test of the immune system, there are not many options. Some of the most common standard tests are C-reactive protein (CRP) and erythrocyte sedimentation rate (ESR). While these are useful markers if elevated, in many cases they appear normal despite the fact that it is clear that dysregulation and dysfunction of the immune system is present.

In contrast, this study used >20 measurements of the immune system (such as cytokines and chemokines) to allow researchers to evaluate the effects of the dietary changes on the person's immune system in detail. Nineteen of these inflammatory immune markers decreased as a result of the fermented foods intervention, showing the marked benefit of fermented foods for immune function and inflammation.

It's true that for certain people, fermented foods are not a viable option. For example, people with histamine intolerance or sensitivity to certain foods may not be able to tolerate fermented foods. In such cases, addressing the underlying imbalances that prevent the intake of fermented foods first is a necessity. Working with a practitioner to resolve the dysbiosis or other factors that contribute to these issues would be a good next step, if the protocol in chapter 8 was not sufficient.

Sugar

While we'll focus mostly on what you can eat to improve your health, it's important to review some foods to avoid as you work through the protocol. Refined sugars are at the top of that list. Fructose can impair barrier function and worsen permeability, increasing LPS in the blood by as much as 40 percent.[25] For this reason, it is essential to avoid sugar, high fructose corn syrup, and other processed sweeteners. Doing so also makes sense from an evolutionary perspective, because our bodies just did not evolve to process these foods—they are a new and hazardous addition to our food supply.

Fat

In general, I do not recommend a diet high in fats or saturated fats for patients with autoimmune disease. Most of the research in this regard comes from animal studies, but some human research confirms that a high-fat diet can have a negative impact on intestinal permeability. One in particular found that people consuming a high-fat meal had higher serum levels of LPS (correlating with intestinal permeability) and elevated inflammation afterward as measured by interleukin-6 levels.[26]

INTERMITTENT FASTING AND CROSS-FEEDING

Intermittent fasting has many benefits, but less well-known is its positive effect on the microbiome. One study showed that fasting increased gut microbiota diversity and the levels of the keystone species Akkermansia and Faecalibacterium prausnitzii.[27] A trial of Chinese males practicing 16-hour intermittent fasting over 25 days found enhanced gut microbial richness with enrichment of prevotella and Bacteroides species; the men also had metabolic benefits such as significantly lower total cholesterol, triglycerides, and liver enzymes, and higher beneficial HDL cholesterol after the fasting.[28]

In a study of around 17 hours of intermittent fasting daily for a month, levels of Akkermansia and Bacteroides were increased.[29] In a study of patients with metabolic syndrome, fasting led to beneficial changes in the microbiome (and reduction in blood pressure).[30]

The way bacterial networks interact in the microbiome to produce beneficial metabolites is called cross-feeding.[31] Our gut bacteria have "primary fermenters" which are the first responders that spring into action when food first enters our digestive tract. These bacteria begin processing and breaking down fiber and other components from our diet. As they do this, they release certain metabolites. Then, other bacteria known as "secondary fermenters" take up and thrive on these primary metabolites.

For example, Bifidobacteria are primary fermenters and produce the short-chain fatty acids acetate and lactate; these metabolites are utilized by the beneficial secondary fermenters Eubacterium and Anaerostipes to produce butyrate.[32] Faecalibacterium can function as a secondary fermenter and metabolize acetate as well. Faecalibacterium is also a primary fermenter that can produce butyrate from the prebiotic fiber inulin. This goes to show the complex web of interconnections in the microbiome.

Cross-feeding may be one of the ways that intermittent fasting helps raise the levels of the diversity in the microbiome.

SUPPLEMENTS

Although I believe in primarily using food to heal the gut, certain supplements can be beneficial. Let's look at how certain supplements can be beneficial toward healing increased intestinal permeability.

Curcumin

I reviewed the many benefits of curcumin in the previous chapter. It does have an additional benefit for intestinal permeability, which is another reason why I consider it a core supplement for patients with autoimmune disease. A study showed that supplementation with 500 mg of curcumin per day over just three days normalized intestinal permeability that was disrupted by exercise under extreme heat, which is known to cause leaky gut.[33]

If you opt to use "straight" curcumin, I recommend a dosage of 500 mg twice a day with food. If you use one of the forms of curcumin that I reviewed in-depth in chapter 8, specially modified to increase absorption, follow the dosage recommendations on the bottle.

Glutamine

Glutamine is an amino acid that can be helpful in healing leaky gut. In a randomized, placebo-controlled trial of adults with impaired barrier function (as part of postinfectious irritable bowel syndrome), 5 g of glutamine taken three times a day was effective at normalizing intestinal permeability as measured by lactulose/mannitol ratios; in this study, it also improved bowel movements, stool consistency, and IBS symptoms.[34]

In patients with elevated intestinal permeability from Crohn's disease, oral glutamine over two months led to improvement in barrier function as measured by lactulose/mannitol ratios.[35] Glutamine reduced intestinal permeability in ICU patients over ten days, as measured by serum lipopolysaccharide (LPS) and zonulin levels.[36] In a placebo-controlled trial with burn patients, oral glutamine lessened intestinal permeability over 14 days.[37]

I typically recommend a dosage of 2–3 g twice a day of glutamine, on an empty stomach at least one hour before meals. If you are working with a practitioner, they may suggest higher doses.

Colostrum

Research indicates that colostrum can be beneficial for improving intestinal permeability. Bovine colostrum is derived from the milk produced by cows for a few days after they give birth; it is rich in antibodies, growth factors, and proteins, and has been used for hundreds of years in complementary medicine.[38]

A randomized, double-blind, placebo-controlled trial found that 500 mg of freeze-dried bovine colostrum twice a day was able to normalize elevated intestinal permeability in adults in just three weeks.[39] In this study, they assessed athletes during peak training (known to increase gut permeability), and colostrum led to improvement in both stool zonulin levels and lactulose/mannitol ratios.

PROBIOTICS

Probiotics have a wide variety of benefits, but function more as immunomodulators and a support to your own beneficial bacteria rather than long-term quantitative boosters of your own microbiome. In the past, the thinking was that if you were low on bacteria, you could take probiotics to "fill up the tank" and raise levels.

In reality, probiotics typically stay in your gut only during the period of supplementation but then are gradually excreted and typically no longer detectable after about two weeks.[40] Therefore, supplemented probiotics rarely colonize and become permanent residents of the microbiome, but this does not detract in any way from their potential benefits.

So, there are plenty of beneficial foods and supplements in the TIGER Protocol that are sufficient for healing intestinal permeability in most people. I tend to add in probiotics for autoimmune patients who have significant gut symptoms. If you suffer from persistent digestive issues such as abdominal pain, constipation, or diarrhea, then you might consider incorporating one of the probiotics mentioned below.

Check the Strain

Probiotics are typically named by genus and species, followed by the strain designation which is a series of letters and/or numbers, e.g., Bifidobacterium Lactis HN019. In this example, the genus is Bifidobacterium, species is Lactis, and the strain is HN019.[41] Sometimes, a further distinction called subspecies is also designated—this same probiotic is sometimes called Bifidobacterium animalis subspecies lactis HN019. Most strains have multiple names, which adds to the confusion.

It is critical to understand that two probiotics from the same exact species but from different strains can have completely different properties.[42] I think of probiotic strains as specializing in certain functions. We want to use them for targeted benefits, such as increasing transit time or healing intestinal permeability.

In the way that all dogs are from the same species but each breed can specialize in a certain thing—a border collie would be far better at herding sheep than a pug—each probiotic strain has a certain "skill set" and excels at some tasks but not others. We always want to make sure we are selecting the right strain from the right species to accomplish the goals we desire.

This is crucial when selecting probiotics in the marketplace. Unfortunately, I find that some brands still do not specify the strain on their product label. Companies that are aware of their product's strain, and the research behind its benefits, will likely include that information in their messaging.

Lactobacillus GG

Lactobacillus rhamnosus GG (LGG) is a probiotic that has substantial research behind it, with over 600 published papers. It was the first Lactobacillus strain to be patented in 1989 due to its survivability in culture. Multiple animal[43] and human studies[44] have shown its ability to normalize elevated intestinal permeability.

LGG has been shown to be beneficial in alleviating diarrhea, irritable bowel syndrome, and other conditions by producing a biofilm that protects the gut mucosa, inhibits pathogens, and creates an anti-inflammatory immune environment; recommended dosage for adults is 10–20 billion CFUs (colony forming units)/day.[45]

Other Lactobacilli

Other lactobacilli have also been shown to be beneficial. A study found that supplemental lactobacilli can reduce elevated intestinal permeability (and GI symptoms) in children with eczema, an autoimmune skin condition associated with impaired barrier function.[46] The strains that were used were Lactobacillus rhamnosus 19070-2 and Lactobacillus reuteri DSM 12246; these are part of Flora-Active, a group of probiotics supplied globally by the Danish company BioCare Copenhagen.[47]

Bifidobacterium Lactis HN019

This probiotic (also called Bifidobacterium animalis subspecies lactis HN019) has been shown to speed up transit time (how efficiently food moves through your GI tract) and relieve constipation as well as improve host immune function and reduce infections; it also supports gut barrier integrity and increases the production of beneficial short-chain fatty acids.[48] It is typically included in combination products along with other strains. Examples of products that include this strain are NOW Clinical GI Probiotic and Optibac Every Day MAX.

Bifidobacterium Longum

Among Bifidobacteria, another well-researched strain is Bifidobacterium longum subspecies infantis 35624 (also known as Bifidobacterium infantis 35624). Randomized, double-blind, placebo-controlled trials show that it reduces serum biomarkers of inflammation such as C-reactive protein, tumor necrosis factor-alpha, and interleukin-6; this was shown in ulcerative colitis and psoriasis (autoimmune disorders), and chronic fatigue syndrome (which may have an autoimmune component).[49]

In patients with irritable bowel syndrome (IBS), this strain was effective when compared to placebo in improving pain, bloating, and digestive function regardless of IBS subtype—constipation or diarrhea predominant or mixed; recommended daily dosage is at least 100 million CFUs/day.[50] Examples of available brands are Align or Bare and Better.

Beneficial Yeast

Although I could devote an entire chapter (or book!) to probiotics, in the interest of time I must move on, but not before mentioning one of my favorite probiotics. Saccharomyces cerevisiae boulardii (also known as Saccharomyces boulardii CNCM I-745 or HANSEN CBS 5926), a strain manufactured by Biocodex Laboratory in France, is actually a beneficial yeast that has potent gut-healing properties. It was discovered by and named after French scientist Henri Boulard in 1920; he isolated the yeast from certain tropical fruits that appeared to protect people from diarrhea during a cholera outbreak.[51]

Over 80 randomized, controlled trials have proven the efficacy of this strain.[52] In patients with Crohn's disease and elevated intestinal permeability, taking Saccharomyces boulardii over three months led to a decrease in permeability as measured by lactulose/mannitol ratios.[53]

This probiotic improves outcomes in IBS, traveler's diarrhea, H. pylori infection, and antibiotic-associated diarrhea (since it is a yeast and not affected by antibiotics); its mechanisms of action include strong anti-inflammatory effects, improved digestion, enhanced gut repair, broad antimicrobial activity, and increased butyrate production.[54]

Multiple brands of probiotics feature this health-promoting yeast, a well-known example being Florastor. Recommended daily dosage is 5 billion CFUs.

How and When to Take Probiotics

You might hear conflicting information about whether to take probiotics with food. However, the science is clear. The pH of your stomach is low when empty (average of 1.7 in one study); this low pH is more likely to kill oral probiotics when taken on an empty stomach.[55]

After a meal (especially one that contains some fat), pH rises up to around 4–5, thus ensuring a higher probability for oral probiotics to pass through the stomach safely.[56] Studies show that probiotics survive best when they are given either with a fat-containing meal or shortly before the meal; taking them 30 minutes after eating reduces survival, because that is when the stomach pH drops again (with secretion of acid) during the digestive process.[57]

I recommend incorporating healthy fats with each meal, as you'll learn in chapter 10. This amount of fat should be sufficient to ensure the survival of oral probiotics after meals.

ADVANCED TIP: WHEN PROBIOTICS DON'T WORK

Often, I see patients that come to me after having tried probiotics. They took them for a long time, perhaps months or years, and did not feel any benefit, and thus concluded that they "didn't work." There could be many reasons for this. Each probiotic has a different set of skills and abilities, so individual patients may have chosen a strain that was not the right match for their needs. Or maybe they selected certain bacteria that they already had plenty of. For example, perhaps they already had plenty of Bifidobacteria in their microbiome and therefore would not have benefited from a probiotic containing Bifidobacteria.

But perhaps the most common reason I see in practice is that they have underlying infections that were not addressed. Probiotics have some antimicrobial activity but are rarely sufficient to resolve infections commonly found in autoimmune patients. Once all the pathogenic bacteria, yeast, and parasites have been cleared out, it is much more likely that probiotics could exert their beneficial effects. That's why infections are addressed before targeting gut health in the TIGER Protocol.

THE ORAL MICROBIOME

As we work to heal the gut microbiome and reduce intestinal permeability, we also have to attend to the oral microbiome. This pivotal factor is often overlooked in autoimmune conditions (and other chronic diseases), even though it has powerful effects on dental health and diseases, the gut microbiome, and systemic inflammation.

Through multiple mechanisms, oral bacteria can play a role in disparate conditions such as cardiovascular disease, diabetes, colon cancer, lung infections, brain abscesses, and autoimmunity.[58] For this reason, the oral microbiome has a substantial impact on the immune system and can sometimes be the missing link in terms of helping a patient with autoimmunity to achieve remission.

The oral microbiome contains the second largest collection of bacteria in the body after the gut, harboring around 6 billion bacteria and over 700 different species.[59] Although this microbiome is relatively well-studied, newer more advanced techniques have found that these numbers are likely underestimating the quantity and diversity of bacteria.

We swallow a whopping 1–2 L of saliva per day. Assuming on the low end that we swallow only 1 L per day leads to an interesting calculation. Considering that saliva contains between 800 million to more than 1 billion bacteria/mL,[60] that works out to an incredible 800 billion to >1 trillion oral bacteria swallowed per day—more powerful than almost any probiotic available on the market. And there are no breaks or "days off" from this influx of bacteria—it is a constant and daily occurrence. From this, we can understand how the oral microbiome could have such a significant impact on the gut microbiome and overall systemic inflammation.

A Key Player in Autoimmunity

Porphyromonas gingivalis (P. gingivalis) is an oral bacterium that is involved in the pathogenesis of periodontitis, an inflammatory disease that destroys the gums and can lead to tooth loss. It also plays a key role in rheumatoid arthritis, as these bacteria are potent inducers of immune-mediated proinflammatory responses leading to bone damage and systemic inflammation.[61] P. gingivalis is also implicated in rheumatoid arthritis through molecules known as "citrullinated proteins."

Accumulating evidence suggests a role for autoimmunity against these citrullinated proteins in the development of rheumatoid arthritis. By driving the production of these proteins, this bacteria may contribute to the development of RA. In fact, anti-cyclic citrullinated protein antibodies (anti-CCP antibodies) are the most common rheumatoid arthritis biomarker, found in the blood of most patients with RA. A more recently discovered bacteria, Aggregatibacter actinomycetemcomitans, is also an inducer of citrullinated proteins and is being studied for its role in RA.[62]

Leaky Mouth Syndrome

The epithelial cells lining the mouth maintain a strong barrier, limiting the entry of microbes and toxins, because the mouth is the gateway to the world and the first line of defense against pathogens. Just as dysbiosis in the GI tract contributes to impaired barrier function, oral dysbiosis can lead to increased permeability and the condition of "leaky mouth," in which inflammation in the oral mucosa caused by dysbiosis and other factors damages the normal barrier, allowing for the entry of bacteria, toxins, and other microbes into the bloodstream.

Because the mouth and gums are highly vascular, anything that slips through can easily travel to other parts of the body and cause complications—as with P. gingivalis. A striking example of this permeability was seen in a nine-year-old with celiac disease (an autoimmune disease exacerbated by gluten exposure) who struggled with abdominal pain despite a strict gluten-free diet. She was symptomatic and had positive serum markers for active disease, which indicated she was somehow getting exposed to gluten. The cause for this turned out to be her orthodontic retainer—gluten is a common additive in plastics, and she was absorbing trace amounts orally. Discontinuing use led to resolution of her symptoms and her celiac markers returned to normal.[63]

Oral Dysbiosis in Autoimmunity

Dysbiosis in the oral microbiome has been discovered in patients with a number of autoimmune diseases. For example, patients with autoimmune liver diseases such as autoimmune hepatitis and primary biliary cirrhosis exhibit signs of dysbiosis in their oral microbiota with increases in the levels of certain pathogens (overgrowth of harmful bacteria in their mouth).[64] Other autoimmune conditions in which changes in the oral microbiome have been identified include Sjogren's syndrome, systemic sclerosis, systemic lupus erythematosus (SLE), and Crohn's disease.[65]

As we've learned, rheumatoid arthritis is also cor
biome; studies from Europe, Asia, and Canada ha
rheumatoid arthritis have a distinct oral (and gastrc
pared to healthy controls.[66]

Strengthen Your Oral Microbiome

To support the health of the oral microbiome, teeth, and g
nutrition is essential. A balanced diet rich in micronutrients, minerals, and
essential fatty acids, like the food plan offered in chapter 10, is the foundation.
Adequate intake of calcium, vitamin D, and vitamin K_2 support healthy teeth.

Avoid processed sweeteners such as sugar or high fructose corn syrup because
simple sugars feed the growth of bad bacteria in both the oral and gastrointestinal microbiome. Processed fructose (anything not found naturally in fruits)
increases LPS and intestinal permeability, as we discussed earlier in this chapter.

Good dental hygiene, including daily brushing and flossing, is important.
Avoid commercial mouthwashes, because the repeated exposure to antibacterial
compounds can have detrimental effects on the oral microbiome. Instead, I recommend the Ayurvedic practice of oil pulling, as described below.

Prevent Dry Mouth

Maintaining adequate levels of saliva is crucial because saliva contains enzymes,
antibodies, and proteins that help maintain a healthy oral microbiome. Scientists have discovered many vital salivary components that both directly and indirectly prevent dysbiosis in the mouth.[67] This is why people with dry mouth from
insufficient saliva are at higher risk of tooth decay, bad breath, and dysbiosis. In
such cases, chewing gum with xylitol, sucking on ice cubes, and increasing water
intake can help increase salivary production. A humidifier, especially in your
bedroom while you sleep, may help as well.

Breathe Right

Chronic mouth breathing is a major cause of dry mouth. We were designed to
breathe through our nose, which will filter and humidify the air we take in.
Mouth breathing increases the odds of snoring and dries out the mouth, which
can contribute to dysbiosis—especially if it occurs for prolonged periods such as
during sleep. If you regularly wake up with bad breath or dry mouth, it's likely
you are breathing through your mouth overnight.

he case, you might try mouth taping, which is a simple solution that big benefits. Immediately before bed, apply petroleum jelly to your lips ace a piece of hypoallergenic tape horizontally across both your lips. There brands of tape made specifically for this purpose; however, you can also use paper tape, the kind you might find in a first-aid kit. Many of my patients swear that this technique dramatically improves their sleep quality. There aren't many available studies on mouth taping, but it is inexpensive and easy to try, and relatively safe. I recommend it only because it can reduce dry mouth as well as gum disease, throat infections, bad breath, and oral dysbiosis.

Green Tea—A True Superfood

When it comes to supporting the oral microbiome, one beverage requires special mention: green tea. Most widely known for its antioxidants and cardiovascular benefits, green tea contains polyphenols (dietary antioxidants) that serve as beneficial prebiotics for both the oral and intestinal microbiota. Studies show that drinking green tea regularly improves heart disease risk profiles and reduces the risk of dying from cardiovascular disease by up to 31 percent.[68] It also has benefits in preventing diabetes, metabolic syndrome, and colon cancer.[69]

But green tea also has numerous benefits for the oral and gut microbiome. Studies show that two cups of green tea daily improve the diversity of the salivary microbiome in healthy adults and increase Ruminococci and Bifidobacteria in the gut as well as Roseburia, Faecalibacterium, and Eubacterium—which produce short-chain fatty acids (SCFAs).[70]

The medicinal properties of green tea likely stem from antioxidants known as catechins; to boost your daily intake of these powerful compounds, add a quarter teaspoon of matcha green tea powder—which is very high in catechins[71]—to your daily cup of green tea.

Lab studies have confirmed that green tea inhibits the growth of oral bacteria.[72] Likely as a result of this, studies also show that it reduces bad breath.[73] Swishing green tea around your mouth before swallowing is a good way to add oral pluses to the many systemic benefits of this healthy beverage.

Oil Pulling and Tongue Scraping

There are a variety of other practices that can be beneficial to your oral microbiome. Oil pulling, in which you swish oil around in your mouth for about 5–10 minutes and then discard it, is an Ayurvedic practice that supports the oral microbiome. Ayurveda believes that oil pulling can prevent tooth decay, gum disease, and bad breath. Studies have confirmed that regular oil pulling with coconut oil is able to significantly reduce levels of bacteria in the saliva, and also reduce plaque levels, thus improving dental health and cutting down on the harmful bacteria that can lead to autoimmunity.[74]

Tongue scraping, another traditional technique, is also beneficial. This can be done with either a toothbrush or a tongue scraper and helps to clear excess bacteria from the tongue, also removing the buildup of tongue coating, if present. Tongue scraping has been shown to improve periodontal markers and reduce markers of inflammation in the gum tissues.[75]

In Ayurveda, the tongue is a microcosm for the entire GI tract, so in that tradition, tongue scraping is believed to provide a gentle stimulation and "internal massage" to all the digestive organs.

Testing for and Treating Dysbiosis

Caring for the oral microbiome and preventing dental dysbiosis is important for helping to keep the immune system balanced. If you suspect you might have oral dysbiosis, look for the following clues: bad breath, gingivitis, tooth decay, or other periodontal diseases.

If you are asymptomatic but suffer from autoimmunity, it's still a good idea to test your oral bacteria. Newer salivary tests for pathogenic bacteria such as P. gingivalis are available from companies like OralDNA and others—but talk to your dentist about whether such a test is right for you. If you do have high levels of potentially deleterious oral bacteria, consider using antimicrobial toothpastes such as Dentalcidin or PerioBiotic to help address the dysbiosis.

Dental Fillings

If you require dental fillings, avoid silver fillings which contain mercury. Instead opt for composite materials, which are safer. If you already have silver fillings, work with a functional medicine doctor to determine whether they should be replaced.

If you require an implant, it is possible to perform allergy testing before the procedure to determine the optimal metal. Typically, titanium alloy is used for dental implants, and it contains small amounts of nickel, which is often the culprit when patients are allergic to titanium implants. If you are tested and found to have an allergy to nickel or titanium, for example, zirconium can be used instead.

Root Canals

In terms of dental care, root canals can also be problematic. While they are not an issue in every case, sometimes they can serve as hiding spots for infections that can contribute to low-grade inflammation in the body, potentially impacting autoimmune disease.

If you're unfamiliar, a root canal is a procedure in which the soft center of the tooth, the pulp, is removed and replaced with a dental filling. The main indication for this is if the center of the tooth is infected.

Some endodontists believe that it's not possible to remove all the infection from the affected tooth with the current technique. As a result, cellular debris and pockets of infection can persist within the treated tooth, silently irritating and triggering the immune system. It's recommended that any person with a root-canaled tooth get a special three-dimensional cone beam x-ray to assess for problems that may be missed by traditional x-rays.

If issues are identified on this x-ray, a variety of newer regenerative technologies can be used to address them by "biological" endodontists, who take a more holistic approach. These include low-level laser treatment for better debridement of the area, ozone therapy for disinfection, and minimally invasive procedures such as GentleWave. Consulting with a qualified endodontist with experience in some of these techniques would be a good place to start.

Now that we're armed with knowledge about improving our gut health, let's revisit Karina.

> It turned out that Karina had long-standing digestive issues that she had never complained about, including bloating, constipation, and episodic abdominal pain. Detailed microbiome testing revealed severe dysbiosis with low keystone bacteria and overgrowth of candida and the potential pathogens Citrobacter and Proteus. Intestinal permeability was markedly increased and inflammation was very high. She also had a number of food sensitivities.
>
> I had Karina go through the TIGER Protocol. We focused a lot on healing her gut and clearing out the potentially pathogenic bacteria and yeast. We rebuilt her microbiome with prebiotics and probiotics. I had her follow the Phase I Diet, eliminating the foods that she was sensitive to while incorporating bone broth and fermented foods.

At her follow-up appointment, Karina spoke animatedly about what she was noticing. Translating, her daughter explained that this was the first time in decades Karina's digestion was working normally. She no longer had pain or bloating and was having regular bowel movements.

Subsequently, her muscle pain and weakness started to improve. Follow-up testing after six months revealed that her creatine kinase (CK) level had returned to normal, for the first time in several years. Eventually she was able to discontinue the prednisone and maintain her remission with diet, lifestyle, and supplements.

CHAPTER 10

Eating—Prebiotic Foods and the Phase 2 Diet

A 33-year-old physician, Mark, came to see me after receiving a diagnosis of psoriatic arthritis. He had dealt with psoriasis, an autoimmune skin disorder, for over a decade. He controlled the rash with topical steroids, though it would never fully go away.

After a few years of hectic ER practice, he started experiencing joint pain and swelling. His rheumatologist diagnosed him with the arthritic component of psoriasis, which can be debilitating. He was started on immune-suppressing drugs that reduced but did not remove the severe pain. Having heard about my practice, he came to see me even though he knew nothing about integrative medicine.

We quickly discovered that Mark had a lot of room for improvement in his diet. On good days he would eat a sandwich or bagels during his busy ER shifts. On bad days it was ice cream sandwiches and soda.

I had difficulty trying to get Mark to improve his diet. Since he was skeptical, I thought getting some data might help convince him. I did food sensitivity testing on him and showed him elevated antibody levels indicating his sensitivity to gluten, dairy, and beef. Seeing the numbers convinced him to change, and we began to work on his diet.

Diet is fundamental to health and plays a critical role in the development of autoimmune diseases, which brings us to the "E" in the TIGER Protocol: eating right. We'll get into how you can create a detailed nutrition plan to further optimize digestion and keep the immune system functioning at its best. Based on my clinical experience, I will present a diverse and balanced plant-based diet that is sustainable.

WHY DIVERSITY MATTERS

In *The Paleovedic Diet*, I explained that our ancestors evolved eating up to 100 different plant foods every single week. Each plant food contains different types of fibers, polyphenols, and micronutrients that each feed different types of bacteria in your microbiome. This is essential to maintaining a rich and diverse microbiome. I recommend you try to eat at least 30 to 40 different types of plant foods every week—this includes fruits, vegetables, grains, legumes, nuts and seeds, and spices.

While this number might seem daunting, it is achievable. A red apple contains different polyphenols and has a distinct microbiota effect from a green apple—so those would count as two different foods. If you had white rice one day, brown rice another day, and wild rice the next, that would count as three distinct foods. White quinoa and red quinoa can be counted separately.

Spices also have powerful prebiotic properties. Each spice is distinct and feeds slightly different bacteria in the microbiota. Therefore, a meal containing turmeric, ginger, black pepper, fenugreek, and garlic would contain five additional plant foods in the form of spices. Increasing the diversity of spices used in your meals is one of the best ways to add new and different plant foods to your diet.

Once you track this carefully for a week or two, you will get a sense of what is necessary, and it will be naturally incorporated into your eating plan.

MY PHILOSOPHY ON FOOD

Before the specific recommendations, I want to share my general philosophy about diet. Ayurveda reminds us that we should "eat to live" and not "live to eat." While it is critical to plan meals carefully and try to eat as well as you can, it is important not to become fanatical about eating the perfect food all the time.

The 90:10 Rule

As you maintain your new habits, I recommend the 90:10 rule. Ninety percent of the time you stick to your prescribed diet and do the best that you can to eat healthy. Ten percent of the time, which translates to once—or a maximum of twice—per week, you can give yourself a treat and consume foods that are not part of your usual diet—perhaps going out to a restaurant for a meal, when you have less control over all the ingredients that go into your meal anyway.

During the Phase I Diet, I take a stricter approach while we are improving the overall function of the digestive tract. However, once things are stable, if you are not struggling with gastrointestinal issues or major food allergies, you should be able to broaden and expand your diet.

How to Eat

A second important aspect is how you eat. It is important to eat your food in a mindful, unhurried state. Try not to eat when you are rushed or stressed out. Always try to sit down while eating and do not stand up and eat. Minimize distractions such as TV, Internet, and the use of other screens. Chewing your food thoroughly and paying attention to your meal will make you less likely to overeat.

If possible, try to enjoy at least one meal each day sitting down together with family or friends, not only for the social connection but because studies suggest that this helps control portion size. Many people eat for psychological reasons such as loneliness, anxiety, and emotional stress; if you find you are reaching for food for one of these reasons and not due to genuine hunger, seek out an alternative outlet.

Eat Slowly

I want to reiterate the importance of this powerful but seemingly simplistic advice, which was tested in a novel study. Subjects were randomly instructed to eat the same meal either slowly or quickly. Those who were told to eat slowly ended up consuming significantly less food and fewer calories—but, in a true win-win, reported feeling fuller and more satiated![1]

I believe this is because eating more slowly allowed time for their brains to receive the signals from their stomachs that they were full and satisfied—we may miss or blow past these signals if we are gulping down food quickly. Although I know many of us have developed the habit of eating quickly, there is great benefit in consciously trying to eat more slowly. Based on the research, you will likely eat less but feel fuller, and your digestion will be better as well.

With all that in mind, let's get to the specific dietary recommendations.

FOODS TO AVOID IN THE PHASE 2 DIET

Refined gluten-based grains such as white flour or wheat flour. When wheat is refined, the whole grain is pulverized and the most nutritious components of the grain, such as the bran and the endosperm, are removed. What's left is the calorie-rich, nutrient-poor staple of the Western diet—flour. Studies have documented that consumption of excess refined grains is associated with higher risk of obesity, diabetes, elevated blood pressure, high cholesterol, and several cancers.[2] In contrast, consumption of whole grains is beneficial. In my view, even gluten-containing whole grains should be limited in autoimmune disease—more on this later.

Vegetable seed oils. These include all vegetable oils made by industrial processing, such as soybean oil, corn oil, canola oil, safflower oil, cottonseed oil, and a few others. The only healthy vegetable oils are olive oil and coconut oil.

Trans fats. Trans fats are made by hydrogenating vegetable oils to make them solid at room temperature. It is well known that trans fats promote inflammation and have a strong connection with heart disease.[3] Even large food manufacturers are removing trans fats from their products. Avoid any food that contains hydrogenated or partially hydrogenated oils.

Refined sugar. Added sugar, especially white sugar, is associated with negative outcomes in autoimmune disease—likely due to inflammatory properties, a tendency to feed harmful bacteria and yeast, metabolic disruption, and other negative effects. For example, in patients with lupus, dietary intake of added sugars was directly correlated with disease-related damage and complications.[4] In addition, sugar consumption worsens numerous metabolic markers,[5] promotes inflammation,[6] and has been associated with obesity, type 2 diabetes,[7] and heart disease.[8]

PREBIOTIC FOODS

The foundation of this diet is a rich and diverse balance of prebiotic foods. This will help cultivate an equally rich, multifaceted microbiome which is the key to a healthy immune system for all people. Following, you'll find a list of the top prebiotic foods to help optimize your gut microbiota. All of these foods should be eaten as frequently as possible, at least several times a week or even daily.

Polyphenols

Polyphenols are a class of antioxidants that are proven to improve the diversity of the microbiome and feed several keystone bacteria.[9] They generally achieve this without creating a lot of gas or bloating, and therefore are usually tolerated by even the most sensitive patients. People living with SIBO or who have intolerance to high-fiber foods are usually able to tolerate foods that contain polyphenols.

So we begin our discussion about what foods to start adding to the diet with the polyphenol-rich prebiotic foods. If you have found that your diet has become overly restrictive and you don't know where to start in terms of expanding your diet and reintroducing foods, this is a good place to begin.

Many polyphenols in foods are large molecules that are poorly absorbed but require metabolism by gut bacteria in order to exert their favorable health effects. For example, 90 to 95 percent of polyphenols from berries are not absorbed and travel to the large intestine, where they are fermented and modified by bacteria into smaller compounds that can then enter the general circulation and effect positive changes.[10]

Polyphenols from berries have been linked to systemic improvements in blood pressure, cardiovascular status, cancer risk, memory, attention, and other cognitive functions—but they require processing by our gut bacteria into smaller molecules that we can absorb in order to reap these benefits.[11] The old saying, "you are what you eat," can be expanded: you are what you eat, digest, and absorb (as long as you have the right gut bacteria).

Polyphenols are also relatively heat stable; although there is some amount of loss from heating, it is minimal and most of the prebiotic effects are preserved. Therefore, it is completely fine to use cooked versions of the following foods if necessary. After the descriptions of the foods are some tables that detail their polyphenol content.[12]

Clove powder. Clove is actually the richest food source of polyphenols in existence. Add a quarter teaspoon to a smoothie or other beverage, or to any meat or vegetable dish that you are cooking.

Berries. All berries are excellent sources of polyphenols, including blueberry, blackberry, cranberry, strawberry, and elderberry.

Other fruits. This includes cherry, plum, red or black grapes, and red apples (the skin contains the polyphenols).

Nuts and seeds. Especially good sources include ground flaxseed, chestnuts, hazelnut, pecan, and black sesame seed.

Vegetables. More intensely colored vegetables such as black or purple carrot, red loose-leaf lettuce, purple cauliflower, red cabbage, and purple potatoes are good sources. Other good sources are spinach, broccoli, onion, and orange carrot.

Tea. Green or black tea are great sources of polyphenols, antioxidants, and other phytochemicals. Green tea is especially beneficial because of its positive impact on the oral and gut microbiota, as we discussed in chapter 4 and further in the previous chapter. EGCG is one of the most abundant polyphenols in green tea, and regulates inflammation. As I mentioned in the previous chapter, adding a quarter teaspoon of matcha powder—which is very high in EGCG and other polyphenols—to your daily cup of green tea is a great way to boost your polyphenol intake.

Cacao powder. Studies show that cacao powder has unique prebiotic antioxidants called flavanols that increase levels of Lactobacillus and Bifidobacterium and decrease levels of potentially pathogenic bacteria such as clostridia; they also reduce inflammation as measured by serum C-reactive protein, and have the metabolic benefit of reducing triglycerides.[13] Cacao also contains magnesium and zinc and is a rich source of polyphenols. Dark chocolate is an option here since it is made from cacao powder. Aim for a minimum of 70 percent (ideally >85 percent) cocoa. As I mentioned in chapter 2, cacao can contain high levels of lead and cadmium. To find brands that have been independently tested to be low in toxins, visit my website at http://doctorakil.com/toxic-chocolate/.

Grains. More colorful grains such as red rice, black rice, and red or black quinoa (technically a legume but often consumed like a grain) have high levels of polyphenols.

Dried peppermint. Peppermint leaves are another exceptionally rich source of polyphenols.

Culinary herbs. Most culinary herbs contain some degree of polyphenols. Especially good sources are star anise, celery seed, sage, and rosemary.

In the following tables, you'll find detailed information from scientific literature about the polyphenol content of the most common foods. They are broken down by different categories such as vegetables, fruits, nuts and seeds, etc.

POLYPHENOL CONTENT IN FOODS

The following charts illustrate the polyphenol content of different categories of foods.

POLYPHENOL CONTENT IN HERBS, SPICES, AND SEASONINGS

Food	Polyphenol content, mg per 10 grams (3.5oz)
Clove	1519 mg
Dried peppermint	1196 mg
Star anise	546 mg
Cocoa powder*	345 mg

Celery seed	209 mg
Sage	120 mg
Rosemary	101 mg
Spearmint	95 mg
Thyme	87 mg
Basil	32 mg
Curry powder	28 mg
Dried ginger	20 mg
Vinegar	13 mg

*Cocoa powder does not fit neatly into any categories but I intend for it to be used as a seasoning so I have included it here.

You may wonder exactly how much is 10 g of the herb or spice? While it varies depending on the specific herb, 10 g is equivalent to approximately 2 teaspoons. Note that this table lists the polyphenol content for just 10 g because that is more realistic in terms of what one would typically consume in terms of the quantity of a spice. The other tables list polyphenol content for 100 g of food because that is a typically consumed quantity for those foods.

POLYPHENOL CONTENT IN FRUITS

Food	Polyphenol content, mg per 100 grams (3.5oz)
Black elderberry	1359 mg
Blueberry	836 mg
Black currant	758 mg
Plum	377 mg
Cherry	274 mg
Blackberry	260 mg
Strawberry	235 mg
Raspberry	215 mg
Black grape	169 mg
Apple	136 mg
Peach	59 mg
Apricot	34 mg

How large is a portion of 100 g of fruits? It varies, but it is equal to 3.5 ounces, which may consist of half a medium-sized apple, one average-sized banana, approximately two-thirds of a cup of berries, etc.

POLYPHENOL CONTENT IN VEGETABLES

Food	Polyphenol content, mg per 100 grams (3.5oz)
Capers	654 mg
Black olive	569 mg
Green olive	346 mg
Globe artichoke	260 mg
Red onion	168 mg
Spinach	119 mg
Shallot	113 mg
Yellow onion	74 mg
Broccoli	45 mg
Asparagus	29 mg
Potato	28 mg

How large is a portion of 100 g of vegetables? While it varies based on the type of vegetable, 100 g is equivalent to 3.5 ounces (one-fifth of a pound)—e.g., two medium carrots, three cups of raw spinach leaves, half a medium-sized baked potato, etc.

POLYPHENOL CONTENT IN BEANS, NUTS, AND SEEDS

Food	Polyphenol content, mg per 100 grams (3.5oz)
Ground flaxseed	1528 mg
Chestnut	1215 mg
Hazelnut	495 mg
Pecan	493 mg
Soybean	246 mg
Almond	187 mg
Black bean	59 mg
White bean	51 mg
Walnut	28 mg

How much is 100 g of nuts or seeds? This is equivalent to 3.5 ounces, which is about three handfuls of nuts (one handful of nuts is approximately 1 ounce).

POLYPHENOL CONTENT IN BEVERAGES

Beverage	Polyphenol content, mg per 100 grams (3.5oz)
Coffee	214 mg
Black tea	102 mg

Red wine	101 mg
Green tea	89 mg
Apple juice *	68 mg
Pomegranate juice	66 mg
Grapefruit juice	53 mg
Orange juice	46 mg

*All juices listed assume 100 percent of the pure fruit juice.

How much is 100 g of a beverage? This is equivalent to 3.5 ounces, which is a little under half a cup of most beverages (approximately 100 mL, depending on the density of the liquid).

FEEDING AKKERMANSIA

We know that Akkermansia is one of the most important keystone species for people on the autoimmune spectrum, because of its ability to help normalize intestinal permeability, reduce inflammation, and promote healthy metabolism. Studies have shown that certain foods that contain red polyphenols are especially beneficial for supporting the growth of this bacteria.[14] In terms of fruits and their juices this includes red grape, cranberry, red apple (skin), pomegranate, and dragonfruit. It also includes red rice, red quinoa, and red potato (eat the skin).

Inulin

Inulin is a beneficial prebiotic that has been shown to raise levels of the keystone species Faecalibacterium prausnitzii, Bifidobacteria, and Lactobacillus; intake of inulin has additional benefits including strengthened gut barrier function, improved transit time, increased insulin sensitivity, decreased triglycerides, increased absorption of calcium and magnesium (by acidifying intestinal pH), and improved satiety.[15] Maximizing intake of the prebiotic inulin is one of the single most powerful things you can do to improve the health of your gut microbiome. This section includes data from published literature on the inulin content of certain plant foods.[16]

Inulin is fermented by the gut bacteria to produce beneficial short-chain fatty acids and other postbiotic compounds—and gas. One has to be careful to start with very small quantities of each of these foods and not overdo it in the beginning, otherwise there could be bothersome gas and bloating. If you have SIBO, these foods probably would not work well for you—in this case, focus on the foods high in polyphenols that we discussed above.

Cooking does slightly reduce the prebiotic content by breaking down some of the inulin, but also makes these foods easier to digest, so there is a trade-off. Lightly cooking or steaming would work well. In cases where you can consume some of these foods raw and tolerate them without any issues, that is an excellent option.

Chicory or Dandelion root. These are grouped together because they are commonly consumed as coffee substitutes. Chicory, a plant from the daisy family, is the richest food source of inulin, containing 36–48 percent inulin by weight. Dandelion is also an excellent source of inulin. Consuming chicory root raw, however, can cause GI distress. For that reason, it is often roasted. Chicory is commonly found in coffee substitutes, where it functions as a caffeine-free herbal beverage that has a flavor comparable to coffee. Unfortunately, not much of the prebiotic content makes it into the coffee because the inulin fibers are filtered out while brewing—but a small amount still does. Another option is to use powdered inulin, which is often derived from chicory root as a healthy prebiotic addition to smoothies and shakes, but that is not essential.

Jerusalem artichokes. Also known as sunchokes, these are the kings of prebiotic vegetables, boasting 16–20 percent inulin by weight. These knobby light brown tubers are quite versatile in the kitchen.

Artichokes. These are another good source, containing up to 10 percent inulin. In addition, artichokes are nutrient-dense and highly beneficial for the liver; they contain a unique antioxidant called cynarin, which helps stimulate bile production, improves gut motility, and aids the digestion of certain fats.[17] While they may seem intimidating, especially with their sharp spines, artichokes can be prepared quite easily, as I will share in my Recipes section.

Garlic. A constant cooking companion, this is a good source of inulin, containing 9–16 percent by weight.

Onion. Also regularly found in recipies, onion is a fairly good source, with raw onion containing up to 7 percent inulin by weight. The inulin is broken down by cooking so minimally cooked onion is more effective as a probiotic.

Asparagus. This is a good option, containing 2–3 percent inulin. Asparagus is also exceptionally nutrient-dense, anti-inflammatory, and helps regulate your blood sugar. It is rich in glutathione, the most important antioxidant in your body, which supports detoxification and other essential functions. You want to cook it "al dente," where it is still crisp, in order to retain the prebiotic properties. Overcooking asparagus will break down much of the inulin, so enjoy it raw or lightly cooked.

Bananas. If they are a little on the green side and not too ripe, bananas contain higher levels of prebiotics. As bananas ripen, the prebiotic fibers break down and convert into simple sugars, which do not have the same benefits—so enjoy them before they become too ripe.

Leeks. They contain up to 16 percent inulin by weight.[18] Related to the onion family, leeks can be substituted in any recipe where you would otherwise be using onions (check out my "Artichoke and Leek Soup" in the Recipes section).

Jicama. This starchy root vegetable, which resembles a potato but has the crunch and taste of an apple, is an excellent source of inulin and fiber. It is a more popular vegetable now and thus has become more widely available.

Taro root. In the next section, we'll learn about resistant starch; taro root is a good source of this and other prebiotics that make it comparable to inulin in its prebiotic effects.[19] This starchy tuber is not well-known in the West but commonly used in Asia and often available in Asian markets.

Resistant Starch

Resistant starch refers to a type of starch that "resists" digestion by our enzymes but can be broken down and metabolized by bacteria. It does not get absorbed or provide any calories to you but does get utilized as a prebiotic. Bacteria in the microbiome ferment resistant starch to produce a range of beneficial postbiotics (and gas, as a side effect).

Resistant starch has some major metabolic benefits—it improves blood sugar parameters, promotes weight loss, increases insulin sensitivity, and provides cardiovascular benefits.[20] Researchers found adding resistant starch to the diet can help optimize triglyceride and cholesterol levels while decreasing fat mass.[21] There are five different types of resistant starch, but types four and five require chemical modification so we will only discuss the first three types.[22]

Type I Resistant Starch

This type is found in the cellulose cell walls of certain grains, legumes, and seeds. Because we cannot break down cellulose, this starch is partly hidden and inaccessible to us—the starch component that is not broken down by our digestive enzymes and makes it to the colon then feeds our gut bacteria. Whatever starch we can break down, we will absorb—the rest will be utilized by our bacteria. If the grain or legume is finely milled or made into flour, then the starch becomes accessible to us and we can digest and absorb more of it; consequently, the resistant starch content goes down.

Legumes, including peas, lentils, and beans. When cooked as whole legumes, and not as a refined flour or in other processed form, legumes contain significant levels of type I resistant starch. The way in which you prepare legumes can impact their resistant starch content. If you soak dry beans in water before cooking, the process does not negatively impact the resistant starch levels and will help reduce levels of anti-nutrients. However, if you are sprouting them, that does significantly reduce levels of resistant starch (which is why sprouting reduces the amount of gas that beans cause). Sprouting makes the beans more easily digestible, and thus more of the starch is absorbed, but sprouting has the downside of lowering prebiotic levels.

Legumes may contain both type I resistant starch and type III resistant starch, depending on how they are prepared. If they are cooked and cooled, some type III resistant starch will form as well, as we will discuss below. Canned beans are a good option because they are pressure-cooked in the can and then cooled, leading to the formation of type III resistant starch (look for cans that are BPA-free as sometimes the lining of cans may contain BPA). Most beans are also high in polyphenols and galactooligosaccharides (GOS) which are an additional source of prebiotics, making beans the unrecognized "triple threat" of prebiotics.

Oats. An excellent source of type I resistant starch, whole oats also contain another beneficial prebiotic known as beta-glucan. Cooking reduces the resistant starch content, so a better approach is overnight oats. Simply soak the oats overnight in almond milk, coconut milk, or other nondairy milk, and enjoy them in the morning without cooking. For overnight oats you may want to use rolled oats or quick oats, as they absorb the liquid better than steel-cut oats (check out my instructions on how to prepare overnight oats in the Recipes section). Overnight oats are more digestible because soaking reduces levels of the anti-nutrient phytic acid. Another option for raw oats is to add them to a smoothie. If you do prefer to cook them, I recommend steel-cut whole oats, which are low glycemic.

Millet, buckwheat, and sorghum. These gluten-free grains are good sources of type I resistant starch.[23] Whole-grain versions have higher levels of resistant starch than processed forms like refined flour made from these grains. Wheat, barley, and certain other gluten-containing grains also contain some type I resistant starch, but because of their potentially inflammatory effects on the body (as discussed earlier) I do not recommend them for people on the autoimmune spectrum.

Sweet potatoes and yams. They contain a significant amount of type I resistant starch. Sweet potatoes are rich in nutrients and antioxidants and also contain both soluble and insoluble fiber. In addition, they are low-glycemic when compared to regular potatoes.

Taro. It is a rich source of antioxidants and fiber and has a mild, nutty flavor. Up to 12 percent of the starch in cooked taro root is resistant starch.[24]

ADVANCED TIP: LEGUMES FOR LONGEVITY

Legumes are actually the superstars of the prebiotic world. Not surprisingly, an interesting study on longevity found that legumes were the single most important dietary predictor of a long life in older people from around the world.[25] The study followed populations in Japan, Sweden, Greece, and Australia and found that every 20 g increase in the daily intake of legumes was associated with a 7–8 percent reduction in mortality.

Type II Resistant Starch

Type II resistant starch refers to starch with a high content of a specific carbohydrate known as amylose. It is not easily broken down by our digestive enzymes and is found in certain raw foods. If these foods are cooked, then the starch can be broken down by our enzymes and absorbed, so the resistant starch is no longer present. This is also the form found in certain supplements as well, such as potato starch and green plantain flour, which you'll learn about in this section.

Because the supplements are more concentrated products than food sources of prebiotics, be careful when considering whether to take them. A caveat is that patients with overgrowth of microbes such as in SIBO or yeast should avoid prebiotic supplements as they can exacerbate the conditions. Before taking any supplement, I recommend consulting with your practitioner.

Plantains. Plantains are fruits that resemble bananas but are a bit larger and more fibrous. They are very popular in the Caribbean and certain African and Asian countries. Green plantain is the richest source of resistant starch and is often made into chips or cooked in other ways. The cooking process does break down some of the resistant starch, but a significant amount remains. They are also an excellent source of potassium and magnesium.

Bananas. As we discussed earlier, bananas contain inulin and they do also have appreciable amounts of resistant starch. In this case, the greener the banana, the higher the resistant starch content. Very ripe bananas have probably lost most of their prebiotics, which have become converted to sugars.

Potato starch. The starch, not the flour, is an excellent source of resistant starch. It is tasteless and dissolves easily in water. If you are using it as a resistant starch supplement the trick is to consume it raw. If you cook potato starch it will be absorbed and metabolized in your body. If you are going to take it as a supplement, I would recommend starting very slow, perhaps with a quarter teaspoon dissolved in four ounces of water once per day after a meal. You may have digestive symptoms such as gas or bloating as your gut bacteria changes. If this occurs, try lowering the dose.

If you tolerate a quarter teaspoon, stay on this dose for three days and monitor for any side effects like gas, bloating, or change in stool consistency. If no major side effects occur, gradually increase by a quarter teaspoon every three days up to a dosage of one teaspoon per day. You do not want the dosage of resistant starch to be too high, at the exclusion of other prebiotics. The key thing with prebiotics is to have a diverse blend, including all the different types of prebiotics that we are discussing, in small quantities—but consistently. Again, use caution if you have SIBO or overgrowth of harmful bacteria in the large intestine, as prebiotic supplements may worsen symptoms in these cases.

Green plantain, cassava, or green banana flour. These are raw, powdered versions of these prebiotic foods. If they are cooked, they lose their prebiotic properties. Again, if you are going to take it as a supplement, I recommend starting very slow, and following the same instructions as above for potato starch. Resistant starch supplement powders can also be blended in a smoothie or protein drink—any food product in which they are not heated will work.

Type III Resistant Starch

Type III resistant starch, also known as retrograde starch, is formed when certain plant foods are cooked and then cooled. The cooling process changes the chemical structure of some of the starches to form resistant starch. If it is reheated just to room temperature, the resistant starch is preserved, but if it is cooked at high heat again, the resistant starch is broken down.

Potatoes. Cooked and chilled potatoes are the most well-known source. Any traditional potato, like white, brown, red, or even purple can be used for this purpose. Potatoes that have been cooked and then chilled in the refrigerator for twenty-four hours undergo a transformation that leads to the production of resistant starch. After twenty-four hours, the potatoes can be reheated to room temperature without any loss or damage to the resistant starch. Potato salad is a great option here.

Rice. Surprisingly, certain forms of rice contain resistant starch. Cooking and cooling white rice produces a modest amount. Studies have found that if you add 2 teaspoons of coconut oil for each 1 cup of white rice while cooking, and then chill the cooked rice for twelve hours, you can significantly increase the resistant starch content and decrease the calories of the rice by at least 10 percent.[26] Another option is parboiled white rice, which has more resistant starch and fiber than regular white rice. Not everyone tolerates grains because of their glycemic effects and other factors, but if you do, cooking white rice in this way is a good option. Be sure to wash the rice well and drain the water in order to reduce arsenic levels before cooking.

Legumes. As mentioned, legumes are a good source of type I resistant starch and prebiotics. If they are cooked and cooled, they also develop significant levels of type III resistant starch.

ARABINOGALACTAN

Arabinogalactan is a prebiotic fiber that improves microbial diversity and benefits the growth of keystone species such as lactobacillus and Bifidobacteria; it has antibacterial properties against harmful *E. coli* and a potential pathogen known as Klebsiella which is implicated in a number of autoimmune diseases.[27]

Arabinogalactan enhances immune function and reduces the incidence of colds and upper respiratory infections.[28] It increases the activity of so-called "natural killer cells," immune cells which help fight off pathogens and microbial threats to your body.[29] A randomized, double-blind, placebo-controlled trial found that arabinogalactan extract significantly increased antibody response against pneumococcal vaccine.[30]

Food sources include **carrot**, **radish**, **pear**, **tomato**, and **coconut meat** and **milk**.[31] I am often asked about whether immune-stimulating agents can exacerbate autoimmune conditions. When consumed in food sources, I don't believe there is a risk of this prebiotic overstimulating your immune system and worsening autoimmune disease.

ALL OTHER PREBIOTIC FOODS

We have covered some of the major categories of prebiotics and the foods that contain them. Now we will go through some other foods that have unique but lesser-known prebiotics. You will notice that legumes are repeated here because they have an additional prebiotic called GOS that I have not reviewed yet.

Leafy green veggies. Make sure you include plenty of nutrient-dense leafy green vegetables in your diet almost every day. They contain unique prebiotics known as sulfoquinovose sugars or SQ sugars, which selectively feed certain beneficial gut bacteria in the microbiome.[32] All greens such as spinach, kale, romaine lettuce, and bok choy are recommended; exceptionally nutrient-dense options include arugula, radicchio, and loose-leaf lettuce. Dandelion greens deserve special mention because they are high in prebiotics, as both the root and the greens are rich in inulin. Avoid iceberg lettuce, which is low in nutrients.

Mushrooms. They contain types of fiber that are completely unique in our food supply (chitin, chitosan, alpha- and beta-glucans) and are thus exceptionally beneficial for improving the health and diversity of the microbiome. Studies show that they can raise levels of Faecalibacterium prausnitzii, Bifidobacteria, Lactobacillus, Akkermansia, and Roseburia (a key butyrate producer), decrease levels of harmful bacteria, and increase production of anti-inflammatory compounds and beneficial short-chain fatty acids.[33] Some compounds in mushrooms, such as polysaccharides and beta-glucans, are able to directly modulate the immune system and improve gut barrier health. The humble white button mushroom has even been shown to improve microbiota diversity and reduce the levels of pathogenic gut bacteria.[34] All mushrooms are excellent but the true superstars are Asian mushrooms such as **shiitake, maitake, enoki, lion's mane**, and **reishi**.

Apples. Apples are a rich source of pectin, a beneficial prebiotic fiber. Red apple skin contains proanthocyanidins, which feed keystone bacteria such as Akkermansia. In addition, their skin contains a compound called querce-tin, which may help support immune system health. Consume a variety of nutrient-dense apples such as Gala, McIntosh, Braeburn, Granny Smith, and Honeycrisp—and be sure to eat the skin.

Apple cider vinegar. Raw, unpasteurized apple cider vinegar (known as ACV) is a rich source of pectin, derived from the apples it is made from. In addi-tion, it contains acetic acid and other beneficial acids that help with maintaining an acidic stool pH, which, as we know, is crucial for making your gut inhospi-table to pathogens and bad actors.

Legumes. Beans, lentils, peas, and all legumes are a good source of galacto-oligosaccharides, or GOS. GOS are short-chain carbohydrates made up of the sugars galactose and glucose. Legumes should be properly prepared by soaking overnight, sprouting, and/or fermenting before they are cooked. I know that some people cannot tolerate legumes for various reasons. In that case, try to incorporate some of the other foods from this section. For example, Jerusalem artichoke is one of the few foods that is not a legume that is also a good source of GOS.

PREVENTING LEAKY GUT

If, after completing the gut healing part of the protocol, you experience a recurrence of leaky gut, many of these foods will help to repair it. Studies show that supplementation with GOS reduces intestinal permeability in adults with obesity, a condition known to cause impaired barrier func-tion.[35] In children, the addition of beans to the diet led to a reduction in lactulose/mannitol ratios.[36] Legumes and beans are one of the best food sources of GOS and are a key part of my Phase 2 Diet. As we discussed in chapter 9, my eating plan includes many foods clinically proven to help normalize gut permeability. It is crucial to maintain a healthy gut barrier once you achieve normal intestinal permeability. This does not mean that you will never again have any degree of leaky gut. Sometimes you might need to take antibiotics, NSAIDs, or other medicines that affect the gut negatively, or permeability might increase from alcohol or dietary factors. As long as you return to the Phase 2 Diet as your baseline, you will auto-matically be incorporating all of the foods that help restore healthy gut function and heal any increased permeability that has developed.

FERMENTED FOODS

We reviewed a lot of research about fermented foods in the previous chapter; they appear here again because studies show that they are anti-inflammatory, boost the diversity of the microbiome, and can actually modulate the immune system—all three effects are hugely beneficial for patients with autoimmune disease, particularly when these foods are eaten daily.

If this is your first experience with fermented foods, be sure to increase your consumption very gradually. Start with, for example, just 1 tablespoon of sauerkraut per day with a meal. If this causes bloating, abdominal distress, or other gastrointestinal symptoms, you may need to start with a lower dose, a teaspoon or lower. I've had some patients who can only tolerate a quarter teaspoon of sauerkraut juice initially (they could not take any of the actual vegetable). After building up their tolerance to the sauerkraut juice over time, they were eventually able to begin taking the actual sauerkraut and increase that dosage gradually. Similar experiences have been reported with kefir. Some patients only tolerate a quarter teaspoon of kefir once a day and it can in fact take many months for them to build up tolerance to the point where they can eventually increase the dosage up to 1 tbsp per day.

I encourage daily consumption of fermented vegetables, because they are rich in probiotics and healthy acids. Sauerkraut is an excellent option. Experiment with different brands to see what you like. Choose a brand that is prepared in a traditional manner and does not contain preservatives like sodium benzoate.

The advantage of sauerkraut pickled in water is that more of the probiotic bacteria will survive. Sauerkraut in vinegar does not contain many live bacteria (which are killed by the vinegar) but it does have the advantage of the organic acids that help maintain a healthy intestinal pH. We alternate between both. Choose whatever is available. It is also not difficult to make your own sauerkraut or other pickled vegetables at home—for detailed instructions, please see my Recipes section.

South Indian cuisine includes *dosa* and *idli*, which are made from a fermented mixture of rice and lentils, and *appam*, which is made from fermented rice and coconut milk. *Lassi* is a widely available fermented dairy beverage that is typically consumed after meals. India features a rich variety of traditional fermented foods that are derived from many different food sources, including *khalpi* (cucumber), *dhokla* (rice and lentil), *sinki* (radish), *ghungruk* (green leafy vegetables), *kanjika* (millet), and *iromba* (fish).[37] African cuisine also features a variety of fermented foods, such as bread made from fermenting grains like sorghum or teff.

Here are some examples of fermented foods to include in your diet:

- sauerkraut
- kimchi
- pickled ginger
- fermented cucumbers
- pickled vegetables of any kind
- yogurt (if you tolerate dairy)
- almond, coconut, or other nondairy yogurt
- kombucha
- dairy or non-dairy kefir
- beet or fruit kvass
- fermented cod liver oil (reviewed below)

FOODS TO EAT EVERY DAY

In addition to prebiotic and fermented foods, here are the main foundational foods that should be consumed every day and comprise the core of your diet:

Vegetables, at least nine servings per day. Vegetables are far and away the most important part of your diet. The phytochemicals and nutrients in vegetables are your primary defense against autoimmunity. As you'll see below, studies show that consuming vegetables at this level offers the maximum reduction in the risk of heart disease, stroke, cancer, and all-cause mortality.[38] I highly recommend cruciferous vegetables (broccoli, brussels sprouts, cauliflower, cabbage, kale, bok choy, etc.), which protect against cancer and support healthy liver function.

Broccoli sprouts, at least half a cup daily. Broccoli sprouts are the richest food source of sulforophane, one of the most beneficial anti-inflammatory plant-based nutrients. You'll learn more about sulforophane in chapter 12.

Fruits, up to two servings every day. Fruits are a great source of fiber, phytochemicals, and antioxidants. Because fruit is much higher in sugar than vegetables, I recommend limiting it to two servings per day for most people.

Root vegetables. You may liberally eat root vegetables such as potatoes, sweet potatoes, beets, carrots, etc.

Healthy fats. These include extra-virgin olive oil, coconut oil, avocado, and ghee (if you have reintroduced it successfully). Coconut oil contains beneficial fats known as medium-chain triglycerides that can inhibit the growth of harmful gut microbes, improve lipid profiles, promote weight loss, and improve neurological function.[39] Flaxseed oil and hemp seed oil are good options for occasional use, but should never be heated.

Spices. All spices are acceptable, especially those we've been discussing throughout this book, including turmeric, clove, ajwain, black cumin, garlic, and ginger.

Legumes. For the multiple prebiotic (and longevity) benefits that I outlined earlier in this chapter, beans, lentils, peas, and all legumes are highly recommended. If you do not tolerate legumes, be sure to include plenty of the other foods listed above.

ADVANCED TIP: FOOD AS PREVENTATIVE MEDICINE

My recommendation of nine servings of vegetables and up to two servings of fruit every day is not arbitrary. Both foods in these groups have mutiple benefits for supporting autoimmunity, and there are key benefits reached at these levels that impact our biggest chronic diseases, the biggest killers worldwide today. A meta-analysis of two million people concluded that the greatest reduction in risk for heart attack, stroke, cancer, and early death came from eating ten servings of fruits and vegetables per day.[40]

The Healthiest Fat

Not all fats are created equally, and some are particularly beneficial. Extra-virgin olive oil (EVOO) is one of my favorite fats, and it is the best choice for people with autoimmunity for a few reasons. EVOO has strong anti-inflammatory properties, mediated by the potent compounds oleic acid and oleocanthal.[41] It is rich in antioxidants, which can counteract the high levels of oxidative stress seen in autoimmune disorders.[42] In rheumatoid arthritis, olive oil (together with fish oil) significantly improved pain and stiffness.[43] It blunts the inflammatory response of immune cells in patients with lupus.[44]

Some of my patients have followed autoimmune protocol diets that suggest all oils are harmful because they are processed. While I agree that many vegetable oils are harmful, I believe that olive oil is the exception, and the scientific literature confirms this.

In addition to anti-inflammatory benefits, olive oil is associated with a lower risk of heart disease, the number one killer of people worldwide.[45] A study that followed 90,000 women over the course of 28 years found that those who consumed the most olive oil had significantly lower risks for death from cancer, neurodegenerative diseases, respiratory diseases, and heart disease.[46]

Cooking with Olive Oil

It is a common myth that you cannot cook with olive oil. The main factor that determines stability of a cooking oil is whether the oil is high in polyunsaturated fats, which are unstable when heated.[47] Studies show that when these oils (like soybean and canola) are heated, they degrade and form harmful compounds like aldehydes which can contribute to cancer.[48]

In contrast, oils that are high in monounsaturated fats, like olive oil, are stable when heated. Because olive oil is low in polyunsaturated fats and high in antioxidants, it can be exposed to high heat without breaking down. In fact, the antioxidants and vitamin E in EVOO protect it from oxidative damage during long periods of heating, even up to 36 hours in one study.[49]

This is why I recommend using olive oil for most of your cooking. If you are cooking at very high heat, you can consider using coconut oil.

OLIVE OIL VS. COCONUT OIL

Coconut oil contains beneficial fats known as medium-chain triglycerides that can inhibit the growth of harmful gut microbes, improve lipid profiles, promote weight loss, improve neurological function, and possibly protect against heart disease.[50]

Are you concerned about the saturated fat in coconut oil or worried about how it might impact cholesterol or heart disease? A randomized controlled trial found that people advised to consume 50 g of coconut oil or olive oil daily had no significant difference in their LDL-cholesterol over time—and, those consuming coconut oil saw significant improvement in their beneficial HDL.[51]

However, because saturated fat may have a less beneficial impact on the microbiome than other fats, as I reviewed in chapter 4, I recommend using olive oil preferentially compared to coconut oil.

FOODS TO EAT FREQUENTLY FOR ALL PEOPLE, AT LEAST FOUR TO FIVE DAYS PER WEEK

These are very healthy, nutrient-dense foods that should be consumed frequently if possible, depending on your preference and tolerance of the foods.

Eggs, including the yolks (which are the most nutritious part). You may eat up to two eggs with the yolks every day. An exception here is for those who have elevated cholesterol. Eating too many foods, like eggs, that are high in cholesterol may further spike cholesterol levels in some people. Exercise caution here.

Meat and poultry. Grass-fed, organic, and/or pasture-raised meats and free-range poultry, including organ meats such as liver, at least once per week.

Fish. Wild-caught oily fish, especially salmon, sardines, anchovies, and mackerel, for a total of up to a pound per week.

Beets. These root vegetables have remarkable benefits. Both the roots and the greens are incredibly nutritious. Beet greens, the leafy tops of beets, are the richest food source of betaine (also known as trimethylglycine), which helps your body to detoxify by supporting methylation and Phase 2 liver detox pathways. Beet greens are one of the most powerful unheralded superfoods that can aid in detoxification. However, if you have a history of oxalate kidney stones, use caution with beets as they are high in oxalates.

Bone broth is rich in minerals, amino acids, and gelatin, which are all very healing for the gut.

Gluten-free grains like white rice, quinoa, millet, wild rice, amaranth, buckwheat, teff, and arrowroot, as well as products made from these grains, are acceptable if you tolerate them well. I do not typically recommend brown rice because it is harder to digest (and tends to be higher in the heavy metal arsenic).[52] It is higher in fiber but there are plenty of other fiber sources in the Phase 2 Diet.

Sprouts such as clover and alfalfa offer a cornucopia of different nutrients and phytochemicals, in addition to broccoli sprouts, which are nutritional powerhouses. Consuming all sprouts as often as you can will be highly beneficial. The only exception is bean sprouts, which are less nutrient-dense.

Fermented cod liver oil (FCLO) is processed at cold temperatures, prepared in a traditional fermentation process, and is rich in vitamins A and D, in addition to containing omega-3 fats. It is also rich in vitamin K_2, which is important for cardiovascular health. If you don't care for the taste of FCLO, regular cod liver oil is an excellent option as well and has all the same benefits without being fermented.

Seasonings. Make liberal use of spices whenever you can. Other seasonings that are beneficial for digestion include apple cider vinegar, lemon juice, lime juice, balsamic vinegar, and green onions. A good substitute for soy sauce is coconut-based alternative Coconut Secret Raw Coconut Aminos.

Pickled ginger. We learned about the power of ginger in chapter 8. In pickled form, it has the additional benefits of a fermented food. I recommend that you try to consume pickled ginger regularly. You might know pickled ginger from sushi restaurants, and while this food might be available in Asian markets, it usually has synthetic food dye to give it that familiar pink color. Natural markets typically stock pickled ginger without artificial colors or preservatives. As a condiment, enjoy two or three pieces with meals as often as you like. For my instructions on how to make your own homemade pickled ginger, check out the Recipes section.

FOODS TO EAT FREQUENTLY FOR SOME PEOPLE, UP TO FOUR TO FIVE DAYS PER WEEK

These are gray-area foods that were eliminated during the Phase 1 Diet. You can try to reintroduce these foods according to the instructions at the end of chapter 5. Based on your individual tolerance and experience, these foods may be beneficial. You can consume these foods frequently if you tolerate them well.

Dairy products. I recommend only full-fat dairy products like yogurt, kefir, and cheese. However, these should not be consumed in excess because of the potentially negative effect on the gut microbiome of saturated fat (as I explained in chapter 4). I typically recommend up to five servings per week of dairy products for patients with autoimmune disease. Avoid low-fat dairy products because of the increased risk of negative health effects as we've discussed.

All nuts and seeds except peanuts. Choices include almonds, cashews, walnuts, pumpkin seeds, sunflower seeds, ground flaxseed, etc. Macadamia nuts, hazelnuts, and almonds are excellent choices because they are low in omega-6 fats. Pumpkin seeds are among the richest food sources of zinc. Flaxseed is an excellent source of polyphenols, as discussed above. Nut butters are acceptable as well. If you have difficulty digesting nuts, you can soak or sprout them. Avoid any nuts you are allergic to.

Gluten-free grains like white rice, millet, wild rice, amaranth, buckwheat, teff, quinoa (actually a legume), and arrowroot, as well as products made from these grains, are acceptable if you tolerate them well.

FOODS TO EAT RARELY (ONCE A WEEK OR LESS FREQUENTLY)

These foods may be the most likely to contribute to inflammation and other disturbances in the body. If you do elect to eat them, I recommend eating them no more than once a week.

Gluten. This includes gluten-containing grains such as wheat, barley, rye, kamut (an ancient form of wheat), spelt, and others. As I explained in chapter 5, I have concerns about the potential inflammatory effects of gluten on patients with autoimmune disease. For the many reasons I outlined earlier, I believe that people on the autoimmune spectrum may be better off not consuming it. If you did reintroduce it successfully after the Phase 1 Diet, I would still recommend eating it no more than once a week.

Corn. The great majority of corn in this country is genetically modified, nutrient-poor, and excessively high in carbohydrates and sugar. Typically, corn is processed heavily before entering the food supply. An occasional corn product made from organic stone-ground whole cornmeal, such as a taco or cornbread (without added flour or sugar), would be acceptable.

Soy. The only type of soy that I recommend eating is fermented soy like *natto* (an incredible source of vitamin K_2) or miso. If you can tolerate *natto*, you only need to eat it once or twice per week to get its health benefits. Technically, tofu and tempeh are also fermented, but I do not recommend regular consumption unless you are vegetarian.

Peanuts. Peanuts are highly allergenic, often genetically modified, prone to mold, and have a less favorable fatty-acid profile than other nuts. I recommend limiting peanut intake to once a week.

Sweeteners. Occasional sweets made with natural sweeteners like raw honey, molasses, maple syrup, or stevia are acceptable. Avoid white sugar and high fructose corn syrup. Also stay away from artificial sweeteners such as aspartame, sucralose (Splenda), or acesulfame potassium, because these promote weight gain (despite having zero calories) and may negatively impact your microbiome by feeding the growth of harmful bacteria.

Processed red meats. The evidence suggests that frequent consumption of processed red meats may raise the risk of colon cancer and cardiovascular disease.[53] Studies seem to indicate that processed red meats are harmful whereas unprocessed meats are not.[54] Processed red meats are made from beef, lamb, or pork, and may include ham, bacon, deli meats such as bologna and salami, hot dogs, and pepperoni. Because all types of processed meats are lumped together in most studies, we don't know which processed meats are better or worse than others. Nitrites or nitrates, preservatives frequently put in processed meats, are potential cancer-causing compounds and may comprise a significant portion of the increased risk; cooking meat at high heat may create other harmful substances—it is unclear how much of the risk might come from these factors versus from the meats themselves.[55]

HOW MUCH TO EAT

This protocol doesn't count calories; nor do I find it necessary to recommend a certain number of calories for each person. What really matters is the *quality* of the food we eat. Calorie requirements vary widely based on genetics, metabolism, activity level, and other factors.

Ayurveda does not recommend tracking calories, and I align with this approach. The important recommendation is to eat until you are about two-thirds full. To use a simple example, if three portions of food would make you full, then eat two portions. It is important to learn to pay attention to signals of satiety and fullness, if you are not doing so already.

How to Make Your Plate

I've made a lot of sugestions on what foods to eat as you take on the Phase 2 Diet. They may seem overwhelming, and some could be unfamiliar and appear to be out of reach. I want you to think of this diet as an ideal to strive toward. Don't feel bad if you are not able to follow it perfectly—allow yourself time to ramp up to this way of eating, especially if many of these foods are new to you.

I have included a comprehensive list of prebiotic and fermented foods, not with the expectation that you will be able to eat all of them every day, but to give you choices on what to add in. You don't have to be perfect in following the diet in order to start receiving benefits from these foods.

With this in mind, I'll provide you detailed instructions on making your plate for each meal, to help you incorporate all these foods into your diet. This is not a contest; do the best that you can as you work to implement these changes. Even moving in the direction of this diet with some initial changes will be highly beneficial as you increase your intake of anti-inflammatory and gut-friendly nutrients. Here are my guidelines:

- Fill half of your plate with a heaping portion of non-starchy vegetables. Aim for three cups of vegetables (measured raw) per meal, which equals three servings, in order to get nine servings of vegetables daily over three meals. You can consume them cooked or raw. You may need to add a side of salad or veggies to achieve the three servings per meal; add a generous amount of broccoli sprouts. Include at least 1 tablespoon of fermented foods with each meal, or work up to it, as we've discussed.
- Fill one-quarter of your plate with protein-rich foods, such as eggs, wild-caught fish, grass-fed beef, organic poultry, organ meat from any animal, or legumes of any type. Aim for about 4 ounces in size, the equivalent of a palm-sized portion or a deck of playing cards.
- Fill one-quarter of your plate with a fiber-rich carbohydrate. This could be either starchy root vegetables, or gluten-free grains as described above. You can include whole fruits here, or have fruits as dessert. Fruit can also be incorporated as a snack, up to two servings per day total.
- I want to highlight the importance of legumes. To reiterate, legumes contain multiple different types of prebiotics and are excellent for the microbiome. If you tolerate them, I would recommend incorporating a half cup of legumes with at least one meal daily. Even if you are getting plenty of protein from animal foods, there is great benefit from eating legumes regularly. If you are having a side salad, you can put the legumes on it as a convenient way of adding them to the meal.
- Include healthy fats, the equivalent of 1–2 tablespoons per meal. Be sure to incorporate plenty of healthy fats, such as extra-virgin olive oil and coconut oil, while cooking each meal. If you are having salad, you can combine olive oil with balsamic vinegar and spices to create a tasty dressing. Avocado can be consumed regularly as well.

- For beverages, consider bone broth, cabbage juice, caffeine-free herbal tea, or 100-percent fruit juice (limited to 8 ounces per day).

GUIDANCE FOR VEGETARIANS

If you are vegetarian, I want to offer some guidance on modifying the eating plan. The basic template for the diet will remain the same, with plenty of vegetables, fruits, legumes, fiber-rich carbohydrates, healthy fats, and an emphasis on prebiotic and fermented foods as outlined in this chapter.

To make your plate with protein-rich foods, you may substitute beans of any type, lentils, eggs (if you eat them), or soy products such as tofu, edamame, or tempeh for the meat and fish.

LAST WORDS ON DIET

I hope you have a clear idea now about the Phase 2 Diet. Strive to vary the foods you are eating each week, and try at least one new plant food each week. Remember that your diet might change over time depending on changes in body composition, health status, fitness goals, and other factors. It is important to remain flexible and work on continuously optimizing and improving your nutrition plan.

Also, it is understandable that you might veer off the diet from time to time. The diet includes plenty of foods that help restore intestinal permeability. If barrier function weakens from alcohol, gluten, other dietary indiscretions, or stress, returning to the Phase 2 Diet will ensure that intestinal permeability will be normalized once again.

Let's check in with Mark, the ER doctor who was reluctant to change his eating habits.

Mark was struggling with psoriatic arthritis despite being on immune-suppressing medications. He had not paid much attention to nutrition previously and was eating the "Standard American Diet." I talked to him about dietary change, but he was skeptical and said that he was data-driven and needed to see some test results. He was willing to take vitamin D and fish oil based on blood tests indicating deficiencies.

I tested him for food sensitivity and showed him the numbers indicating his sensitivity to gluten, dairy, and beef. Stool testing revealed markedly increased intestinal permeability, and inflammation that was raging in his GI tract even though he did not have digestive symptoms.

Convinced, Mark began to make major dietary changes. Being rather Type A, he completely eliminated the foods he was sensitive to, started incorporating salads daily, and even added broccoli sprouts and fermented foods. I put him through the TIGER Protocol, with an emphasis on the gut-healing regimen.

After four months, Mark was eager to do repeat stool testing. We identified major reduction in GI inflammation and improved but not normal gut permeability. After continuing his protocol for two more months, he finally experienced resolution in his leaky gut—and his joint pain and swelling. He was surprised to see that his psoriasis, which had been refractory for a decade, also began to clear up.

The steroid creams he was using began to work better, and their effects lasted longer. He was able to eventually reduce and come off his medications, and control his symptoms with diet, exercise, vitamins, and stress management.

CHAPTER 11

Rest—Tools For Optimizing Rest

Hannah was a 35-year-old attorney who came to see me after she was diagnosed with mixed connective tissue disease (MCTD), a rare autoimmune disorder. For over five years, she'd struggled with symptoms including fatigue, joint pain, swollen fingers, and a rash, before eventually connecting with a specialist who diagnosed her correctly. Although she was prescribed an immune-modulating medication and high doses of ibuprofen, Hannah had not seen significant improvement in her symptoms.

During our visit, Hannah expressed discouragement because the medications were just not helping. I started her on the TIGER Protocol and she faithfully followed the complete program of detoxification, dietary changes, and gut healing. We also replenished certain vitamins that were low.

Her symptoms did not improve. We attempted curcumin and glutathione, but she could not tolerate either. She reported that she was highly sensitive to all supplements and an increasing number of foods. She tried to open the capsules and take a few sprinkles of each supplement—but her extreme sensitivity made that impossible.

As we continued working together, Hannah shared that she had survived a number of Adverse Childhood Experiences (ACEs) in life. I suspected that addressing this trauma would play a major role in her recovery—and might even be the single most important thing we could do to turn her health around.

Tending to your diet, detoxifying, and healing your gut are perhaps the main aspects of this protocol, but some pieces extend outside our physical selves. To that end, we'll spend some time exploring mind-body strategies to reduce stress and optimize rest.

STRESS DRIVES AUTOIMMUNITY

Stress plays an undeniable role in autoimmune conditions; it is a key root cause for the initial occurrence of autoimmunity, and a driver of flare-ups and exacerbations of autoimmune illnesses. Research has found that stress is involved in the development and progression of multiple sclerosis, rheumatoid arthritis, lupus, inflammatory bowel disease, and Graves' disease[1], as well as autoimmune hepatitis.[2]

Our bodies are always trying to balance sympathetic (fight-or-flight) and parasympathetic (rest-and-digest) physiology. Seeking to increase parasympathetic activation is an important goal for all people, especially those dealing with autoimmunity, to counteract the chronic sympathetic arousal that stress causes. In this chapter, we'll learn some of the best ways to achieve this.

Science has elucidated the exact pathways through which stress can aggravate autoimmunity. Stress activates the sympathetic and downregulates the parasympathetic nervous system. Reduced parasympathetic signaling via its main nerve, the vagus, leads to greater production of the inflammatory cytokines interleukin-6 and TNF-alpha, which drive the maturation of immune progenitor cells into Th22 cells. These recently discovered Th22 cells produce interleukin-22, which causes increased molecular modification of autoantibodies, making them more reactive and therefore likely to spark tissue damage and autoimmune flare-ups.[3]

Simply put, stress causes sympathetic activation and increased inflammation, driving a cascade that increases the aggression of autoimmune antibodies and makes them more likely to trigger an attack on body tissues.

Tackling Stress Improves Autoimmunity

We have consistent evidence that taking steps to address stress improves outcomes in autoimmunity. A variety of approaches have been shown to be beneficial, including counseling, psychotherapy, and mind-body techniques such as mindfulness and meditation.[4]

In patients with rheumatoid arthritis, the practice of Mindfulness-Based Stress Reduction (MBSR) over a six-month period led to a 35 percent reduction in psychological distress and depressive symptoms, and improved parameters of well-being.[5] Autoimmune hepatitis patients who achieved long-term remission incorporated coping strategies such as mind-body therapies that helped them manage stress.[6]

In those with inflammatory bowel disease (IBD), relaxation training reduced abdominal pain (and stress and anxiety), while improving quality of life and mood.[7] Meditation in particular has epigenetic power—a study in IBD patients found that nine weeks of mindfulness meditation training caused changes in the expression of genes involved in inflammation, cell growth, and oxidative stress— revealing how meditation can favorably alter gene expression in autoimmunity.[8]

MULTIPLE BENEFITS OF MEDITATION

I am a big proponent of meditation. The practice has been shown to lower stress levels and anxiety, and increase feelings of well-being; meditation also leads to improved concentration skills and mental sharpness, which can translate to better intellectual performance.[9] Research has found that those who practice meditation regularly develop longer attention spans and faster cognitive processing.[10]

Research even shows that meditation has a beneficial impact on obesity, likely by reducing levels of the stress hormone cortisol (which promotes weight gain, especially around the abdomen) and improving eating patterns and behavior.[11] If there was a pill that had all these benefits, it would probably be the most valuable and sought-after medicine ever created.

Meditation and Autoimmunity

For autoimmune conditions specifically, meditation has many benefits. It can positively impact inflammation and the gut barrier.[12] A review of 45 studies concluded that meditation is able to lower markers of inflammation such as C-reactive protein and tumor necrosis factor-alpha.[13] Research on patients with IBS found that meditation reduced abdominal pain and bloating; this is likely mediated via effects on the gut-brain axis, the two-way interface between the brain and the GI tract.[14]

When it comes to the immune system specifically, meditation is salutary as well. For example, one study found that those who completed an eight-week clinical training program in Mindfulness-Based Stress Reduction had a stronger immune response to flu vaccine.[15] Another study on those who practiced meditation regularly found lower levels of the cytokine interleukin-6, an immune signaling compound tied to inflammation and chronic disease.[16]

Transforms Your Brain

Meditation has positive effects on neurotransmitters, the molecules that brain cells use to communicate with each other. Meditation has been shown to raise levels of beneficial GABA, acetylcholine, serotonin, and dopamine, and lower levels of stimulatory compounds like cortisol, epinephrine (also known as adrenaline), and norepinephrine.[17]

Additionally, meditation can change not only the function but also the structure of the brain. Research on neuroplasticity has demonstrated that regular practice can create measurable transformations in a short period of time.

The aforementioned Mindfulness-Based Stress Reduction or MBSR is one such example—it's one of the most common meditation programs and was initially created to help patients with chronic pain, who reported significant reductions in pain after regular practice.[18] These improvements correlate with tangible brain changes. Research on participants undergoing a MBSR program found increased gray matter in the hippocampus and the cingulate cortex—areas involved in learning, memory, and emotional regulation—after just eight weeks.[19]

Studies have shown that meditation can increase the size of the prefrontal cortex, the part of the brain that is involved in cognition and rational decision-making.[20] Meditation also appears to shrink the amygdala, known as the fear center of the brain; this is likely how it reduces stress reactivity and enhances emotional control.[21]

The brain can be divided into two basic components, white matter and gray matter, which differ based on their content of a key protein called myelin. Meditation increases the amount of gray matter and reduces typical age-related atrophy and loss of brain cells, suggesting that it can diminish the negative impact of aging on the brain.[22]

White matter also benefits from meditation practice, which leads to enrichment of white matter brain regions that govern emotional reactivity (correlating with improved emotional regulation).[23] Finally, meditation appears to increase beneficial gamma brainwaves, which have been associated with improved attention and awareness.[24]

For all these reasons, I believe meditation is unsurpassed in its health-promoting effects and therefore indispensable for people with autoimmune disease—and for those at any point on the autoimmune spectrum. One type of meditation does not appear to be superior to another, and I will teach you several options. Whether it is MBSR, simple breathing exercises, or loving-kindness meditation, the most important thing is that it be practiced consistently. At least ten minutes a day is recommended. Below, I've offered five techniques for you to try.

Diaphragmatic Breathing

One of the simplest meditation practices is diaphragmatic breathing (also called "belly breathing"). This is a great way to begin if you are new to the practice.

You can do this in any position, but I suggest sitting comfortably in a chair, with your spine upright but relaxed. Place one hand on your abdomen and notice how it moves along with your breath. You want to have your abdomen rise when you breathe in and fall when you breathe out. This engages the diaphragm, a large, dome-shaped muscle at the base of your lungs.

This is in fact opposite to how many people breathe. Generally, when you intentionally take a breath in, your chest and shoulders rise and your abdomen is drawn inward. If you look at how newborn babies breathe, they usually breathe using their diaphragms, which is a healthier way to breathe because it leads to deeper, fuller breaths.

Diaphragmatic breathing has been shown to activate the parasympathetic nervous system. To begin, try to practice for about five minutes or so. You can practice this technique any time—while stopped at a red light in the car, while waiting in line at the grocery store, or at night before you are going to sleep.

Breathing Awareness Meditation

This practice uses your breath as a focus for awareness during meditation. Again, sit with your spine upright but relaxed. You can also lie down if you prefer (but you might fall asleep—although this can be helpful if you have trouble falling asleep at night).

Become aware of your breathing, wherever you notice it in your body. You might feel the air moving in and out of your nostrils or notice the rise and fall of your abdomen. Try not to breathe in any particular way. The goal here is simply to observe the breathing. If you prefer you can say something to yourself, like "breathing in" as you breathe in, and "breathing out" as you breathe out.

Your mind will definitely wander. It is a misconception to think that this means you are "not good at meditation" or that you are doing something wrong. This is, in fact, the very nature of the mind. When that happens, gently bring your mind back to your breathing. The goal is not to eliminate thoughts or keep your mind completely still. If your mind is constantly wandering, this does not mean that you "can't meditate"—that is completely normal.

The process of bringing your awareness back to your breath, over and over, is what defines this practice of meditation. Begin with about 5 minutes and then you can gradually increase to 10 to 15 minutes daily.

Minute Meditation

The preceding two methods are designed for a block of time at least 5 to 10 minutes long. If that feels like a lot, try this one-minute meditation. It can be used anytime during the day when you feel like you need a break. If you are in a state of distress and feel like you need to calm your mind or center yourself, this is a valuable yet quick practice. I designed this exercise for my busiest patients, who could at least set aside sixty seconds a day. Although it might seem like an insignificant amount of time, this brief meditation still has benefits, and can be a good entry point.

It can be done in any position, wherever you are. Take a deep breath in through your nose and exhale out through your mouth. Let go of any thoughts about what has happened earlier in the day, or what you need to do after the minute has passed. You can either take a few diaphragmatic breaths or practice breathing awareness (as discussed in the first two techniques).

Try to ground yourself in your physical body and bring your awareness down out of the busyness of the mind and into your body. This helps to create a little distance from the maelstrom of thoughts. Direct your attention inward and try to feel your body from within. If it is helpful, you can focus on physical sensations such as your feet touching the floor, or your back resting against the chair. This facilitates a return of awareness into the present moment, which is one of the goals of meditation.

Continue to take a few more slow, deep breaths until the minute has passed. You can do this multiple times throughout the day as needed. I often use this as a more productive and restful moment of pause during the day instead of reaching for my phone reflexively whenever I feel like I need a quick break.

Body Scan

This body-based meditation is an aspect of mindfulness, which is non-judgmental awareness of the present moment and all its aspects. You will scan your body from head to toe and release tension in each area. If you notice discomfort or pain anywhere, do not judge it or get caught up by it. Try to observe the sensation and then move on.

You can practice this either sitting or lying down. Begin with a couple of slow, deep breaths. Continue breathing rhythmically throughout this process. Notice the toes of your left foot by wiggling them a little and releasing any tension they might have. Bring your attention in turn gradually upward to your left foot, lower leg, knee, and thigh, focusing on any tension in those areas and trying to release the tension as you exhale.

Repeat this exercise with your right leg, starting with the toes and working upward. After you have completed both legs, shift your focus to your back, abdomen, and chest, feeling your body from within and softening those areas as much as possible.

Next, observe the muscles in your neck, shoulders, and head, and try to let go of any tightness in those areas. As you exhale, focus on releasing muscular tension. The forehead may carry tightness, so relax that area if necessary. Once you reach the top of your head, visualize your body as an integrated whole. Imagine your entire body completely relaxed, and take some slow, long breaths to conclude.

This practice usually takes around 5 to 10 minutes, but you can go as quickly or as slowly as you like.

Loving-Kindness Meditation

In medical school, one of my professors, a trained Buddhist practitioner, taught me the practice of loving-kindness (also known as "metta"). In the Buddhist tradition, metta meditation is encouraged to help cultivate a kind attitude toward oneself and others. She shared with me a basic loving-kindness exercise in which I would close my eyes and silently repeat the following four phrases, spending about a minute on each one before going on to the next:

1. May I be safe and protected.
2. May I find real happiness.
3. May my body be healthy and strong.
4. May I find inner peace.

I found this practice to be valuable in coping with the turmoil of medical school. In a more advanced version of the meditation, one can then direct the four phrases in sequence and address other people (i.e. "May you be…").

Studies show forgiveness can help improve physical and mental health and increase well-being.[25] To cultivate some of that and tap into the healing power of forgiveness, direct these phrases toward someone with whom you are having issues, a person who is challenging in your life.

A traditional way to conclude this meditation is by expanding your good wishes to include all beings. If you like you may choose a statement such as, "May all beings be safe and protected."

Using an App for Meditation

There are many smartphone apps that can be used to help facilitate meditation. They offer meditations that are guided by others, and therefore make it easy to get started. I recommend Smiling Mind, which is free, and has guided mindfulness meditations. I also like Headspace, Insight Timer, and Calm. If you are so inclined, try out different apps to see what works well for you.

Alternatives to Meditation

I want to acknowledge that meditation may not be for everyone, and is not the only option. However, if you have not attempted to meditate before, I encourage you to try each of the techniques you learned above a few times, even if they feel peculiar or foreign.

Do not expect immediate results. Meditation is like working out a muscle—it requires regular practice to deliver results. If you still feel like it's not for you, seek out other rituals to manage stress.

For some people, spending time in nature, exercise, prayer, or journaling may be preferable. Listening to soothing music can be a great way to relax. Bringing mindful awareness to any activity you perform can return your mind to the present moment, reducing anxiety and tension. The most important thing is to set aside time daily for an activity that helps you relieve stress and improve your state of mind.

MEDIA OVERLOAD

A sometimes unrecognized source of stress is our constant exposure to media through our smartphones. A recent survey found that the average American checks their phone 96 times per day, which works out to once every 10 minutes or so. Technology is a double-edged sword; it connects us with other people, but also can hijack our attention and create unease and tension. Obviously, we rely on our phones and cannot abandon them, but here are some tips on developing a healthier relationship with technology:

- Schedule times during the day to check your email, rather than having it open constantly. I set aside time every four hours or so during the day to open my email and respond.
- Turn off all notifications except for the most critical.
- Be mindful of social media. I log in once a day to create content but seek to minimize the number of times I browse social media to consume content.
- If you feel like you need a break, take a walk, have a cup of tea, daydream, do some stretching, or practice the minute meditation discussed above instead.
- Periodically schedule a "technology fast" where you can disconnect from your laptop and phone for a certain period of time, at least 24 hours if possible.
- Avoid using electronic devices for at least one hour before bed. These devices emit blue light, which can impede production of melatonin, which is necessary for sleep.
- While there is no conclusive evidence linking the electromagnetic radiation from cell phones to health issues, I take precautions and do not leave the phone on my bedside table while I sleep. We also have our Wi-Fi on a timer that shuts off at night.

HEART RATE VARIABILITY (HRV)

For those who love data, heart rate variability, a measurement of the time between your heartbeats, is a good marker with which to track your progress in parasympathetic activation. A higher HRV reflects greater parasympathetic activation (of the calming and restorative aspect of your nervous system), and a low HRV is associated with sympathetic dominance (chronically being in fight-or-flight mode), and some of its resulting negative health effects.

Studies show that a low HRV is associated with hypertension, stress, and an elevated risk of heart disease.[26] Research also indicates a possible link between low HRV and depression.[27] If you want to get a sense of how effective these mind-body practices are, measuring HRV is the best way to do it, besides the changes you'll notice in your life over time.

Tracking and Raising HRV

HRV responds quickly to changes and can be measured by devices like the Oura ring, Apple Watch, or the HeartMath device used in my clinic. It is a form of biofeedback—a technique that uses monitoring devices to help you gain more control over body functions such as your heart rate or breathing. Free apps like Elite HRV can be used in combination with various products, such as a heart rate monitor that you strap around your chest, to measure HRV accurately.

In chapter 6, we looked at research showing that patients with autoimmunity generally have lower HRV, and likely would benefit from approaches that have been proven to increase HRV, such as diaphragmatic breathing and supplementation with fish oil.

Meditation has been shown to help raise HRV in those who are stressed.[28] Of course, exercise is one of the best ways to improve many aspects of cardiovascular health, including HRV; sauna use has also been shown to boost HRV.[29] To this end, multiple elements of the TIGER Protocol have the capacity to enhance your HRV.

PLACEBOS—NEUROPLASTICITY IN ACTION

In chapter 6, you were introduced to the concept of neuroplasticity, the science of how you can rewire your brain and literally change its structure. The discovery of neuroplasticity—showing that thought and mental experience can change brain structure and function—has revolutionized our understanding of the brain.

Here, you'll find some visualizations that utilize these principles. These are real, evidenced-based practices that will allow you to harness the power of neuroplasticity. So, while they may feel foreign, like meditation practice, I assure you that practicing them can only do you good.

To help you better understand how visualization works, I'll first share some research about the incredible power of placebos, to illustrate the powerful link between mind and body.

All About Placebos

While the definition of a "placebo" is an inert substance that has no effect, studies show that placebos have a real and measurable therapeutic effect. There are many factors that can contribute positively to the placebo effect, such as a doctor's white coat or a patient's expectation about a medication.

In fact, some conventional treatments may work mostly as a result of the placebo effect. For example, in patients with mild to moderate depression, the effect of antidepressant medication is comparable to a placebo (but they both work).[30]

How Placebo Affects the Brain

Studies on the placebo effect reveal that it is not just a relaxation response but a tangible effect that causes neuroplastic alterations in the brain. MRI scans demonstrate that when the placebo effect occurs, measurable shifts occur in the brain.

In one study, researchers applied an inert "placebo" cream to participants' skin before delivering a painful electrical shock. Half the people were told it was an inert lotion, and half were told that it was a highly effective painkiller. Patients who believed that they had received a pain-numbing cream actually reported less pain than the control subjects; interestingly, these patients were found to have significant reductions in activity on MRI scans in brain structures related to pain perception.[31]

Follow-up research discovered that placebo treatment causes a release in endogenous opioids called endorphins—compounds produced within the brain to erase pain.[32] Your body can synthesize various molecules that impact pain perception. Placebos activate this "internal pharmacy." This suggests that beliefs can directly cause chemical and functional changes in the brain. Therefore, placebo cures are no less real than cures by medication or other interventions.

One caveat is that placebos are not a panacea—they are not going to be beneficial in really serious health issues. My goal here is for you to take advantage of whatever benefit they can provide, even if it is just in your pain level or quality of life.

Placebo Precision

Placebos are precise and targeted in their effect. The placebo response does not broadly affect the entire nervous system, the way relaxation might. It targets only what the patient is focusing on with pinpoint accuracy.

In an ingenious study, scientists applied painful stimuli to both index fingers of study participants. Then they applied a "pain-relieving cream" which was actually a placebo to only one index finger—people receiving the inert cream actually experienced pain relief—but only in the index finger with the cream.[33] This suggests their minds were pinpointing the exact location of treatment to ease the pain, and then causing a reduction in pain in just that spot.

The Size of the Effect

Placebos can vary in terms of perceived degree of effect. Someone who believes they are getting a high-quality treatment rather than a low-quality treatment will likely have a greater degree of improvement, even if both treatments are placebos.

For example, in a study of patients with Parkinson's disease, participants were told that they would receive either an expensive or cheap new medication; both "medications" were plain saline injections. Patients who were told they were receiving the expensive treatment exhibited greater improvement in tremor and muscle stiffness than patients who were told they were receiving the low-cost medicine.[34]

To take it further, "placebo surgery" was shown to be as effective as regular surgery in some cases. To study the effects of arthroscopic surgery of the knee for osteoarthritis, researchers randomized patients to receive either traditional knee arthroscopy with debridement (removal of damaged tissue) or a sham surgery in which the usual knee incisions were made under anesthesia and all aspects of the regular operation were simulated. At the end of two years, pain reduction and improvement in physical function were identical in patients who received actual knee surgery and patients who received sham surgery.[35] According to follow-up surveys, patients really could not tell whether they had received the surgery or not—but they got better either way.

The fascinating lesson here is that your body has an incredible ability to heal itself, especially when it believes that it should be healing, such as after surgery. The power of belief, expectation, and hope to translate into measurable physical differences is profound. I find it awe-inspiring that the mind has the capacity to impact the physical body in such a significant way.

Lessons from Placebo Science

Instead of rejecting placebos as useless, we should take advantage of them. We should use every opportunity we can to cultivate the belief that we are going to get better, and that we should in fact expect ourselves to improve and feel better.

Of course, as mentioned above, placebos are not a cure for everything.

However, it is worthwhile for you to do whatever you can to feel good about your body and expect that it will work to heal itself as much as possible from afflictions. The body has a phenomenal self-healing capacity.

It's worthwhile to examine the beliefs you have about your body and your health. Simply having a conviction that you will recover can be powerful medicine, as can using tools such as visualization and imagery to help focus these efforts.

GUIDED IMAGERY AND VISUALIZATION

As a physician, I must admit I was initially skeptical about the capacity of guided imagery and visualization to have real benefits. However, as I reviewed the research, I became convinced. Research documents the beneficial effects of guided imagery on reducing postoperative pain and anxiety.[36] Another study centered on those who performed motor imagery, wherein they imagined making various movements in an arm that had to be immobilized, and had less harmful impact from disuse of their arm than those who did not perform imagery.[37]

These methods can be especially powerful in dealing with pain, as pain may be produced in the body but ultimately is experienced in the brain.

Using the Brain to Reduce Pain

Dr. Michael Moskowitz is a pioneer in this field. He is a physician and pain specialist who developed neuroplasticity-based exercises as a last attempt to cure himself after suffering from 13 years of chronic pain after a spinal injury.[38]

Dr. Moskowitz used the concept of "competitive plasticity" to his advantage. Specific regions of the brain, like the posterior parietal lobe, normally process both pain and visual perception. If they are occupied by one process, the other is diminished. Through continuous visualization, Moskowitz was able to shift the focus of the brain cells in that region to visual activity and away from their habitual activity of processing pain, which eventually reduced the brain's overall perception of pain.[39]

I have included an exercise below to illustrate how this works. This technique required discipline and repeated focus over several weeks before he started seeing improvement. It took several months for significant change. After applying the practice for a year and essentially curing himself, Dr. Moskowitz began treating others. He has created a website, neuroplastix.com, which compiles his teachings and techniques; it features a *Neuroplastic Training Workbook* which, if you're interested in pursuing this type of healing, could be helpful.[40] This can be valuable if you are dealing with chronic pain as a part of, or in addition to, autoimmunity.

Our discussion of these techniques is not meant to diminish the impact of pain caused by a genuine physical injury. Nerve damage or joint destruction can be caused by autoimmune (or other) conditions and can contribute to chronic pain.

But even in these cases, there is at least some degree of brain sensitization, where the brain has inadvertently become adept at tuning in to the signals of pain and thus amplifying them to an extent—especially if the pain has lasted more than three months. Incorporating these exercises allows you to desensitize your brain to pain, and then observe what is left in terms of actual physical pain coming from the body. This allows one to reduce the brain intensifying component and see what is stemming just from the affected body parts.

Brain on Fire

Based on Dr. Moskowitz's work, I developed a brief guided imagery exercise you can use to deal with pain. If you experience pain from an autoimmune disease (or any other condition) this is worth trying. It can be used in acute painful episodes and to attempt to reduce chronic pain:

- Begin in a comfortable position, sitting or lying down if you need to. Take a couple of slow, deep breaths. Notice the pain, wherever it is in your body. Then, visualize your brain. Imagine that there is a part of your brain that is receiving the signals of pain from your body, and that this region of the brain is on fire. You can picture some small flames or embers in that part of the brain to deepen your perception of this fire.
- Now, imagine that this fire has been extinguished. It is suddenly put out. Perhaps you picture taking a fire extinguisher and completely putting out the fire or throwing on a thick blanket that fully snuffs out the flames. Now you are seeing your brain in a state where it is not receiving any pain signals. Focus on the image of a brain that is not getting any messages of pain, and therefore completely free of pain. This brain—your brain—is in a state where it is completely free of pain signals.

- Check in with your body and notice if there is any change in the pain you are experiencing. If not, imagine your brain again and picture a new region of the brain that is on fire due to your pain signals. Then repeat the practice of extinguishing the fire. Continue the practice for at least a few minutes. Repeat this method several times throughout the day as needed, until you notice consistent reduction in your pain levels.

Body Image Tricks

The theory that body image affects pain perception was tested in a study of patients with hand osteoarthritis, where damaged joints serve as undeniable physical sources of pain. Researchers used a computerized device that displayed distorted images of the subject's own fingers in real-time, to make them appear smaller or thinner than they really were; subjects held their hands under a screen which displayed the distorted image. Remarkably, scientists found that almost all the patients had a 50 percent or greater temporary reduction in pain, and for a third of them there was complete elimination of pain for some time.[41]

Another study looked at patients with chronic hand pain and swelling and had them trick their brains into modifying their mental image of their hands.[42] Participants watched their hands performing certain movements either without binoculars, with binoculars (so their hands appeared bigger), or with inverted binoculars (so their hands appeared smaller). Researchers found that pain levels increased when participants viewed their hands as magnified and decreased when they saw their hands as smaller than they really were—more interestingly, they observed that *physical swelling* became measurably greater almost immediately in the patients' fingers when they saw their hands magnified, and significantly less when they saw their hands miniaturized.

The Shrinking Body Part

These experiments show that modification of your mental image of painful body parts can reduce the experience of pain in those areas. Here is an exercise that takes advantage of this principle:

- If you're experiencing pain in a certain part of your body, close your eyes and visualize it in your mind. First notice it as regular life-size and then imagine that the body part starts to become increasingly small. Imagine that it is shrinking, until it becomes microscopic. Imagine that the signals from that body part to your brain are getting correspondingly smaller and fainter. Practice for a few minutes and repeat this exercise as needed during the day. Eventually, you may notice that you have the capacity to reduce your experience of pain, at least to a certain extent.

Visualization for Fitness

A mind-boggling aspect of visualization is that studies show that people who imagine themselves flexing a muscle achieve actual physical strength gains in that muscle.

In an extraordinary experiment, scientists compared a group that did physical exercise with one that only imagined doing exercise. Both groups either actually did or imagined doing 15 contractions of a finger muscle daily. After four weeks, those who had done physical exercise increased their strength by 30 percent; those who had only imagined performing exercise also increased their muscle strength by a respectable 22 percent, while a control group that did not exercise had only a 3 percent change.[43]

This was replicated in another study where physical training increased strength by 53 percent, visualized training increased strength by 35 percent, and a control group showed no change.[44] This works because the same neural pathways are activated in visualizing exercise and exercise itself. Through neuroplasticity, those neuronal connections are primed and strengthened, leading to better real-world performance. This is the reason why world-class athletes sometimes incorporate visualization. It should be said that while visualization can lead to improvement, it's not a replacement for exercise. Instead, you can use this skill if you're unable to move your body, for whatever reason, or to help manage chronic pain from your autoimmune disorder.

VAGUS NERVE ACTIVATION

Let's switch gears and discuss how to enhance your parasympathetic response by targeting its main conduit, the vagus, your body's longest nerve. Vagus means "wanderer" in Latin, and this nerve meanders throughout your entire body, allowing your brain to have constant two-way communication with all your organs and tissues.

As we discussed, the parasympathetic nervous system is the "rest-and-digest" antidote to chronic stress. Helping to activate the vagus nerve can help support the parasympathetic nervous system to attain benefits such as decreasing inflammation, lowering blood pressure and heart rate, and lessening stress and anxiety.

Most mind-body practices, such as deep breathing, meditation, and yoga are believed to create their beneficial effects at least partially through stimulation of the vagus nerve.[45] Because the vocal cords are connected to the vagus nerve, singing or chanting is also an effective way to strengthen it. These are all accessible practices that activate your vagus nerve.

Immersing yourself in cold water or splashing cold water on your face can also galvanize the vagus nerve.[46] This is part of a repertoire of treatments in conventional medicine called "vagal maneuvers," often used in children to treat conditions that would benefit from activating the parasympathetic nervous system. These include applying ice or other cold stimulus to the face, stimulating the gag reflex with a tongue depressor, or techniques that create abdominal pressure, such as pressing the knees to the chest or having the child try to blow through an obstructed straw.[47]

The first time I witnessed the power of the vagus nerve in action was during a pediatric shift in a hospital, part of my medical training. A young child came in with an arrhythmia, for which vagal maneuvers are first-line therapy before going to pharmaceuticals. A senior pediatrician took a plastic bag filled with ice and placed it over the child's forehead and eyes for 30 seconds. Immediately, the heart rate slowed to normal—and stayed that way. I was stunned.

Vagus Nerve Electric Stimulation

Direct electrical stimulation of the vagus nerve is a promising new therapy. While this is a more invasive treatment, initial research is promising. A study of "drug-refractory" rheumatoid arthritis patients (not improving despite trying several conventional drugs for the disease) implanted a small vagus nerve stimulator in each of their chests and found that 80 percent of them had decreased markers of inflammation and improved symptoms. It significantly reduced signs and symptoms and was free of side effects, a remarkable result for a non-drug intervention in autoimmune patients who had not responded to multiple pharmaceutical treatments.[48]

Early evidence for using vagal nerve stimulation to treat autoimmune bowel diseases such as Crohn's disease or ulcerative colitis is also promising, leading to less inflammation and fewer hospital admissions.[49] It appears to work by activating the potential of the vagus nerve to trigger anti-inflammatory pathways and reduce levels of incendiary cytokines, immune system messengers that generate an inflammation response. Many clinical trials testing this therapy are ongoing; if you have failed multiple medications and are still struggling with severe auto-immune symptoms, ask your physician if this may be an option for you.

Vagus nerve stimulation with an implanted device is already an established therapeutic option for patients who fail traditional drug treatment of depression; this highlights the two-way signaling of the vagus, because the electrical impulses transmitted from the nerve back up to the brain can relieve symptoms of depression.[50]

Portable Electric Stimulation

A related tool that takes advantage of the principles of neuroplasticity is a portable, non-implanted device that provides very mild electrical stimulation to the tongue through a mouthpiece.[51] Now FDA-approved for improving balance and gait in multiple sclerosis (MS), the Portable Neuromodulation Stimulator (PoNS) device works by sending signals back through the nerves that supply the tongue, into the brain, where they can activate brain areas that regulate movement, sensation, sleep, and other functions.[52] Two small randomized, placebo-controlled trials showed that the PoNS device significantly improved balance, gait, and working memory in MS patients.[53]

This illustrates the neuroplastic concept that the brain has a huge network of self-regulating systems, which when activated by electrical signals or other means can help the brain to rebalance itself and positively impact many different functions. Thus it makes sense that the device is also showing benefits for patients with other neurological disorders, such as Parkinson's disease, stroke, and traumatic brain injury.[54] This device is FDA-approved for use in multiple sclerosis, so talk to your neurologist if you have MS to see if it is right for you. This is a promising therapy, but more research is needed to confirm its benefits and optimal usage in other conditions.

EMOTIONAL FREEDOM TECHNIQUE

Now we go from high tech to decidedly low tech, and review some techniques that rely on wisdom from Traditional Chinese Medicine. Emotional Freedom Technique (EFT) is a practice which seeks to defuse painful emotions associated with stress and trauma. It utilizes tapping on specific acupuncture points while repeating certain phrases to retrain the nervous system to reduce the emotional intensity associated with prior stressors or traumatic experiences (detailed instructions are available online in various sites such as https://www.thetappingsolution.com/).

I recommend EFT frequently as an adjunctive therapy for my autoimmune patients who are recovering from or dealing with ongoing stress. Many of them find it to be an effective treatment that helps them to reduce the negative effects of stress on their bodies.

Harvard Medical School psychiatrist Rick Leskowitz calls EFT "the most impressive intervention I've encountered in 25 years of work."[55] Research has confirmed its efficacy. A randomized controlled trial with war veterans found that EFT was 80 percent effective in treating the symptoms of PTSD as a stand-alone therapy, a remarkable success rate for a drug-free approach to a complex and challenging condition.[56]

A modified, simpler version of EFT, known as the First Aid Stress Tool (FAST), relies on the same principles (instructions available at https://firstaidstresstool.com/). EFT and FAST are completely free but highly effective treatments that you can do on your own at home.

Eye Movement Desensitization and Reprocessing (EMDR)

EMDR was developed in the 1980s, based on the observation that certain repetitive eye movements could reduce the intensity of troubling thoughts. Multiple randomized controlled trials have shown its efficacy as a supplemental therapy for the treatment of trauma in Post-Traumatic Stress Disorder (PTSD).[57]

Research has also documented the efficacy of EMDR to treat trauma from adverse childhood experiences (ACEs).[58] As we discussed in chapter 6, ACEs create an outsized risk for the development of autoimmunity and are often present in patients with autoimmune disorders.

Studies have also shown that EMDR can be a useful adjunctive treatment in various other conditions such as anxiety, depression, pain disorders, and chronic stress.[59] To find a therapist who practices this technique, you can either ask your psychotherapist for a referral (if they do not already practice it), or visit the EMDR International Association directory (https://www.emdria.org/find-an-emdr-therapist/).

COGNITIVE TOOLS

As mentioned in chapter 6, it is important to learn tools for working with your thoughts and emotions. While this is an area that most of us do not receive training in, I believe it can be a rewarding and productive domain to attend to in order to reduce the impact of stress on autoimmunity and enhance your mind-body resilience.

I resonate with these words from the Indian author and spiritual teacher Paramahansa Yogananda: "Watch your thoughts. All your experiences come percolating through your thoughts. It is the company of your thoughts that uplifts or degrades you."[60] There's also this pertinent message from the Buddha: "We are what we think. All that we are arises with our thoughts. With our thoughts, we make our world."[61] Both these statements highlight the importance of working with our thoughts. The goal is not to suppress or deny your thoughts but to develop some detachment from them, which can lead to improved emotional self-regulation.

When we tie together a series of thoughts, we create a story in our mind. The stories that we tell ourselves about our mind, body, and life constitute a big part of our identity. Dealing with your autoimmunity, you might have created a negative self-image or story about yourself based on the disease that caused you to limit yourself, or feel like you had to. Shifting our thoughts can change our story and transform how we think about ourselves—which can have a ripple effect on multiple life domains.

To help accomplish this, I'll share with you an eclectic set of tools compiled from my studies in mind-body medicine and psychology.

Upleveling

This approach draws on the work of self-help author Ken Keyes, Jr. In writings about "The Mechanism of Unhappiness," he spoke about this concept of changing our mental "addictions" to preferences.[62] In this case, what Keyes means by addiction is not what we usually think of, such as dependence on a drug, but rather, something you believe you *must* have in order to be happy. When you don't have it, you feel resentful, negative, or irritated. This increases your suffering and detracts from your ability to be happy.

In this technique, you try to become aware of the unfulfilled expectation that is triggering you to feel offended, upset, or angry—and work on shifting it to a preference. He described this approach as Upleveling.

Let's look at an example. You're dealing with a new diagnosis of lupus, and among other symptoms, you've found a troublesome new sensitivity: if you are out in the sun for more than a few minutes, even with sunscreen, you develop an itchy, red rash. You used to be an avid gardener, spending hours outside on most days, and suddenly this is no longer an option. You might become frustrated and annoyed. In this case, you are "addicted" to the idea that you should not be sensitive to sun exposure.

If you practice Upleveling, you can change that to a preference. You would rather not be sensitive to sunlight—it's not something anyone would wish for—but since this is part of the disease, you can still accept it without negativity. It is what it is, just the reality of the situation. Then, you can make the best of things and possibly come up with creative solutions. For example, you might purchase long sleeves and long pants with a high sun protection rating, and shift your gardening to short sessions either at dawn or dusk. You realize that you can do things in a new and different way—and still be happy.

Let's take another example. You are in a meeting at work, and someone criticizes one of your ideas. Your immediate reaction might be to become upset and annoyed. How dare this person question an idea that you came up with! In this case, your "addiction" is to not have anyone criticize your ideas. When that occurs, you immediately experience some frustration and, perhaps as a result, other negative feelings.

The alternative is to practice Upleveling, shifting that addiction to a preference. So, you might prefer that no one criticize your ideas, but if they do, you are still okay with it—because it is only a preference. This removes the emotional charge from the experience. You might even be able to objectively determine whether that person had a valid criticism, and whether you can take something positive from it. This way, you don't lose your peace of mind. Most importantly, you don't trigger internal mental stress, and its associated harmful physiology.

As I began to practice his technique, I realized I had a lot of addictions! My mind had so many needs and requirements about wanting everything to be a particular way. As is the way life usually works, things happened all the time that did not align with my "addictions." In becoming aware of these, I was able to gradually practice Upleveling those addictions to preferences, and increase my sense of peace and ease while navigating the challenges of everyday life.

Reframing

Reframing is a well-known approach that is part of Cognitive Behavioral Therapy (CBT). Essentially, it involves taking a curious, questioning perspective on unconstructive thoughts and reframing them into more useful thoughts. While CBT is often administered by a professional, these methods of examining and challenging negative patterns of thought can be implemented on your own.

There are a multitude of different methods under this umbrella, but here are a few examples:

- Positive Reframing—this involves consciously thinking about the upsides to a negative situation that you may not have focused on. It does not mean you are in denial about what's happening, but perhaps you think about lessons to be learned from a challenging situation or something related to it that you could be grateful for, no matter how small.
- Not Personalizing—in this method, you remind yourself not to take things personally. We often think that others act or behave the way they do because of us, but in reality, their actions may not have anything to do with us. Whatever someone does, thinks, or says, remind yourself not to take it personally. Also, do not blame yourself for things that you have little or no control over.
- Modifying Language—you might find yourself thinking in absolute terms, such as "things will never get better" or "I will always feel like this." Simply rephrasing those thoughts with less extreme words can be a good starting point. Reflecting on examples in your life that disprove these blanket statements can be helpful.
- Avoiding All-or-Nothing Thinking—in this pattern, we tend to think of situations as black and white with no gray in between, as either a complete success or a total failure. In reality, life is full of gray and focusing on the nuance in any scenario can help to avoid catastrophizing.
- Questioning Expectations—sometimes if we set rigid expectations for ourselves, we can become disappointed if those expectations are not met. Perhaps you're stressed out by the expectation that you should always be making more money, without realizing that this is a notion you have created, perhaps from earlier life experiences, but that you do not need to hold onto if it does not serve you.

Choosing Better-Feeling Thoughts

Borrowed from neuroscience, this technique takes advantage of the concept that every thought is associated with a certain feeling or emotion—we touched on this in chapter 6. To gain insight into the nature of the thoughts you might be having, you can delve into the way you are feeling.

Esther and Jerry Hicks discuss this approach in their book *The Astonishing Power of Emotions*. The theory is that you should be feeling good most of the time, and if you are not, you can look to your feelings to guide you as you gradually shift your thoughts; if your thoughts begin to change in a positive direction, you should notice an improved feeling.

The Hickses acknowledge that it is not possible to switch immediately from a completely negative thought to a fully positive thought, but even changing to a thought that is slightly less negative can help you feel a little bit better—and that is a move in the right direction. They write: "So, start where you are (since you have no other choice), and try to find increasingly better-feeling thoughts... It is your work to continue to reach for thoughts and feelings of greater relief and comfort..."[63]

Here's an example of this process in action in someone who just received a diagnosis of multiple sclerosis, and was further disturbed by seeing a patient in a wheelchair on their way out of the clinic:

> *"This is a very scary diagnosis.*
> *I should've taken better care of myself.*
> *Why did this happen to me?*
> *I hope that's not where I'm headed... [shifting thoughts]*
> *I don't know what that person's story is.*
> *That person may be better today than a month ago.*
> *That person's experience and my experience are unrelated.*
> *This diagnosis has caused me to ask for even more wellness.*
> *On a vibrational level, I am at my greatest state of wellness."*[64]

SOCIAL CONNECTION

Something often overlooked as part of an overall health program is the importance of community. A meta-analysis of 148 studies with over 300,000 people concluded that having strong social support has a bigger impact on longevity than physical activity, toxin exposure, and even smoking 15 cigarettes a day![65] This is a startling illustration of the profound impact that our social connections have on our health.

The quality of your social relationships is one of the most fundamental determinants of health. With the recent COVID pandemic and many things shifting to online, an epidemic of isolation and loneliness has become greatly exacerbated. This is critical in autoimmunity because researchers have shown that the experience of loneliness can lead to changes in gene expression that increase inflammation and negatively impact the immune system.[66]

The ways in which we might find meaningful connection may differ greatly. I encourage you to try to enhance your social connections in multiple ways, to bring more richness and depth to your relationships, because a strong, diverse network of social integration is the best way to optimize your immune function and overall health.

Here are some ideas to explore:

- Join a group of people with like-minded interests. Websites such as meetup.com or citysocializer.com can provide local options.
- Plan activities with your loved ones. We sometimes take for granted the people closest to us. Scheduling specific activities where you can spend quality time with your loved ones is a great way to strengthen those relationships.
- Take a class. Your local civic center, YMCA, or community college can be good starting points.
- Send a thank-you note. This could be to someone whom you are grateful for but have not recently expressed your feelings. You will get the additional benefit of gratitude which is a powerful practice in its own right and can potentially improve sleep quality, blood pressure, eating behaviors, and even inflammation markers.[67]
- Volunteer. Studies show that doing volunteer work in any form that appeals to you can be beneficial for health.[68]
- Get to know your neighbors. Since my family moved to a new home, we have made extra effort to get to know our neighbors, and the rewards have been home-grown vegetables, shared desserts, and new friendships.
- Invest some time in your coworkers. This might entail joining company get-togethers, spending some additional time talking to those you work with, or meeting with them outside of work to grab a tea or coffee.

For those who can't be fully mobile, the following strategies can be especially helpful.

- Get a pet. Animals can often provide companionship without judgment (and can provide some additional bacterial exposure to help your microbiome!). Studies show that having a dog or cat in the household improves the microbiome, especially in children.[69]
- Reach out to a family member or friend that you have lost touch with.
- Become more active in your church or spiritual/religious organization if this is meaningful to you.
- Connect with others online. While it is imperative to meet people in person, there are myriad ways to connect with folks online as well.

We met Hannah at the beginning of the chapter; she was struggling with Mixed Connective Tissue Disease despite being on anti-inflammatories and an immunosuppressant medicine.

Hannah shared that her childhood had been difficult. Her father had been an alcoholic and was abusive toward her mother. She had witnessed domestic violence at home and suffered from physical abuse herself. She described being in a state of constant vigilance for years, which led to chronic insomnia as well as what she described as "always feeling on edge."

Her escape had been academics—she focused all her energy on doing well in school. She won a scholarship to college in a neighboring state—and left home, never to return. Later, Hannah graduated law school at the top of her class. She had created her own path and been doing well at a top-tier law firm for the past few years.

Hannah had worked hard to distance herself from her past and was not eager to dredge things up. I told her that while it was not necessary to relive her traumatic experiences, giving attention to them was essential because I suspected that they were holding her back from healing in the present moment. She agreed to work with a trauma-focused therapist, who also referred her to a bodyworker trained in working with patients who had experienced abuse. In addition, she practiced Emotional Freedom Technique (EFT) and found restorative yoga to be very helpful. Her therapist recommended a weighted blanket (a blanket with weight added to it to help a person feel calm and soothed) and introduced her to the First Aid Stress Tool (FAST), which she found comforting.

As she incorporated several of these techniques daily to activate her para-sympathetic nervous system and reduce the amount of time she spent in chronic "fight-or-flight" mode, Hannah noticed that her sensitivity began to reduce. She became able to tolerate more foods, and could take low doses of some supplements.

She found that her sleep was slowly improving, and her joint swelling and rashes became less frequent. She eventually started a daily meditation practice, which was very beneficial for her in addition to the yoga. Her symptoms eventually normalized, and she was able to discontinue the ibuprofen and achieve remission with just the Plaquenil.

PART THREE

REACH THE NEXT LEVEL OF HEALTH

CHAPTER 12

Modulate the Immune System

After delivering her first child, 34-year-old Jada was struggling with severe ulcer-ative colitis. During the stress and sleepless nights of her baby's first year, she began noticing the GI symptoms. When she finally received a diagnosis, she was started on an oral medication called mesalamine, but this didn't relieve her symptoms. That's when she came to see me.

With specialized testing I discovered Jada had sensitivities to gluten and dairy, and severe GI inflammation. I started her on an elimination diet and high doses of curcumin and another anti-inflammatory supplement called Boswellia.

After a few months, she reported significant improvement, but felt like she could not continue the strict diet. With a young child at home and a busy job, she was not able to manage a restrictive diet and returned to consuming gluten and dairy. Her symptoms worsened. She asked me if there was any option for a "permanent fix"—one that would allow her to return to eating the diet she had been previously.

In this chapter, we'll talk about strategies that can help modulate the immune system now that some of the root causes for autoimmunity have been addressed. Many techniques in this chapter rely on the principle of hormesis (a beneficial stress that triggers favorable body changes), which I introduced in chapter 7.

In my experience, these techniques work better after tackling the five driv-ers of autoimmunity we discussed earlier in the book. Trying to modulate your immune system while these factors are simultaneously driving autoimmunity is less effective.

We begin by investigating some supplements. In chapters 7 and 8 you were introduced to glutathione and curcumin, which I consider to be core supple-ments for patients with autoimmunity. Vitamin D is also essential, and we'll explore why in chapter 14. Another compound I consider invaluable as part of the TIGER Protocol is sulforaphane.

SULFORAPHANE

Sulforaphane is a compound found in broccoli that was discovered by researchers at Johns Hopkins University. There are over 2,000 research studies documenting its benefits, which include reducing inflammation by activating the Nrf-2 pathway, boosting the immune system by increasing activity of natural killer cells, crossing the blood-brain barrier (many compounds are unable to) and optimizing brain function, combating oxidative stress, and exerting antimicrobial activity.[1] Like curcumin, this phytochemical appears to have multiple benefits across diverse organ systems.

While sulforaphane is present in cruciferous vegetables, which should be consumed often, the single best food source is broccoli sprouts—that's why they are an integral component of both the TIGER Protocol Phase 1 and Phase 2 Diets.[2] In case broccoli sprouts are not available to you in your local stores, you can sprout your own at home from broccoli seeds purchased online. It's important to note here that *alfalfa* sprouts may worsen lupus and other autoimmune conditions because they contain L-canavanine, which could contribute to inflammation.[3] For this reason, I suggest you avoid them. They are unique among sprouts in terms of autoimmune risk, as other sprouts have not been shown to be harmful.

Food Hacks to Maximize Sulforaphane Levels

The research showed that eating raw broccoli led to faster absorption and higher blood levels of sulforaphane when compared to eating cooked broccoli.[4] The reason for this is that an inactive precursor compound in broccoli needs to be converted by the enzyme myrosinase into sulforaphane, but this enzyme is inactivated by heat.

A trick to increase sulforaphane in cooked cruciferous vegetables is to add a source of this myrosinase enzyme, such as mustard seed powder, to them. Per one study, when 1 g of brown mustard powder was added to cooked broccoli, the bioavailability of sulforaphane was increased by more than 400 percent.[5]

BAKING SODA IN AUTOIMMUNITY

Yes, this same inexpensive powder you might use to control the odor in your fridge can also help to modulate your immune system. Consuming baking soda reduces inflammation via positive effects on your nervous system and your spleen, an organ in your left upper abdomen that filters your blood and regulates immune function. You probably haven't heard of the power of baking soda as there is little financial incentive to promote such a low-cost item.

The mechanism behind this is intriguing. One study found that ingesting baking soda shifted the pattern of immune cells known as macrophages in the spleen from pro-inflammatory M1 cells to anti-inflammatory M2 cells; there was also an increase in the number of T-regulatory cells, which calm autoimmune activity, and triggering of anti-inflammatory pathways through the vagus nerve.[6] The dose used in the study was 2 grams (around half a teaspoon) dissolved in 8 ounces of water daily.

This humble additive has been studied for improving exercise performance for over 50 years.[7] Research consistently shows benefits for enhancing endurance in high-intensity workouts (weight training or resistance training), interval training, and in aerobic exercise.[8]

It also can be beneficial for the kidney. In patients with chronic kidney disease, supplementation with baking soda may slow the decline in kidney function usually seen in the condition.[9] These other benefits are due to its positive effect on acid/base balance in the body.

Dosing and Contraindications

Baking soda contains sodium, which can be problematic if you maintain a low-sodium diet due to high blood pressure. It can also cause gastrointestinal side effects such as gas, abdominal pain, or diarrhea. Baking soda can interact with medications like aspirin and prednisone. Consult with your physician before beginning use. It should not be given to children or pregnant women. Do not take baking soda without diluting in water, because it can irritate the mouth and throat. Avoid *baking powder*, which is not the same as baking soda.

I suggest starting with a quarter teaspoon dissolved in 8 ounces of water once a day on an empty stomach and increasing as tolerated to the dosage of half a teaspoon daily. Since we do not have long-term safety data in autoimmune disease I would suggest a regimen of periodic use, e.g., one month on/two months off.

OTHER SUPPLEMENTS

There are some other supplements that show promise for autoimmune patients, although more research is needed to verify. One example is the herb Rehmannia glutinosa, which is often used in Chinese medicine.

Among patients with lupus in Taiwan, rehmannia use was one of the herbs that comprised an integrative medicine strategy associated with decreased risk of lupus nephritis, a common kidney complication of lupus.[10] In animal studies, catalpol, a key component of rehmannia, was found to have beneficial effects in models of rheumatoid arthritis and multiple sclerosis.[11] In Korean women, rehmannia was also shown to have prebiotic effects, increasing levels of Bifido-bacteria and Actinobacteria after eight weeks.[12]

Another example is black cumin. You may recall in chapter 8 I suggested incorporating black cumin for its antimicrobial activity. It also has potent anti-inflammatory potential. A randomized placebo-controlled trial in 40 patients with Hashimoto's thyroiditis found that black cumin reduced levels of anti-thyroid peroxidase antibody and increased levels of thyroid hormone.[13] In women with rheumatoid arthritis, black cumin significantly reduced joint pain and inflammation and morning stiffness over one month when compared to placebo.[14]

Both of these herbal supplements are promising, but more clinical trials are needed to investigate their efficacy.

COLD EXPOSURE IMPROVES IMMUNITY

Intermittent cold exposure is a simple and free hormetic therapy (where a beneficial stress triggers favorable body changes) that may strengthen immunity. A study of 3,000 people who took a hot shower followed by a cold shower for 30–90 seconds found that those who took cold showers were 29 percent less likely to call in sick.[15]

Research also suggests that cold showers may have some antidepressant and pain-relieving properties.[16] There is evidence to support the use of cold-water therapy in fibromyalgia and other chronic pain conditions.[17] A meta-analysis of 23 studies found that cold water immersion is effective for enhancing recovery and reducing fatigue after sports, which is why many athletes use it.[18]

A bonus is that exposure to cold speeds up metabolism and fat burning through beneficial effects on hormones such as adrenaline; one caveat is that shivering is a necessary mechanism to activate fat breakdown, so if you're seeking to promote weight loss, do not resist the urge to shiver.[19] Another study found that cold exposure increased resting energy expenditure, glucose utilization, and insulin sensitivity by having beneficial effects on a beneficial type of body fat known as brown fat. Brown fat regulates body temperature and impacts metabolism.[20]

An easy way to incorporate cold exposure is to turn the water as cold as you can handle for the final 30 seconds of your shower. Per the research, exposing yourself to more than 90 seconds of cold doesn't increase the efficacy. If it appeals, and you have access to one, you can soak in an ice bath; going outdoors without a jacket on a cold day (briefly), also encourages hormetic stress.

In chapter 7, I reviewed the health benefits of sauna therapy in detail; it can help with detoxification, immunity, inflammation, pain reduction, heart health, and cellular repair. I mention it again here as a reminder that I consider this an essential practice for patients on the autoimmune spectrum.

The combination of frequent cold exposure and sauna therapy is a very powerful one. Both strategies rely on hormesis to fire up multiple health-promoting mechanisms in the entire body.

INTERMITTENT FASTING (IF)

Fasting can help modulate the immune system and induce fundamental changes in immune cells. You were introduced to IF in chapter 9; if you recall, IF enhances diversity and boosts the levels of certain keystone species in the microbiome. Studies show that fasting can also quell inflammation, which is key for autoimmune patients.

In a study with rheumatoid arthritis patients, fasting was linked to reductions in the inflammatory markers C-reactive protein (CRP), interleukin-6 (IL-6), and erythrocyte sedimentation rate (ESR), which correlated with reduction in joint pain and disease activity.[21] Another study in overweight individuals found that fasting shifted the makeup of circulating immune cells to a more anti-inflammatory pattern by increasing the levels of the beneficial T-regulatory cells that quell autoimmunity.[22]

Researchers who study fasting sometimes direct their focus toward practicing Muslims during Ramadan; the holiday involves intermittent fasting for around 17 hours daily for a month or so. Studies have shown that IF during Ramadan leads to reduction in inflammatory markers such as CRP, IL-6, leptin, and tumor necrosis factor-alpha.[23]

When it comes to autoimmune conditions, fasting can be particularly beneficial, as it reduces the antigenic load in the diet—an antigen is a protein that your immune system is exposed to (and could react negatively to in some cases). By fasting, you drastically reduce the number of food antigens encountered daily. As we discussed in chapter 5, the immune system can react negatively to certain foods via food sensitivities and allergies, which can play a key role in autoimmunity (for example, MS patients are more likely to harbor food sensitivity antibodies against dairy proteins than healthy controls.)[24]

If your immune system happens to be overreacting to several foods as part of food sensitivity and/or allergy, removing these from your diet temporarily can help calm the immune system. This is the basis for the elimination of certain food groups in the TIGER Protocol Phase I Diet, but is also another mechanism that can be helpful for anyone on the autoimmune spectrum.

Fasting Across the Autoimmune Spectrum

Fasting has its benefits, but there are three autoimmune conditions where it can be particularly useful.

Rheumatoid Arthritis (RA). If you're living with RA, fasting may be the right strategy for you. A review of four controlled studies concluded that fasting followed by a vegetarian diet for at least three months in patients with RA is likely to have a clinically significant benefit.[25] In my own practice, I usually will suggest a trial of a vegetarian diet in patients with RA at least once to see if it is helpful.

Psoriasis. If you struggle with this painful skin condition, you may be motivated to learn that a study of 108 people doing IF during Ramadan found that their skin significantly improved over that time.[26]

Multiple Sclerosis (MS). In a small, randomized study of 16 MS patients, intermittent fasting over 15 days induced significant changes in the microbiota and beneficial changes in the number and function of certain immune cells.[27] Dr. Valter Longo, a researcher from the University of Southern California, has popularized the idea of a Fasting-Mimicking Diet (FMD), a 3–5 day reduced-calorie eating plan designed to replicate the benefits of fasting. A randomized trial in 60 patients with MS found that FMD was safe and associated with improvements in quality-of-life measures, showing that it has the potential to improve autoimmunity, as has been shown in animal studies.[28]

Fasting Improves Metabolic Profiles

In addition to the immune modulating and anti-inflammatory effects that are especially helpful in autoimmunity, fasting has other health-promoting benefits. Chief among these are metabolic improvements, such as reduced blood pressure, cholesterol, and blood sugar—and weight loss through the promotion of fat burning.[29]

IF has also been shown to normalize metabolic hormones such as insulin, leptin, and ghrelin[30]—and increase levels of growth hormone, a key compound produced by the pituitary gland in the brain that supports muscle, bone, and metabolic health.[31]

Fasting in Practice

When it comes to autoimmunity, there is not one type of fasting that has been proven superior to another. Several different types of fasting have been researched and shown potential in the studies above. My recommendation is that you experiment with different types to see what works well for you. It is best to begin with shorter, less frequent fasts and then build up as tolerated. Drinking lots of water to make sure you are well-hydrated is important. Here are a few options for getting started.

Time-Restricted Eating (TRE). TRE is a variant of IF in which you restrict your eating to a certain window of time, typically eight hours or less. For example, you might consume your food within an 8-hour window from 11 a.m. to 7 p.m., and fast for the other 16 hours (this has also been called 16:8 intermittent fasting). To begin, try this on two nonconsecutive days of the week, such as Monday/Thursday. As you gain experience with this, you can gradually increase the frequency of the practice (# days/week) and shorten the daily window of time during which you are eating.

Fasting-Mimicking Diet (FMD). As discussed above, FMD involves periodically cycling through days of limited caloric intake. A pilot study looking at FMD over three months found weight loss of about five pounds and reductions in abdominal fat, cholesterol, and blood sugar.[32] Animal studies suggest a rejuvenating effect and positive impact on the immune system, including reduced autoimmunity.[33] A commercially available product called Prolon[34] provides all the food necessary to complete a 5-day cycle of FMD; it is also possible to make your own version at home with comparable foods using online instructions.

Alternate-Day Fasting (ADF). ADF involves alternating days of regular calorie consumption with low calorie days, where you might consume one-third or less of your usual caloric intake. This strategy can be helpful especially if you also want to lose additional weight, according to one research review of over 100 studies.[35] If trying ADF, I suggest practicing for a couple of weeks at a time, then take a break for a few weeks if necessary to prevent excessive weight loss.

Fasting Contraindications

Fasting is not recommended for children, people with a history of eating disorders, or those who are pregnant or breastfeeding. Use caution if you are underweight or taking any prescription medications.

I recommend avoiding vigorous exercise especially while you are new to fasting. Drinking plenty of water, perhaps with added electrolytes, is essential. Avoid exposure to temperature extremes such as the heat of a sauna during a fast. Consult your physician before beginning any fasting regimen.

PHOTOBIOMODULATION

Photobiomodulation (PBM), the application of light for therapeutic effect, can be an effective tool to modulate the immune system. PBM—also called Low-Level Light Therapy (LLLT)—has been used since the 1960s in clinical practice and is FDA-approved for the relief of muscle and joint pain.[36]

PBM can be performed using either lasers or LED lights. The use of low-level lasers has been studied in various conditions, with red light being the most common therapy.

How Light Heals

To understand how light therapy works, you need to know about mitochondria. These are the microscopic but potent structures (often called your "power generators") present within every single cell of your body. They are responsible for making energy and coordinating cellular activities. Mitochondria are activated by light exposure, which leads to greater energy production and reduced inflammation.

Red light therapy, the most common PBM, does not have the harmful UV rays from sunlight (or lights used in tanning booths)—and so it does not hurt or burn your skin. The lasers that are used do not heat the skin significantly, which is why PBM is also called "cold laser."

There are three well-researched mechanisms of how PBM works that are pertinent for autoimmunity. It combats inflammation by increasing the production of certain anti-inflammatory compounds called cytokines, reducing the number of pro-inflammatory cells, and increasing the number of immune cells that clean up cellular debris and damage and kill pathogens.[37] In addition, PBM reduces oxidative stress, which is typically elevated in autoimmune disease, and can increase the production of ATP, the body's main energy currency (countering the fatigue that is a common symptom seen in autoimmune conditions).[38]

In terms of autoimmune conditions, Dr. Fred Kahn, vascular surgeon and early pioneer in laser therapy, has successfully used laser PBM to treat patients with rheumatoid arthritis, fibromyalgia, and other chronic pain and joint conditions.[39]

Dr. Kahn's work is consistent with research showing that laser therapy successfully reduces pain. In patients with osteoarthritis of the knee, low-level laser therapy was found in one study to significantly improve pain, functionality, and range of motion when compared to a placebo laser.[40] This confirmed an earlier double-blind, placebo-controlled trial showing that low-level laser was an effective treatment for painful knee osteoarthritis.[41]

A meta-analysis of 18 studies concluded that laser therapy is effective for the reduction of pain in a variety of musculoskeletal conditions.[42] The effects may also last for some time after the laser therapy concludes—a review of six studies of PBM for plantar fasciitis, a painful inflammation of the feet, concluded that the therapy could significantly reduce foot pain, and that the benefits lasted for around three months after treatment was completed.[43]

LED Light Therapy

The emergence of LEDs, which are lower in cost and more widely available than lasers, has led to the use of red LED light as a PBM therapy.

When applied to the scalp, LED light penetrates through and causes positive changes in the brain, such as improved blood flow and enhanced brain cell function, and shows promise as an adjunctive therapy for traumatic brain injury, stroke, and neurodegenerative disease.[44] In relationship to autoimmunity, PBM has also been shown to reduce neuroinflammation in animal models of multiple sclerosis.[45]

The Bottom Line

PBM appears to be most effective for reducing inflammation and treating pain, so if you are experiencing pain as part of, or in addition to, your autoimmune condition, this may be a modality worth exploring. If you do want to try PBM, check with your physician first to make sure there is no contraindication. If you can proceed, some doctors offer PBM, as do some salons and spas. You can procure red LED light bulbs to install at home. There are also portable devices available for purchase and home use. When selecting a device, choose one that has been third-party tested for safety.

PULSED ELECTROMAGNETIC FIELD (PEMF) THERAPY

PEMF therapy is another useful approach for addressing pain and inflammation—it uses devices that emit a low-level magnetic field to create favorable changes in the body. It has a substantial body of research to support its efficacy. It has been used in conventional medicine for decades as a noninvasive FDA-approved treatment for poorly healing fractures, where the only alternative is an uncertain surgery.[46]

The use of magnets in Western medicine is well-established but not widely known. Transcranial magnetic stimulation, which uses a pulsed electromagnetic field to stimulate brain regions that regulate mood, is a clinically proven treatment for depression, especially in people who have not responded to other treatments.[47]

In addition to helping wound healing, multiple studies show that PEMF is effective in relieving pain and inflammation. A review of 11 randomized control trials found that it alleviated pain and stiffness and improved function in patients with joint osteoarthritis.[48] A meta-analysis of 14 randomized control trials found that the treatment improved chronic low back pain.[49]

PEMF is generally safe if used as recommended. Side effects include temporary pain, fatigue, or dizziness. People with pacemakers or other implanted devices should not use this therapy because of magnetic interference. It should be avoided by women who are pregnant or breastfeeding.

As with any new treatment, check with your doctor before beginning. Many devices are available including machines of various sizes and shapes and mats that you can lie on. As with all therapies, I recommend starting with the lowest "dosage," which in this case translates to minimal duration and intensity of treatment, and then building up gradually.

LOW DOSE NALTREXONE (LDN)

LDN is a compounded prescription medicine that we use in integrative medicine to regulate the immune system. Although this is a pharmaceutical, it differs from most autoimmune drugs in that it does not suppress the immune system but rather has a modulatory effect and actuates the body's self-healing pathways.

Naltrexone in standard dosages is used for alcohol and opioid abuse disorders. While effective at high doses (50 mg) for addictions, at low doses (5 mg or less), naltrexone has completely different properties—it increases the body's production of endorphins, the so-called "feel-good" hormones responsible for the runner's high. These compounds have anti-inflammatory and immune-regulating properties. The term "endorphin" is derived from "endogenous morphine" (the opioid pain reliever which mimics their effects).

LDN has the effect of blocking opioid receptors in the brain for a few hours. This transient blockade leads to an increase in synthesis of endorphins such as beta-endorphin and met-enkephalin.[50] Endorphins produced by the body modulate the immune system (via both direct and indirect effects on various immune system cells) and reduce inflammation.

Studies show that LDN can help improve symptoms and reduce immunosuppressant medication usage in ailments such as multiple sclerosis, inflammatory bowel disease, and rheumatoid arthritis.[51] It also has been shown to reduce pain and inflammation in a chronic pain syndrome known as fibromyalgia, which is believed to have an autoimmune component.[52]

LDN in Practice

LDN is made and dispensed through specialized pharmacies called compounding pharmacies, which make nontraditional doses and preparations of medicines not available in standard pharmacies. A doctor's prescription is needed. Although it may not be covered by insurance, it can be obtained for ~$25/month for a three-month supply. Compounding pharmacies that offer LDN at affordable prices include CareFirstRx Specialty Pharmacy, Belmar Pharmacy in Colorado, or Skip's Pharmacy in Florida (all three are mail-order pharmacies).

It has minimal side effects and is typically well tolerated. The most common side effect is vivid dreams, which may cause sleep disruption (most of the studies use nighttime dosing of LDN, which can sometimes cause this reaction). If this occurs and persists for more than a few days, switching to take LDN with breakfast instead of at bedtime can resolve the issue.

LDN should not be taken by patients on chronic opiate medicines, because it will limit their efficacy. Check with your physician to see if it is appropriate for you.

EXPERIMENTAL THERAPIES

As the prevalence of autoimmunity grows, so does research into therapies to treat it. These are not ready for prime time, but in the future, they may offer innovative breakthroughs in the treatment of autoimmune disease.

The BCG Vaccine. Commonly used to protect against tuberculosis in the developing world, this vaccine has been shown to have an immunomodulatory effect that suppresses overactive immune systems.[53] It was discovered that it protects against pediatric asthma and is effective when treating bladder cancer.[54] It is being studied for efficacy in diseases like multiple sclerosis and type 1 diabetes.[55]

Chimeric Antigen Receptor T-Cells (CAR-T). Currently in use for certain types of aggressive cancers, this treatment can reprogram abnormal immune cells in the patient's body. It is traditionally used to help the immune system recognize and eliminate tumor cells in leukemia or lymphoma.[56] German scientists employed this therapy successfully in a young woman with severe lupus that did not respond to conventional treatments.[57] The patient saw a rapid reduction of lupus antibodies and an improved immune system, with complete remission in six months.

Stem Cells. All of your body's cells are derived from stem cells. While they can become many different types of cells, stem cells also help to keep inflammation under control and repair and regenerate damaged tissue. Some promising research involves using stem cells to treat autoimmunity.[58] A stem cell infusion in treatment-refractory RA patients (who had not responded to strong drugs called TNF-alpha inhibitors) led to significant clinical improvement compared to placebo; a single IV infusion had benefits lasting at least ten months.[59]

FECAL MICROBIOTA TRANSPLANT

Fecal microbiota transplantation (FMT), may seem unusual, but it can be a potent therapy for resetting the immune system. Stool from a healthy donor is introduced into the digestive tract of the patient, either through a tube passed through the nose into the stomach or directly into the colon through enema or colonoscopy.

FMT has been proven to be the best therapy for recurrent *Clostridium difficile* infection, which is a serious GI infection causing severe diarrhea and colitis. While this can be treated with antibiotics, the recurrence rate is high, and resistance to the antibiotics develops quickly. Remarkably, FMT consistently cures even the most refractory *Clostridium difficile* infections with success rates far superior to any antibiotic.

FMT for Autoimmunity

A meta-analysis concluded that FMT is likely to help induce clinical remission in ulcerative colitis and Crohn's disease, where the immune system attacks and damages the intestines.[60] I have had several patients with ulcerative colitis receive fecal transplant as part of research studies, with generally positive results.

Animal studies and some human case reports suggest that FMT may also be helpful for multiple sclerosis.[61] Clinical trials have also shown benefit in autism disorder in children and for alleviating depression and anxiety through effects on the gut-brain axis.[62] This is an area of active research and I hope that FMT will have more applications for autoimmune conditions in the future.

YOU HAVE OPTIONS

The many evidence-based therapies we covered in this chapter make for a valuable supplement to the TIGER Protocol. Combined with the promise shown in the experimental therapies we touched on above, there's much hope for the future. I hope you will leverage these practices to advance your health even further. To end, let's follow up with Jada, who we met at the beginning of the chapter.

While going dairy- and gluten-free helped Jada relieve her ulcerative colitis symptoms, that style of eating was unsustainable for her. She was looking for a more long-term solution.

At that time, a research study at the University of California, San Francisco (UCSF) was recruiting patients with ulcerative colitis for fecal microbiota transplant (FMT). I had seen some promising initial research for patients with ulcerative colitis and talked to Jada about the opportunity. I counseled her about the risks and benefits. She was interested and decided to enroll in the clinical trial.

A few months later, she received the procedure as part of the study at UCSF. The next day, her symptoms were dramatically better. She received FMT twice within a month as part of the study protocol. Her bowel movements became unrecognizable to her—because they were so normal and so different from what she had gotten used to. She said, "It feels like I am passing someone else's poop." This was not inaccurate, because essentially, she had received a transplant of someone else's optimal microbiome, and that was leading to her new normal bowel movements (stool is mostly comprised of gut bacteria). Under the supervision of her gastroenterologist, she tapered off her oral medication. The gains she had made persisted.

Since then, she has continued to be clinically stable off medications. If she overdoes it on gluten or dairy, she starts to get some GI symptoms, but fortunately they resolve with dietary changes and bone broth. Her primary goal was to have flexibility in her diet, and the FMT allowed her to achieve this.

CHAPTER 13

What to Do If You're Not Getting Better

Brandy was a 43-year-old African American woman with rheumatoid arthritis. She had been diagnosed with the illness in her late 30s during a stressful stretch of her career and learned to manage it with a few different medications. However, her symptoms were never fully gone, and having made a change to a slower-paced job, she was ready to look into things more deeply.

I saw her and put her through the TIGER Protocol. There were not many toxins or infections present, and her gut health was pretty good overall. After completing the protocol, she felt only a bit different and was disappointed. At that point I started to look into other areas.

If you follow the protocol, you should see results; however, there's always a possibility that even after following all the recommendations I've offered so far, you may still experience symptoms. Here, we'll review some potential causes for lingering symptoms, and actions you can take if you aren't feeling better.

SMALL INTESTINAL BACTERIAL OVERGROWTH (SIBO)

In healthy individuals, there are a very small number of good bacteria in the small intestine when compared to the large intestine, where the bulk of the microbiota resides. SIBO is a condition within which there is a shift toward potential pathogens such as Klebsiella and *E. coli* within the small bowel, as well as an overgrowth of these bad actors where they don't belong.[1]

This dysbiosis and overgrowth in the small bowel leads to a number of profoundly negative consequences. They include increased intestinal permeability, impaired absorption of essential nutrients, and various GI symptoms such as gas, bloating, constipation and/or diarrhea; outside the GI tract, SIBO can contribute to immune dysregulation and systemic inflammation.[2]

There is evidence for a high occurrence of SIBO in several autoimmune conditions such as type 1 diabetes,[3] inflammatory bowel disease (Crohn's disease and ulcerative colitis),[4] multiple sclerosis,[5] autoimmune liver disease,[6] and systemic sclerosis.[7] If you're experiencing persistent digestive symptoms, consider asking your physician to test you for SIBO because of its GI, immune, and systemic consequences.

SIBO can be diagnosed by a special type of test known as a breath test, which involves drinking a solution such as lactulose that can be metabolized by bacteria and measuring breath samples over three hours to determine the GI levels of these bacteria. This test can be ordered by a gastroenterologist (in which case insurance coverage may be possible) or by a functional medicine doctor.

The conventional treatment for SIBO is with prescription antibiotics like rifaximin and neomycin; some studies have shown comparable efficacy for herbal antimicrobial supplements as well (from the companies Metagenics and Biotics Research).[8] If you suspect that SIBO may be a factor in digestive symptoms and/or autoimmunity, please consult a gastroenterologist (or functional medicine practitioner) to pursue further testing and treatment.

BALANCING HORMONES

Suboptimal hormone levels can cause an array of disabling symptoms—disrupting energy, sleep, mood, cognitive function, libido, and other key areas—and thus have a major impact on quality of life. Hormones work together synergistically to produce optimal function, just like all the different instruments in a symphony.

Sometimes we measure adrenal hormones that are part of the HPA (hypothalamus-pituitary-adrenal) axis. This circuit can be disrupted by chronic stress, leading to abnormalities in the levels of key stress hormones such as cortisol and DHEA. In autoimmune patients the levels can also be impacted by chronic inflammation or the use of medications like steroids.

If these hormones are either too high or too low, they can wreak havoc in the body and cause diverse symptoms including fatigue, lightheadedness, insomnia, blood sugar issues, brain fog, and more. This is especially common in Hashimoto's hypothyroidism, because the thyroid and the adrenal glands are closely linked, but it can be seen in other autoimmune disorders.

Several options are available for testing these hormones, including blood, saliva, and urine, although I typically use blood tests as insurance is more likely to cover these. If levels are low, we can consider supplementing with herbs or amino acids to regulate glandular function, or with adrenal hormones such as DHEA at a low dose. The goal with either approach is to optimize levels within the normal range and see if this leads to improvement in symptoms and overall well-being—and not to raise levels beyond the normal range.

Studies confirm that this approach may be helpful for some people. A recent randomized placebo-controlled trial found that supplementation with DHEA improved quality of life in female patients with rheumatoid arthritis.[9] Work with your integrative or functional practitioner to optimize your hormones, especially if your quality of life has been impacted.

LYME AND ASSOCIATED DISEASES

Lyme disease is an infection caused by the Borrelia bacteria; it causes acute symptoms including fever, headache, and the classic "bulls-eye" erythema migrans rash. Chronic manifestations potentially include fatigue, joint pain, and neurological symptoms. First discovered in the town of Lyme, Connecticut, the illness is transmitted by ticks. While the CDC estimates around half a million cases of Lyme disease per year in the United States, the actual number is likely higher due to problems with testing and underreporting.[10]

Lyme disease often occurs together with other bacterial infections such as Bartonella, Babesia, or Rickettsia, which are known as "co-infections" and are transmitted by the same organism. While the disease is often suspected due to a history of tick bite, many people with the disease do not recall having been bitten by a tick (they probably never noticed it).

Lyme disease is controversial. Mainstream medical guidelines state that Lyme disease is rare and easy to treat with a short course of antibiotics.[11] The International Lyme and Associated Diseases Society (ILADS) argues that Lyme can be a complex, chronic condition that requires extended treatment beyond conventional guidelines.[12] According to an article published in the prestigious *New England Journal of Medicine*, 10 to 20 percent of Lyme disease patients, even after treatment with antibiotics, develop a clinical condition called Post-Treatment Lyme Disease Syndrome (PTLDS), which can have various nonspecific lingering symptoms.[13] The reasons for this are unclear.

Research has shown that under duress, the Lyme bacterium can change from its usual corkscrew shape to a spherical "round body" that does not have any proteins on its surface, making it much harder for immune cells to identify and destroy it.[14] Also, Borrelia directly weakens multiple facets of the immune system, increasing the likelihood that it can establish a persistent infection within the host.[15] Lyme bacteria can acquire resistance to antibiotics and have been shown to persist in humans even after the government-recommended antibiotic treatment course is completed.[16]

If you suspect that Lyme or one of its associated diseases is contributing to your autoimmunity, consult with a doctor who is trained in the diagnosis and treatment of chronic Lyme disease. It is a complex field, so it is important to work with a practitioner who is up to date with the science.

To find a doctor you can search via the nonprofit organization LymeDisease .org at https://www.lymedisease.org/members/lyme-disease-doctors/ or use the Find a Provider link of the International Lyme and Associated Diseases Society (ILADS) at https://www.ilads.org/patient-care/provider-search/.

MOLD TOXICITY

Mold is a microscopic type of fungus that becomes visible when it grows in colonies, typically in damp or humid areas. Some fungi produce metabolites known as mycotoxins which can have negative health effects. Mold contamination of crops or animal feed can impact agricultural profits or livestock health and is therefore closely monitored in these products.[17] While exposure is typically environmental from a living space, mold or mycotoxins can sometimes inadvertently be ingested through certain foods such as grains.[18]

The most well-known, established effects of mold are on respiratory conditions such as asthma or allergies. However, there is some research showing a connection between mold exposure and autoimmunity. A large multicenter study with 209 people, which analyzed the effects of exposure to mold, found that, in addition to pulmonary effects and allergies, there was an abnormally high level of several autoimmune antibodies known as autoantibodies. These increase the risk of autoimmune disease; mold-exposed people also had other markers of immune dysregulation evident in blood testing.[19]

Another study followed 80 people who had been exposed to a mold-infested building over time and found that they had a greatly increased prevalence of autoimmune conditions compared to the general public.[20]

Some research has investigated the possibility of autoimmune damage to the nervous system triggered by mold. A study found that patients exposed to a water-damaged building were more likely to have neurological autoantibodies (abnormal antibodies directed against components of the nervous system such as brain or nerve proteins) than healthy controls.[21]

In another study, people who were exposed to mold in their homes were more likely to have elevated levels of neurological autoantibodies when compared to 500 healthy controls.[22] An investigation of 100 patients exposed to toxic mold at home found abnormal immune system markers in 80 percent of them and objective findings of neurological dysfunction in 70 percent.[23] More research is needed to investigate the connection between mold exposure and autoimmunity.

If you find that your autoimmune disease is not improving with the TIGER Protocol, and you have been exposed to a water-damaged building or suspect mold toxicity for other reasons, it may be useful to connect with a practitioner who is well-versed in mold toxicity. This is its own subspecialty, as not all functional medicine providers are trained in this. You can look for a medical professional through the International Society for Environmentally Acquired Illness website (iseai.org/find-a-professional/).

If you suspect ongoing exposure to mold, you can test your home for its presence. There are various assessments available. One, developed by the US Environmental Protection Agency, is an Environmental Relative Moldiness Index (ERMI), which analyzes mold found in dust samples from the house.[24] You can perform an ERMI through certain companies such as Mycometrics (mycometrics.com) or Envirobiomics (envirobiomics.com) or a more cost-effective option could be DIY mold testing via Immunolytics (immunolytics .com). If testing is positive, and you suspect you have symptoms related to mold exposure, remediation by an experienced professional is recommended.

CELL DANGER RESPONSE

In a seminal paper,[25] Dr. Robert Naviaux presented the cell danger response (CDR). It reviewed how mitochondria, the powerhouses that produce energy in every cell, sense and respond to cellular danger signals. In the presence of toxins, infections, or other challenges, mitochondria stop producing energy, and no longer synthesize the main energy molecule of our bodies, ATP.

The CDR goes through three distinct stages that are part of normal physiologic response to stressors. Under normal circumstances, mitochondria use a lot of oxygen in the cell to synthesize ATP and produce energy through a process known as oxidative phosphorylation.

Mitochondria are sensitive organelles that are among the first to sense danger and begin to trigger changes in response—the first being to stop utilizing oxygen. This causes levels of oxygen in the cell to rise, which leads to the formation of reactive oxygen species, commonly known as "free radicals." These are used by the cell to neutralize the harmful invaders and hopefully repel them as part of CDR stage I.

If this is successfully completed, the cell moves on to CDR stage II, where it seeks to replace damaged proteins and structures, then eventually to CDR stage III, with a focus on regeneration. In this repair phase, anti-inflammatory compounds are produced to quell the inflammation, and the mitochondria pick up on the signals to resume consuming oxygen and producing ATP.

If this normal cycle goes awry, either due to persistent infections, recurrent toxin exposure, or other factors, then many of the mitochondria remain turned off and this leads to a multitude of negative effects, especially persistent inflammation.

Within the cell, energy production remains impaired, which causes symptoms like fatigue and malaise. The cell signals to others that the threat is still active, leading to a variety of systemic changes in potentially distant tissues and organs. This understanding is increasingly being used by functional medicine doctors who treat patients with complex chronic medical conditions, to help develop a plan for autoimmune patients to stop the cycle of mitochondrial dysfunction and persistent inflammation.

MICROBIOME TESTING

If you are still struggling with refractory autoimmune symptoms and unrelenting digestive issues, consider testing your microbiome with a specialized stool analysis. This can evaluate key markers including:

1. levels of your beneficial keystone bacteria
2. diverse pathogens such as bacteria, viruses, fungi, parasites, and archaea
3. short-chain fatty acid levels, broken down into butyrate, acetate, and propionate
4. inflammation markers such as calprotectin and lactoferrin
5. levels of digestive enzymes such as pancreatic elastase

6. malabsorption and processing of carbohydrate, protein, and fat
7. presence of microscopic blood in the stool (occult blood)

Most of these tests are not available in a conventional lab, with the exceptions of blood in the stool, markers of digestive enzymes, and testing for the most common pathogenic bacteria and parasites.

Labs like Diagnostic Solutions Lab, Doctors Data, and Genova Diagnostics allow you to use a stool sample that you collect at home and ship directly to the lab. Consult a functional medicine doctor who can order the test for you and analyze the results.

This can provide guidance for your practitioner to create a more customized gut-healing protocol, in order to see improvement in your digestive function and symptoms, with the hope of reducing systemic inflammation and eventually improving your autoimmune condition.

ALTERNATIVE MEDICAL SYSTEMS

Other medical approaches like Traditional Chinese Medicine and Ayurveda can complement the conventional care you are receiving, especially if you are not improving. Research is sparse in this area as most research is funded by pharmaceutical companies that stand to make billions for successful drugs, whereas similar financial incentives are not present for holistic therapies. Nonetheless, I believe these modalities have tremendous value to offer, and have seen good results in many patients who have taken advantage of either approach.

Traditional Chinese Medicine (TCM)

Acupuncture is one of the main therapeutic modalities of TCM. The National Institutes of Health (NIH) has compiled research suggesting that acupuncture can help with chronic pain conditions such as low back pain, headache, neck pain, and osteoarthritis; it may also alleviate side effects caused by cancer treatments.[26]

Acupuncture is being studied for its efficacy in multiple sclerosis, rheumatoid arthritis, and inflammatory bowel disease, and initial results are promising.[27] My colleagues who practice Chinese medicine report that TCM can be a helpful adjunctive treatment option for autoimmune conditions, especially those in which pain is a prominent symptom. If you are interested, seek out a practitioner with experience treating patients with autoimmunity.

Ayurveda

The traditional medical system of India, Ayurveda has been practiced for over 3,000 years. Its name is derived from the Sanskrit words "Ayu" meaning "life" and "Veda" meaning "science"—i.e., "The Science of Life." I wrote extensively about Ayurveda in my first book, *The Paleovedic Diet*, so I will review details pertaining to autoimmunity here.

Ayurveda is a wide-ranging system with treatment modalities including the use of diet, spices, herbs, breathing techniques, yoga, massage, and bodywork. It maintains that every person is unique and recommends a diet and lifestyle program customized for each individual.

A small, randomized, double-blind study with 43 people found that Ayurvedic herbal treatment was equal in efficacy to the conventional drug methotrexate in the treatment of rheumatoid arthritis, with fewer adverse events in the Ayurvedic group.[28] A meta-analysis of several studies concluded that Ayurveda may reduce pain and increase function in patients with osteoarthritis.[29]

Of course, curcumin has been extensively studied, as I described earlier, which is why it is an essential component of the TIGER Protocol. Although it is part of the Ayurvedic pharmacopeia, I believe the use of Ayurveda as a comprehensive treatment system would be far more powerful than the use of a single supplement alone.

Panchakarma is an intensive detoxification therapy in Ayurveda, and it has been immensely helpful for a number of my patients with autoimmune conditions. Some case studies report the beneficial use of panchakarma in autoimmune disorders that have not responded to conventional medicine.[30]

This is generally performed on an inpatient basis at Ayurvedic treatment centers, where patients stay for at least 1–2 weeks to receive the therapy. Such Ayurvedic centers are present in a few locations in the United States, and throughout India.

Overall, I believe that Ayurveda has a lot to offer in the area of autoimmunity, and more research is needed to corroborate this.

WHERE TO GO FROM HERE

I hope it has been helpful to review some of the unrecognized barriers to healing autoimmunity, and their potential solutions, in this chapter. Use the additional information here as a guide, especially if you are seeking further improvement.

Overall, getting established with an integrative medicine or functional medicine practitioner is one of the best long-term strategies for getting better (I provide resources for this at the end of the next chapter).

Let's reconnect with Brandy, who, after going through the TIGER Protocol to address rheumatoid arthritis, wasn't seeing the results she expected.

To determine why Brandy wasn't improving, we decided to do further testing and identified mold mycotoxins in her system. It turned out that her home had suffered water damage from a bathroom leak the year before. After investigating and remediating the mold at home, the mycotoxins no longer appeared in her test results. In addition, she had a significant reduction in her symptoms for the first time.

Brandy also had struggled with obesity and metabolic syndrome, and so I decided to put her through some fasting. We agreed to a combination of intermittent fasting and periodic longer fasts. I wanted to address her autoimmune condition but also reduce her high risk of heart disease from the metabolic syndrome (and an increased risk which surprisingly comes from the rheumatoid arthritis).

She noted significant weight loss, improvement in metabolic markers, and reduction in pain and inflammation. In addition, I prescribed her low-dose naltrexone to help modulate her immune system. The naltrexone made a huge difference for Brandy. She felt improved mood and energy and dramatic reduction in her pain levels. She was able to reduce down to just a single immune-modulating drug in addition to the naltrexone, and continued to maintain her remission with a healthy diet and intermittent fasting.

CHAPTER 14

Putting It All Together: Nutritional Supplements and Next Steps

At 31, James was diagnosed with Graves' hyperthyroidism—his thyroid stimulating immunoglobulin (TSI) antibodies were triggering the release of excess thyroid hormones. As a result, he was experiencing classic symptoms like palpitations, weight loss, fatigue, diarrhea, and a tremor.

He was referred to an endocrinologist who recommended immediate radioactive iodine ablation, in which he would be given a radioactive form of the mineral iodine, destroying the thyroid as a result. Subsequently, thyroid hormone levels fall precipitously—but because they are essential for life, James would have to begin lifelong oral thyroid replacement therapy.

James was planning to proceed but sought out a second opinion from me to determine if there was any way to preserve his own thyroid gland. After a first round of tests identified several contributing root causes, such as gluten sensitivity, high toxin levels, leaky gut, and abnormal stress hormones including cortisol, I suggested treatment via the TIGER Protocol, to which he agreed.

As with most health concerns, once you complete the protocol, it will be necessary to maintain your health through some key steps, which I'll outline here.

SHOULD I TAKE A MULTIVITAMIN?

Patients often ask if multivitamins are actually helpful. Most studies that have looked at the effects of taking a multivitamin have found they are neutral or have a modest benefit.[1] These studies usually look at "standard" vitamins instead of "whole food" or full-spectrum vitamins that I believe are of better quality.

Almost all the patients I test—even those with an impeccable diet—have some type of nutritional deficiency. Because of this, I do recommend vitamin supplements, but I suggest either those derived from whole foods or with the full spectrum of the nutrient in question. If you discover a nutrient deficiency and elect to take a multivitamin to bolster nutrient levels, look for either a multivitamin derived from whole foods (offered by New Chapter, Standard Process, Garden of Life, and other brands) or one that contains the full spectrum of each vitamin rather than isolated components. The quality of the product makes a huge difference; the vitamins and minerals available in whole foods (and whole food–based supplements) are often more complete than the vitamins and minerals in certain supplements.

Because most studies look at standard multivitamins—as noted above—I typically do not recommend standard multivitamins. For example, the entire vitamin E complex includes four tocopherols and four tocotrienols. In contrast, what you typically find in a standard multivitamin or vitamin supplement is just alpha-tocopherol, which can legally be labeled "Vitamin E" according to FDA standards.

Alpha-tocopherol is actually associated with a higher long-term risk of cancer and heart disease when taken in supplemental form.[2] In contrast, studies that have looked at more complete versions of the vitamin E complex found that they reduce the risk of cancer and heart disease and may have other benefits, from improving bone health to supporting healthy blood sugar and protecting against oxidative stress.[3]

Depleted Soil = Nutrient-Poor Produce

The prevalence of nutritional deficiencies is increasing significantly, and part of the reason is that even the fruits and vegetables in our diet have fewer nutrients than they did previously. Plants only have as many nutrients as they can absorb from the soil they are grown in. Research from the US Department of Agriculture has shown that crops grown in today's depleted soils, compared to identical produce from the 1950s, are significantly lower in calcium, phosphorus, iron, vitamin B2, and vitamin C.[4] Other studies found that the average mineral content of calcium, magnesium, and iron in cabbage, lettuce, tomatoes, and spinach dropped 80–90 percent between 1914 and 2018.[5] New crop varieties engineered for rapid growth and changes in farming techniques, in addition to soil depletion, are likely responsible for these changes.

Increased Usage of Nutrients and Widespread Deficiency

The stress of modern life and the toxins in our environment also increase the amount of nutrients that our bodies use up every day. Furthermore, illness can raise your nutritional requirements—when your body is trying to heal the chronic inflammation associated with autoimmunity, it uses more essential nutrients. For example, in autoimmune conditions such as RA or MS, zinc may be utilized at a higher rate by cells trying to heal, thus depleting body levels of it more quickly.[6]

These causes are why most of my patients have some type of micronutrient deficiency. Population studies confirm shocking levels of nutrient deficiency among Americans. Recent data shows that 100 percent don't get enough potassium, 94 percent don't get enough vitamin D, 92 percent don't get enough choline, 89 percent don't get enough vitamin E, 67 percent don't get enough vitamin K, and so on for multiple other nutrients.[7]

All of these factors—depletion of nutrients by autoimmune illness, loss of vitamins and minerals from our food, and modern stresses leading our bodies to utilize nutrients faster—make nutritional deficiency an extremely serious issue, and one that patients with autoimmunity would be well-served to address. Moreover, many of these nutrients are crucial for reducing autoimmunity and maintaining normal immune function.

Evaluating Vitamin and Mineral Levels

In the following sections, we'll take a look at the individual vitamins and minerals that can be beneficial to support your journey back to health. In order to determine which supplements you might need, it's best to start by assessing nutrient status—but one has to know the right tests to order.

For example, with magnesium: the vast majority of your body's magnesium is intracellular, or within your cells. Very little (<1%) is circulating in your blood.[8] So, measuring blood magnesium level is often not too helpful in evaluating magnesium status. Studies confirm that intracellular magnesium levels within the red blood cells are a better indicator of true magnesium status.[9]

VITAMIN D

The majority of my patients have some degree of vitamin D deficiency. Vitamin D, which is actually a hormone rather than a vitamin, has many important effects in the body.

For autoimmunity, Vitamin D is crucial because it can favorably modulate the immune system.[10] Studies show that optimizing vitamin D can lessen disease activity in rheumatoid arthritis and lupus.[11] Vitamin D also appears helpful not only when treating autoimmunity but in preventing the development of autoimmune disease. One study showed that supplementing with vitamin D and/or omega-3 fatty acids over five years reduced the risk of developing autoimmune illness by 25–30 percent compared to adults who took neither supplement.[12] This vitamin is also critical for bone health, cancer prevention, and cardiovascular health.

It is important to measure your 25 hydroxy-vitamin D level (25-OH Vitamin D) to see where you stand. This test is widely available at most labs. I have a slightly higher target range for the optimal level based on studies in autoimmune conditions.[13]

25-OH Vitamin D Level	Classification
<20	Low
21–39	Normal but suboptimal
40–60	Optimal
61–99	Only recommended for cancer patients, likely not needed in autoimmune disease
>100	Potentially harmful

You've probably heard it's possible to make vitamin D from sun exposure, but you need considerable full-body sunlight daily without sunscreen, which is hard to achieve. It is present in food sources like seafood, dairy products, and mushrooms, but not in large amounts. This is why most people require a supplement to boost their vitamin D levels.

I suggest you talk to your physician about checking your vitamin D levels. It is important to track your progress by rechecking the levels two to three months after supplementation. I have had patients require high dosages over long periods of time to slowly push up their numbers. In contrast, others have rapidly attained levels that were too high and had to immediately stop taking it, as excess vitamin D can cause toxicity, which may manifest with nausea and vomiting, weakness, or other symptoms.

MAGNESIUM

As with vitamin D, most people are also deficient in magnesium. It can be hard to get sufficient amounts of this mineral through food. It is estimated that 60 percent of US adults do not achieve the recommended daily intake, and nearly half are frankly deficient.[14] Recommended daily intake of magnesium is 320 mg for women and 420 mg for men.[15]

Magnesium affects hundreds of metabolic and cellular processes and is one of the most important minerals for overall health. Potential symptoms of low magnesium include fatigue, poor sleep, migraine headaches, muscle spasms, hair loss, constipation, and anxiety. It is involved in over 600 different enzyme reactions in the body.[16]

For autoimmune disease in particular, magnesium plays an important role. Hashimoto's disease is often accompanied by deficiencies in key minerals such as magnesium.[17] In patients with autoimmune type I diabetes, low levels of magnesium were associated with poorer outcomes and disease complications.[18]

There is also a significant relationship between magnesium and vitamin D. Magnesium is an essential cofactor for vitamin D function within the body. Studies show that combined supplementation with magnesium and vitamin D may be more effective at improving vitamin D status than vitamin D alone.[19]

When working with your doctor, ask for a red blood cell magnesium level test. As discussed above, this is a more accurate gauge than blood magnesium level. Get your levels into the upper half of the normal range defined by your laboratory. Reference ranges can vary, but a typical normal range is 4.0 to 6.4; in this example, you would want your level to be above 5.2.

There are many magnesium-rich foods which you should consume regularly, if you can tolerate them—including green leafy vegetables, nuts, avocados, legumes, and dark chocolate (see table below for details).[20]

Food source with typical serving size	Magnesium content (milligrams)
Spinach, 1 cup	157
Pumpkin seeds, 1 ounce	156
Chard, 1 cup	154
Chia seeds, 1 ounce	111
Almonds, 1 ounce	80
Cashews, 1 ounce	74
Dark chocolate (70-85% cacao), 1 ounce	65
Black beans, ½ cup	60
Avocado, 1 medium	58
Figs, ½ cup	50
Potato, baked with skin, 3.5 ounces	43
Brown rice, ½ cup	42
Yogurt, low fat, 8 ounces	42
Kidney beans, ½ cup	35

Banana, one medium	32
Wild Atlantic salmon, 3 ounces	25
Raisins, ½ cup	23
Chicken breast, 3 ounces	22

There are multiple types of magnesium supplements; it's important to choose the right one. The main difference between them is their bioavailability (how much is absorbed), which can lead to different effects within the body. Magnesium oxide and sulfate have relatively lower bioavailability, which means that less is absorbed and a larger amount stays behind in the intestine (and because magnesium draws water into your intestine, this can lead to loose stools). However, if you suffer from constipation, these may be good options.

Magnesium malate, chelate, and glycinate have higher bioavailability; magnesium citrate also is fairly well absorbed.[21] Transdermal magnesium oils and creams, which are absorbed directly through the skin, may be helpful in treating muscle cramps and spasms related to magnesium deficiency (they sometimes cause itching, however, which is a benign side effect). They can also be used by patients who cannot tolerate oral magnesium.

I recommend taking magnesium at night because it can help with sleep. Start with around 100–200 mg. If necessary and tolerated, it can be increased to 100–200 mg twice a day as long as this amount does not upset your stomach.

ZINC

Zinc is a vital nutrient, essential for hormone production, proper cell growth and repair, digestion, wound healing, and the function of over 300 enzymes in the body.[22] Zinc is commonly thought of as an immune booster, and research shows that it activates your T-lymphocytes, cells which are essential for healthy immunity.[23]

Studies have found that patients with multiple sclerosis have lower circulating levels of zinc than healthy controls.[24] People with Hashimoto's disease are often found to be deficient in zinc.[25] A meta-analysis of multiple studies also found low zinc status associated with other autoimmune conditions such as lupus, celiac disease, autoimmune liver disease, and Sjogren's syndrome.[26]

In patients with chronic inflammation such as in RA or MS, zinc is often used at a higher rate by cells trying to heal, thus depleting body levels—therefore, a secondary deficiency of zinc could also develop in autoimmune conditions.[27]

We talked about intestinal permeability in chapter 9; zinc is helpful here because it can aid in normalizing increased intestinal permeability. A randomized, double-blind study found that 3–6 mg of zinc daily can help improve gut barrier integrity.[28]

To raise your zinc levels, aim for the US government-recommended daily intake of 11 mg for men and 8 mg for women. Consume plenty of foods rich in zinc, such as meat and poultry, nuts, seeds (pumpkin seeds are a great source), legumes, mushrooms, and dark chocolate. Shellfish are high in zinc, with oysters being the richest source, as you can see in the table below.

A blood level of zinc (plasma zinc) is an acceptable way to assess levels if needed—you do not need the intracellular level as with magnesium. I recommend you stay at the upper half of the normal range, which can vary based on the lab.

Here is a list of zinc-rich foods, taken from a government database:[29]

Food source with typical serving size	Zinc content (milligrams)
Oysters, 3 ounces	74.0
Beef chuck roast, 3 ounces	7.0
Crab, 3 ounces	6.5
Beef patty, 3 ounces	5.3
Lobster, 3 ounces	3.4
Pork chop, 3 ounces	2.9
Baked beans, canned, ½ cup	2.9
Chicken, dark meat, 3 ounces	2.4
Pumpkin seeds, 1 ounce	2.2
Yogurt, low fat, 8 ounces	1.7
Cashews, 1 ounce	1.6
Shrimp, 3 ounces	1.4
Chickpeas, ½ cup	1.3
Cheese, Swiss, 1 ounce	1.2
Dark chocolate (70-85% cacao), 1 ounce	0.94
Almonds, dry roasted, 1 ounce	0.9
Kidney beans, ½ cup	0.9
Chicken breast, ½ breast	0.9
Cheese, cheddar or mozzarella, 1 ounce	0.9
Wild Atlantic salmon, 3 ounces	0.54
Mushrooms, white button, 3.5 ounce	0.51

VITAMIN K$_2$

There are two types of vitamin K. K$_2$ is distinct from the more well-known vitamin K$_1$, which is found in many foods, including leafy green vegetables, and primarily involved in blood clotting.

Vitamin K$_2$ is a lesser known but crucial nutrient as it provides myriad health benefits. Studies show K$_2$ has a remarkable array of health benefits across multiple organ systems—it can reduce the risk of heart disease, improve bone health, increase insulin sensitivity, promote healthy skin, prevent osteoporosis, protect against certain cancers, and lower the risk of kidney stones.[30]

This vitamin regulates key proteins that direct your body to put calcium into the bones and teeth—where it belongs—and prevent it from ending up in the blood vessels, where it can raise the risk of cardiovascular disease, or in the kidney, where it can form kidney stones. Deficiency is common because it is not found in high levels in many foods (see table below).

Emerging evidence indicates that this nutrient is important for immune function, and can reduce inflammation and oxidative stress, two key drivers of autoimmunity. Multiple sclerosis patients were more likely than healthy controls to be deficient in vitamin K$_2$, and lower levels correlated with higher risk of MS flare-ups.[31] In patients with eczema, vitamin K$_2$ has been shown to modulate the immune system and reduce inflammation.[32]

While more research is needed in terms of its autoimmunity, in my view this nutrient is critical and underappreciated despite evidence-based benefits for the heart, bones, kidney, immunity, and other systems as described above.

Food sources of vitamin K$_2$ include meats (especially organ meats) as well as egg yolks, grass-fed butter and cheese, and fermented vegetables. Ghee and butter are reasonably good sources. Some amount of K$_2$ can be synthesized by certain gut bacteria in your microbiome, but this is inconsistent, and so getting adequate dietary intake is important. The following table lists the typical vitamin K$_2$ content of various foods, based on published studies of vitamin levels in plant and animal foods,[33] pork,[34] dairy products,[35] meat,[36] and cheese.[37]

Food Sources of Vitamin K$_2$	
Food, per 100g	**Micrograms**
Natto (fermented soy dish)	1103
Pork sausage	383

Beef liver	106
Hard cheese (gouda)	76.3
Soft cheese (brie)	56.5
Ghee	35
Egg yolk	31.4
Butter (grass-fed)	15.0
Chicken liver	12.6
Chicken breast	8.9
Ground beef	8.1
Sauerkraut	5

I recommend aiming for 100 to 200 micrograms daily of vitamin K_2—target the higher end of this range if you have or are at risk for heart disease, osteoporosis, cancer, diabetes, or kidney stones. If you are unable to attain those levels using some of the foods listed above, a supplement is an option.

The richest food source of vitamin K_2 by far is *natto*, a Japanese fermented soybean product, which I like but many find unpalatable due to its strong smell. Even one or two servings of natto per week would meet your intake goals for this vitamin. The bacteria used in fermenting natto synthesize the vitamin K_2; other soy products do not contain it. You can find natto in Asian markets, where it is often sold frozen.

Many vitamin D supplements come combined with vitamin K_2, because both nutrients are important for bone health. In terms of supplemental dosage, it depends on your food intake of this vitamin—aim for a combined K_2 intake from food and supplements of 100 to 200 micrograms daily. Supplemental K_2 should be avoided in patients with blood clotting issues or those taking blood thinners.

IMPORTANCE OF OMEGA-3 FATS IN AUTOIMMUNITY

Most people do not get enough anti-inflammatory omega-3 fatty acids and end up overloaded with pro-inflammatory omega-6 fats, which are found in vegetable seed oils, grain-fed meat, and processed foods. The positive effects of omega-3 fatty acids on autoimmunity have been confirmed in multiple studies looking at the treatment of rheumatoid arthritis, lupus, type I diabetes, and multiple sclerosis.[38]

Omega-3 fats comprise the cell membrane, the vital outer barrier that envelops every single cell in your body. Omega-3s are essential precursors for hormones that regulate inflammation and the immune system, but also blood clotting and arterial function.

Due to these effects, they play a central role in heart health and reduce the risk of cardiovascular disease, especially sudden cardiac death.[39] They are good for the brain too—people with the highest omega-3 levels had a nearly 50 percent reduced risk of developing Alzheimer's compared to those with the lowest levels.[40] Having a high omega-3 index was associated with an increased life expectancy of five years in one large study.[41]

Omega-3 fats lead to the production of a range of bioactive metabolites in the body such as resolvins, protectins, and maresins. As their name suggests, resolvins are critical for resolving inflammation, and they can be divided into two main categories—E-series resolvins, produced from the omega-3 EPA, and D-series resolvins, which are synthesized from the omega-3 DHA.[42] Resolvins and other downstream metabolites of omega-3s (like protectins) in the body are indispensable for resolving the inflammatory cycle and mitigate autoimmune pathways. For all these reasons, it is imperative to ensure optimal omega-3 intake either from food or supplements.

Maintaining a healthy omega-6 to omega-3 ratio in your body of 5:1 or lower is ideal. It is possible to measure this ratio with blood tests, or via an omega-3 index, which analyzes the ratio of omega-6 to omega-3 fats in your blood. Such tests are available through mainstream laboratories such as Quest Diagnostics and Labcorp.

The best way to optimize levels is to decrease your intake of omega-6 fats and increase your intake of omega-3 fats. Omega-3s may be best derived from whole fish rather than from fish oil supplements, although both contain the all-important long chain-omega-3s EPA and DHA. Eating fatty fish at least 2–3 times per week should be sufficient. If you do not eat fish, you may consider taking a fish oil supplement. Vegetarian sources of omega-3s include walnut, flax, and chia. However, these contain the precursor short-chain omega-3 ALA, which needs to be converted in the body to the more beneficial long-chain omega-3s EPA and DHA, and this conversion is typically inefficient in most people.

When choosing a fish oil supplement, there are a few factors to keep in mind. First, choose a brand that regularly tests for heavy metals, PCBs, and dioxins. Good quality brands state on their label that they regularly perform third-party testing for toxins. Secondly, look for products that are molecularly distilled.

This is a purification procedure that produces a more concentrated fish oil and removes contaminants. Third, you want fish oil that has been derived from fish that are low in mercury, such as sardines, anchovies, and salmon.

If you are vegetarian or vegan, or cannot take fish for other reasons, you can opt for algae-based omega-3 supplements. They are superior to plant-based food sources that only contain short-chain ALA. Algae supplements contain more DHA than EPA, but still have adequate levels of both long-chain omega-3s. The main downside is cost, as the supplements tend to be expensive.

GET MOVING

Sustaining your long-term health is an imperative aspect of your journey. I recommend my patients focus on the four pillars—healthy diet, exercise, good sleep, and stress management. Giving attention to these four areas each day is the foundation for a good daily routine. We have talked extensively about all of these except for exercise, so let's turn to that here.

I believe it is critical to move daily. US government guidelines recommend 150 minutes per week of cardiovascular exercise, which works out to about 30 minutes at least 5 days a week, plus at least 2 days a week of activities that strengthen muscles.[43]

Besides the usual positive impacts of exercise for heart health, metabolic fitness, muscle strength, and mood, a noteworthy benefit for autoimmune disease is that exercise appears to improve the diversity of the microbiota, which is key for long-term gut health.[44] This may be one of the reasons why athletes have been shown to have higher microbiota diversity.[45]

Moving daily can take many different forms. Even if you are not able to do vigorous exercise, walking, yoga, swimming, or other low-impact activities make a difference. Do whatever works for you as long as you find a way to move your body every single day. This should be an indispensable part of your daily routine.

Resistance Training

Resistance training, which is exercise that builds muscular strength and endurance, should be an absolutely essential piece of your exercise routine in addition to cardiovascular exercise. I find that patients often do not emphasize this enough in their fitness regimen. You don't have to join a gym to do this type of exercise—you can do body-based workouts such as push-ups, pull-ups, planks and/or sit-ups, or use dumbbells or resistance bands at home.

Resistance training has enormously beneficial effects on hormones such as insulin, growth hormone, and testosterone—which are vital for both men and women.[46] It is necessary for maintaining muscle mass and strength, which are crucial for optimizing metabolism and promoting a long and healthy life—reducing all-cause mortality and preserving quality of life as we age.[47] This is why I refer to muscle as "the organ of longevity." Resistance exercise also has a favorable impact on anxiety and depression, and improves sleep.[48]

Prolonged Sitting

With increased time spent on virtual meetings and computer work, most of us are spending a lot more time at a desk. You might not think much of this. But studies show that if you sit for long periods of time, you have an increased risk of death—even if you exercise regularly.

A study of over 200,000 adults found that sitting for 11 hours a day was associated with a 40 percent greater risk of death over just 3 years than sitting for less than 4 hours per day—regardless of whether the participants did regular exercise.[49] Another study found that women who sit 6 hours a day were 35 percent more likely to die during a 14-year follow-up period compared to women who sit less than 3 hours a day.[50] These findings have been confirmed in multiple studies.

This is of course in addition to the damaging musculoskeletal effects of sitting, which tighten muscles and stiffen joints, often leading to low back pain or achy joints.

Pertinent to autoimmune disease is the fact that sitting a lot is associated with higher levels of C-reactive protein and plasma fibrinogen, both critical markers of inflammation.[51] It also causes declines in multiple cardiometabolic markers by lowering good cholesterol, insulin sensitivity, levels of enzymes that break down fat, and our ability to keep blood sugar in check.[52] Gene expression is markedly worsened by sitting, so the exceptionally harmful epigenetic effects of sitting are likely responsible for the shortened lifespan observed in those who sit too long.[53]

A growing body of research confirms that prolonged sitting actually *cancels out* the benefits of exercise. Exercise is reliably proven to lead to certain metabolic improvements—unless you have been sitting a lot. One study showed that in people who are sitting more than 13 hours a day, one hour of aerobic exercise failed to produce the typical lipid and glucose metabolic benefits that are usually seen after exercise.[54]

Something inherent to sitting makes the body resistant to the benefits of exercise. Consistent exercise does not repair the serious damage caused by prolonged sitting, so we have to separate the two: get sufficient exercise and also minimize sitting.

If you work an office job, using a standing desk is a great way to keep yourself on your feet. For the ambitious, treadmill desks enable one to walk several miles during work. If you can get an adjustable workstation, to alternate between sitting and standing, that would create a good balance. Try to spend more hours standing or moving than you are sitting each day.

Seeking to be physically active whenever possible is key. Find ways to reduce sitting and incorporate activity into your daily routine. Try to get as many steps as you can throughout the day. If you are not able to switch to a standing desk, sit on a yoga ball that forces you to make frequent, tiny movements. The same thing is accomplished by sitting on a "stability balance disc," a firm circular disk that you place on your chair which improves core strength and encourages micro-movements.

Taking frequent breaks to stand up from sitting is another option. A NASA scientist concluded that standing up from a sitting position 35 times per day—about 5 times per hour—can effectively maintain physical conditioning.[55]

NEXT STEPS—FIND A PRACTITIONER

I recommend you find an integrative medicine or functional medicine practitioner to work with more closely. As we've discussed, functional medicine is a subset of integrative medicine that uses specialized lab tests to diagnose and treat imbalances in the function of different organ systems. A good first step is to ask your local primary care physician if he or she can refer you to a provider in your area. If not, I will recommend a few sources.

While there is not a single centralized listing of all functional medicine practitioners, there are multiple online directories, and sometimes a provider is in one listing but not another, so it is a good idea to explore all of the following when you're searching.

The University of Arizona (where I trained with Dr. Andrew Weil) offers an online directory of practicing integrative medicine clinicians, available at https://integrativemedicine.arizona.edu/alumni.html.

The Institute for Functional Medicine (IFM) has a Find a Practitioner database, which is a good place to start: https://www.ifm.org/find-a-practitioner/.

Although these websites are not specific to functional or integrative medicine, you can find clinicians familiar with nutrition and integrative medicine: http://paleophysiciansnetwork.com/doctors and https://re-findhealth.com/.

For help with more specialized issues such as mold or chronic infections, The International Society for Environmentally Acquired Illness (ISEAI) Find a Professional website is a great resource—http://iseai.org/find-a-professional/.

As we end, let's revisit James, who was recommended radioactive iodine ablation for his autoimmune hyperthyroidism.

James began the TIGER Protocol under my supervision. I prescribed propranolol to control his symptoms and buy us some time so we could start tackling the underlying factors. Propranolol reduced some of his hyperthyroid symptoms and made the situation feel less urgent. Toxin testing revealed high levels of toxins including waterborne chemicals and plastic residues, so he installed a home water filter, switched away from plastic, and began the TIGER Protocol detox.

I started him on a gut-healing protocol with the Phase I Diet, bone broth, fermented foods, and L-glutamine. I asked him to maintain a strict gluten-free diet because of his gluten sensitivity. Although he did not have any GI issues initially, he felt this improved his energy levels. He also incorporated regular exercise and a daily ten-minute meditation practice to bring down his elevated cortisol levels. He was able to come off the propranolol within two months as his symptoms improved.

We began testing his thyroid hormone levels every two months and they started to decline. By six months his T3 and T4 thyroid hormone levels had dropped into the high end of the normal range, but he was still having some residual symptoms, namely the tremor, and wanted to accelerate his progress.

I started James on low-dose naltrexone to help modulate his immune system and hopefully speed up the recovery. He noticed further improvement on this, and at 12 months all his thyroid markers had normalized. His thyroid-stimulating immunoglobulin, the autoantibody that is indicative of Graves' disease, also dropped into the normal range for the first time since his diagnosis, indicating a full remission of this condition. He was very grateful to recover without the radioactive iodine ablation and has been in remission ever since with a diet and lifestyle regimen.

The autoimmune realm is complex, but there are significant levers that you have the power to shift by giving attention to the root causes of toxins, infections, gut health, diet, and stress. You now have a framework guided by the latest science and research to understand why autoimmune disease develops and what you can do about it. It's my hope that you feel encouraged by the knowledge and wisdom you have gained from this book. My goal was to empower you with all the tools and techniques I have gleaned during my two decades of caring for autoimmune patients. We covered a lot of ground here; thank you for sticking with me until the end.

The road back from autoimmunity is not straightforward, and there can certainly be bumps along the way. Unfortunately, there's no quick fix or "magic bullet." But, by following the protocol, and with perseverance, it is possible to get better and to feel better.

Autoimmune disease has many facets, and it is best approached with a holistic, integrative medicine strategy. The comprehensive TIGER Protocol can help you to focus on things that you can control, such as diet, lifestyle, and behavioral interventions that could help to improve outcomes—and modulate your immune system for long-term well-being, rather than suppressing it for short-term relief.

In the best case, following the TIGER Protocol can lead you to a place of optimal wellness, where you might feel even better than you felt before you first heard the word "autoimmune." With this book, you are well on your way to transforming your autoimmune condition. At the very least, I hope it serves as a stepping-stone to improved health and vitality, whereby you are able to reduce flare-ups and exacerbations, and move toward remission with the minimum of medications.

As we end, I'd like to return to the definition of health that I introduced at the beginning of the book—"the ability to live your dreams." I encourage you to regularly consider your deeper ambitions, goals, and life purpose. What would you like to use your health for? What would be the equivalent of your "moonshot" in your personal and professional life? For me, it has been the writing of this book, which has been the culmination of my work over the past 20 years (I am looking for my next moonshot now!).

The process of seeking out higher aspirations is critical; doing so infuses our lives with a sense of meaning and direction. The process of cultivating and refining this is usually lifelong—I think of it more as a journey rather than a destination, similar to the practice of living well with autoimmune disease.

It has been my honor to share a little bit of your journey with you through this book. I wish you many blessings and a life full of joy, vitality, and happiness— one where you can live your life to the fullest, as the greatest and healthiest "vision" of yourself possible.

To Your Health,

Dr. Akil

14-Day Meal Plan

This 14-day plan (two plans over two weeks) offers a sample menu for you to follow during the TIGER Protocol. One week covers the Phase 1 Diet, the more restrictive, elimination diet, and the second week includes recipes for the Phase 2 Diet, a blueprint for your long-term eating plan.

The plan is designed to be simple and convenient. You will see that your lunch meals often incorporate leftovers from the previous night's dinner. When a recipe requires use of the oven, I have included multiple components that can be baked at the same time.

The breakfast options are included on a rotating basis with a few simple, easy-to-prepare meals. Snacks are not included here, but they can be incorporated from the "Side Dishes."

TIGER PROTOCOL PHASE 1 DIET SAMPLE MENU

Day 1

Breakfast
Anti-Inflammatory Morning Smoothie

Lunch
Artichoke and Leek Soup

Dinner
Oven-Baked Chicken with Sweet Potato

Day 2

Breakfast
Cinnamon-Raisin Oatmeal

Lunch
Leftover Oven-Baked Chicken with Sweet Potato

Dinner
Salmon Fish Curry and Garlicky Shiitake Mushrooms

Day 3

Breakfast
Golden Green Smoothie

Lunch
Leftover Salmon Fish Curry and Garlicky Shiitake Mushrooms

Dinner
Pumpkin Soup and Roasted Green Beans with Black Cumin

Day 4

Breakfast
Ginger-Cinnamon Tropical Overnight Oats

Lunch
Leftover Pumpkin Soup and Roasted Green Beans with Black Cumin

Dinner
Stir-Fried Ground Beef and Kale over Quinoa

Day 5

Breakfast
Kitcheri

Lunch
Leftover Stir-Fried Ground Beef and Kale over Quinoa

Dinner
Spiced Salmon Burgers in Lettuce Wrap

Day 6

Breakfast
Anti-Inflammatory Morning Smoothie

Lunch
Leftover Spiced Salmon Burgers in Lettuce Wrap

Dinner
Artichoke and Leek Soup

Day 7

Breakfast
Cinnamon-Raisin Oatmeal

Lunch
Ginger-Lime Scallops with Basil Pesto Quinoa

Dinner
Oregano-Thyme Roasted Black Cod over Spinach and Rice

TIGER PROTOCOL PHASE 2 DIET SAMPLE MENU

Day 1

Breakfast
Scrambled Eggs with Leafy Greens

Lunch
Romaine Lettuce-Artichoke Salad with Black Beans

Dinner
Chicken Tikka Masala over Rice

Day 2

Breakfast
Vanilla Chia-Berry Pudding

Lunch
Leftover Chicken Tikka Masala over Rice

Dinner
Macadamia-Encrusted Wild Salmon with Buckwheat

Day 3

Breakfast
"Chaffles"

Lunch
Dover Sole with Red Pesto and Sweet Potato

Dinner
Oven Roasted Artichoke with Avocado Hummus

Day 4

Breakfast
Blueberries with Cashew Cream

Lunch
Black Cumin Shrimp Curry

Dinner
Beef Curry over Rice

Day 5

Breakfast
Chocolate-Hazelnut Overnight Oats

Lunch
Leftover Beef Curry with Rice

Dinner
Coconut Flatbread and Sunflower Seed Hummus with Cumin

Day 6

Breakfast
Golden Green Smoothie

Lunch
Toasted Rosemary Crackers and Sunflower Seed Hummus with Cumin

Dinner
Spiced Turkey Meatloaf with Sweet Potato

Day 7

Breakfast
Scrambled Eggs with Leafy Greens

Lunch
Leftover Spiced Turkey Meatloaf with Sweet Potato

Dinner
Romaine Lettuce-Artichoke Salad with Black Beans

TIGER Protocol Recipes

Cooking has been a lifelong passion of mine, and I'm excited to introduce you to these original recipes.

In my first book, I acquainted readers with my top 13 healing spices, such as turmeric, black cumin, ajwain, cinnamon, and fenugreek, and 53 recipes featuring them as ingredients—and I'm still frequently asked about the best ways to cook with these spices to access their therapeutic effects. To that end, many of the recipes in this book incorporate these marvelous spices—you'll see one or more of them in every dish. For patients with autoimmune disease, the anti-inflammatory, antioxidant, and prebiotic, microbiome-enhancing effects are especially important.

We covered many healing foods throughout the text, and these recipes should provide you with a good starting place. Hopefully, you'll discover some new ideas and ways of incorporating these foods into your diet. All the main ingredients in each recipe have been included for their unmatched nutrient density, such as, for example, fish, shellfish, artichokes, and mushrooms.

I recommend the ingredients be organic if possible, but, if this is not possible, get the highest quality available to you. Other quick notes:

- All recipes are free of gluten, dairy, soy, corn, refined sugar, and alcohol. With each recipe, I will specify whether it is acceptable for the Phase 2 Diet or both diets (anything approved for the Phase 1 Diet can also be used in the Phase 2 Diet).
- Many of the recipes use garlic cloves. As you might recall, I recommend crushing garlic and waiting 10 minutes for the allicin to form before using it in the recipe. I will not be repeating this in each recipe so please keep this in mind.
- The Fermented Foods listed at the end of this section are not specifically mentioned in the Meal Plan. However, I intend for them to be

incorporated on a regular basis alongside your daily meals. A large serving is not required, even a tablespoon per meal will be beneficial.

Bon Appetit!

BREAKFAST

Cinnamon-Raisin Oatmeal

Phase 1 or Phase 2 Diet

If you tolerate it well, oatmeal can be an excellent source of fiber, antioxidants, and prebiotics. It supports healthy levels of cholesterol and blood sugar, thus supporting heart health. Oatmeal contains anti-nutrients like phytic acid that inhibit absorption, but these are inactivated by soaking the oats overnight.

This recipe calls for steel-cut oats, which are minimally processed and low glycemic. In this recipe, the traditional Ayurvedic approach of toasting the oats slightly gives them a rich flavor—coconut is used in place of ghee as a nondairy alternative. Cinnamon and cardamom provide phytochemicals as well as natural sweetness.

Makes two servings

1 cup steel-cut oats
1 teaspoon coconut oil
¼ cup raisins
¼ teaspoon cinnamon powder
⅛ teaspoon cardamom powder
2 tablespoons walnuts (may top with other nuts if you prefer)

Soak the oats in water at least 12 hours overnight. In the morning, discard the water. In a pan, heat the coconut oil until it melts. Add the oats and stir to toast them for about 2 minutes.

Add 2 cups of water and simmer on low heat for about 7 minutes. Cover the pan but leave it slightly open to allow steam to escape so that the water does not boil over. Then add raisins, cinnamon, and cardamom. Stir well and continue to simmer on low to medium heat for another 5–7 minutes, stirring occasionally. Once the oats have softened, remove from heat and top with the nuts.

NUTRITION FACTS, per one serving (recipe makes two servings): 445 cal, 15 g protein, 68 g carbohydrate, 10 g fiber, 14 g fat

Overnight Oats

Phase 1 or Phase 2 Diet

If you are not familiar with overnight oats, they comprise a simple but customizable breakfast that doesn't require any cooking. I recommend using old-fashioned rolled oats as these will impart the optimal texture and consistency. Old-fashioned oats are slightly more processed than steel-cut oats but still low glycemic.

You'll find a few variations on this recipe here. The first uses mango and coconut for a tropical flavor that pairs well with the spices. The second has a Nutella-like flair, the hazelnut spread we often used to enjoy as a treat while growing up. I often top it with strawberry, which pairs well with chocolate.

I did not include any desserts in the meal plan, but these recipes come close— like dessert for breakfast!

Ginger-Cinnamon Tropical Overnight Oats

Makes two servings

½ cup rolled oats (measured dry)
I tablespoon chia seeds
¼ teaspoon ginger powder
¼ teaspoon cinnamon powder
pinch of salt
I cup unsweetened coconut milk
¼ cup fresh sliced mango (may substitute frozen mango)

Add all the ingredients except for the mango to a bowl or Mason jar and mix well. Cover and refrigerate overnight. In the morning, add the sliced mango and serve. You may add a splash of nondairy milk if needed depending on the consistency you like.

NUTRITION FACTS, per one serving (recipe makes two servings): 351 cal, 5 g protein, 26 g carbohydrate, 5 g fiber, 24 g fat

Chocolate-Hazelnut Overnight Oats

Makes one serving

½ cup rolled oats (measured dry)

1 tablespoon chia seeds

⅛ teaspoon cinnamon powder

¼ teaspoon salt

1 tablespoon hazelnut butter (may substitute almond butter if hazelnut is not available)

1 tablespoon cacao powder

1 cup unsweetened almond milk

¼ cup chopped strawberries

Add all the ingredients except for the strawberries to a bowl or Mason jar and stir well. Cover and refrigerate overnight. In the morning, top with the strawberries and serve. Add a splash of nondairy milk if needed.

NUTRITION FACTS, per one serving (recipe makes one serving): 408 cal, 15 g protein, 51 g carbohydrate, 13 g fiber, 18 g fat

Anti-Inflammatory Morning Smoothie

Phase 1 or Phase 2 Diet

This delicious smoothie draws on the anti-inflammatory benefits of turmeric, cinnamon, and ginger, boosted by the antioxidants of cacao powder. Ground flaxseeds provide polyphenols for the microbiome and omega-3 fats, which also help reduce inflammation (but omit these for the phase 1 version of the recipe). MCT oil supports healthy metabolism and blood sugar. It makes a delicious breakfast and a healthy snack later in the day. I use collagen powder but other nondairy protein powders may be substituted.

Makes one serving

8 ounces of filtered water

1 scoop grass-fed collagen powder

1 tablespoon raw cacao powder

1 tablespoon MCT oil

1 tablespoon ground flaxseeds (omit for the Phase 1 version of the recipe)

1/4 teaspoon cinnamon powder

1/4 teaspoon ginger powder

1/8 teaspoon turmeric powder

liquid stevia extract or raw honey to taste

In a blender, pulse all ingredients until smooth. Serve immediately.

NUTRITION FACTS, per one serving (recipe makes one serving and this is for the version with ground flaxseeds and stevia):
290 cal, 31 g protein, 6 g carbohydrate, 4 g fiber, 17 g fat

Golden Green Smoothie

Phase 1 or Phase 2 Diet

This smoothie is packed with powerful anti-inflammatory nutrients to jump-start your day. It combines a few green plants with golden turmeric and ginger to provide a panoply of phytochemicals.

Makes one serving

2 cups spinach

1/2 cucumber, peeled and chopped into 2-inch pieces

1 stalk raw celery

1 inch raw ginger root

1/2 inch turmeric root, or 1/4 teaspoon turmeric powder if the root is not available

5–10 mint leaves

juice of half a lemon, freshly squeezed

half a granny smith (or other) apple, cut into 1-inch pieces

In a blender, combine all ingredients and pulse until smooth. Serve immediately.

NUTRITION FACTS, per one serving (recipe makes one serving):
162 cal, 5 g protein, 36 g carbohydrate, 7 g fiber, 1 g fat

Kitcheri

Phase 1 or Phase 2 Diet

From the Ayurvedic perspective, kitcheri is one of the most healing foods for the gut. It is composed of mung beans, widely considered the most easily digested legume, and white rice, with a powerful blend of therapeutic spices.

We know that many of these spices have prebiotic properties that feed the microbiome, and from the Ayurvedic perspective they are believed to stimulate the *Agni*, or digestive fire. Maintaining a healthy Agni is the key in Ayurveda to optimizing your digestion.

The classical recipe is just rice, mung beans, and ghee. I have added vegetables to this version to provide some additional phytonutrients and fiber. I have substituted coconut oil for the ghee to create a nondairy version.

Makes two servings

¼ cup yellow mung beans (also called split yellow mung dal)

1 cup white rice (measured dry), ideally basmati

1 tablespoon coconut oil

½ teaspoon cumin seeds

½ cup onions, diced

1 clove garlic, minced

¼ teaspoon ginger powder

1 cup zucchini, chopped into half-inch pieces

½ cup carrots, chopped into half-inch pieces

¼ teaspoon turmeric powder

¼ teaspoon of coriander powder

½ teaspoon salt

Soak the yellow mung beans and rice in water for at least 8 hours or overnight. When ready, drain well and rinse with fresh water. In a skillet or pan, melt the coconut oil. Add the cumin seeds and fry for about one minute or until they start to sizzle and pop. Then add the onions and sauté for about a minute.

When the onions become translucent, add the garlic and ginger and sauté for about 1 more minute. Next, add the zucchini, carrots, and remaining spices and salt. Mix well and add in the soaked rice and mung beans.

Add enough water such that the water level is around 2 inches above the top of the rice and beans. Bring to a boil and then cook on low heat, stirring occasionally. Kitcheri is ready when most of the water is absorbed, which usually takes about 25–30 minutes. Allow to cool for 2 minutes and mix well before serving.

Alternatively, you can make this in an Instant Pot or other pressure cooker, in which case the cooking time will be reduced to 10 minutes or so.

NUTRITION FACTS, per one serving (recipe makes two servings): 528 cal, 14 g protein, 99 g carbohydrate, 8 g fiber, 8 g fat

Scrambled Eggs with Leafy Greens

Phase 2 Diet

Eggs are among the most versatile foods and make a convenient breakfast. Rich in choline, vitamin A, B vitamins, and selenium, they truly are nutritional powerhouses. This recipe incorporates Swiss chard and spinach to provide beneficial phytochemicals, and onions for their prebiotic effects.

Makes one serving

1 tablespoon olive oil
$\frac{1}{4}$ medium-sized pink onion, diced into half-inch pieces
one clove garlic, crushed
1 cup spinach leaves
1 cup Swiss chard leaves, chopped into 1-inch pieces
$\frac{1}{4}$ teaspoon sea salt
3 eggs
$\frac{1}{8}$ teaspoon black pepper

Heat 1 teaspoon of the olive oil in a skillet over medium heat. Add the onions and sauté for about 2 minutes until they begin to turn translucent. Then add the garlic and stir fry for another 30 seconds. Add spinach, chard, and salt and cook on medium heat for about 2 minutes.

Move the spinach and chard to one side of the pan. On the other side of the pan add the remaining 2 teaspoons of olive oil, then add the eggs and stir well, until they are fully cooked. Sprinkle the black pepper over the eggs, then mix the spinach and chard with the eggs. Serve immediately.

Nutrition Facts, per one serving (recipe makes one serving):
338 cal, 19 g protein, 6 g carbohydrate, 2 g fiber, 27 g fat

Vanilla Chia-Berry Pudding

Phase 2 Diet

Chia seeds are a rich source of omega-3 fatty acids. They are an excellent source of fiber—this breakfast provides a whopping 20 g to start your day. The addition of berries dramatically increases the antioxidant content of this dish, and cinnamon provides metabolic and glycemic benefits.

I recommend making this the night before and storing it in the fridge because it takes a couple of hours for the chia seeds to be ready. They absorb liquid and swell up to a few times their size when soaked. In the morning, you can add the berries and some almond milk for an easy breakfast with zero prep time.

Makes two servings

3 cups unsweetened almond milk

½ cup chia seeds

1 teaspoon vanilla extract

a pinch of sea salt

1 teaspoon lemon juice

½ cup blueberries

½ cup raspberries

¼ teaspoon cinnamon powder

optional sweetener—monk fruit to taste, or 1 tablespoon honey or maple syrup

In a bowl, pour in the almond milk then add the chia seeds, vanilla, sea salt, and lemon juice. Mix well. Place in the fridge overnight. In the morning, add the berries and cinnamon and, if necessary, a splash of almond milk to loosen things up. I find the berries sweeten the dish nicely, but if you prefer you can add one of the optional sweeteners listed. The dish will keep in the fridge for 3 days if you are not able to finish it at one sitting.

NUTRITION FACTS, per one serving (recipe makes one serving and this is if you had used honey):
369 cal, 11 g protein, 41 g carbohydrate, 20 g fiber, 19 g fat

"Chaffles"

Phase 2 Diet

Chaffles are waffles made from egg and shredded cheese that can be made in any waffle maker. We use nondairy cheese substitutes for this recipe, which are usually made from coconut oil, potato, and similar ingredients. The baking powder is not essential but does improve the texture of the waffles; I recommend including it. These can be savory or sweet; both versions are listed below.

Sweet version:

Makes two servings

2 ounces nondairy cheese
2 eggs
¼ teaspoon cinnamon powder
⅛ teaspoon cardamom powder
2 tablespoons cocoa powder
2 tablespoons almond flour
¼ teaspoon baking powder
fresh berries
liquid stevia, monk fruit extract, or maple syrup, to taste

Shred the cheese into strips or cut into half-inch cubes. In a bowl, beat the eggs. Add the cheese and then all of the other ingredients and mix well to form batter. Pour the batter into a waffle maker (greased with coconut oil if necessary) and cook for 4–6 minutes or until golden brown. Top them with fresh berries of any type, and/or liquid stevia, monk fruit extract, or a bit of maple syrup.

NUTRITION FACTS, per one serving (recipe makes two servings)—might vary depending on the type of nondairy cheese you use:
253 cal, 15 g protein, 12 g carbohydrate, 2 g fiber, 18 g fat

Savory version:

Makes two servings

2 ounces nondairy cheese

2 eggs

2 tablespoons coconut flour

¼ teaspoon baking powder

guacamole or salsa, optional

Shred the cheese into strips or cut into half-inch cubes. In a bowl, beat the eggs. Add in the cheese and the other ingredients and mix well. Pour the batter into a waffle maker (greased with coconut oil if necessary) and cook for 4–6 minutes or until golden. Top with guacamole or salsa for added flavor.

NUTRITION FACTS, per one serving (recipe makes two servings)—might vary depending on the type of nondairy cheese you use:
235 cal, 14 g protein, 12 g carbohydrate, 3 g fiber, 16 g fat

Blueberries with Cashew Cream

Phase 2 Diet

Blueberries are among the richest food sources of antioxidants. They pair really well with this rich cashew cream that is easy to prepare at home.

Makes two servings

1 cup raw cashews

1 cup water

1 tablespoon maple syrup or honey

1 cup blueberries

Soak the nuts in water overnight for at least 12 hours. Drain the nuts and discard the water. Add 1 cup of fresh water, the cashews, and the sweetener to a food processor or blender. Purée until thick and creamy. Add water if needed until desired consistency is achieved.

Top with the berries and serve immediately.

NUTRITION FACTS, per one serving (recipe makes two servings and this is for the version using maple syrup):
461 cal, 11 g protein, 41 g carbohydrate, 4 g fiber, 32 g fat

ENTRÉES

Artichoke and Leek Soup

Phase 1 or Phase 2 Diet

This recipe takes advantage of two vegetables that are exceptionally rich in prebiotics. You can purchase artichoke hearts in cans or bottles—make sure they are packed in brine, not oil. You can also find them in the freezer section. Leeks are related to onions and have a similar, albeit milder flavor, which pairs well with artichoke.

Using bone broth as a soup base is a great way to incorporate it into your diet. It helps to thicken the soup, and the coconut oil gives it added heartiness as well.

Makes one serving

1 leek, white and light green areas finely chopped
1 tablespoon coconut oil
½ teaspoon salt
¼ teaspoon black pepper
2 cloves garlic, minced
14 ounces artichoke hearts in brine
2 cups chicken or beef bone broth (may substitute vegetable broth)
1 tablespoon fresh parsley, chopped
1 tablespoon freshly squeezed lemon juice (from around ½ lemon)

Cut off about 1 inch of the leek at the base along with the roots and discard. At the spot where the light-colored stem intersects with the dark green leaves, make a cut and discard or compost the green leaves (these are quite bitter and usually not used). Finely chop the remaining leek.

Add the chopped leeks to a large bowl filled with water. Mix well with your hands to clean dust and dirt. Drain and pat dry.

In a large skillet over medium heat, melt the coconut oil. Sauté the leeks along with the salt, pepper, and garlic for about 3–4 minutes. Empty the artichokes into a colander, and drain the brine. Add the artichoke hearts to the skillet, along with the bone broth, parsley, and lemon juice. Cook for another 10 minutes or so, until the vegetables are tender.

Allow the soup to cool for a few minutes. Then blend with an immersion blender in the pot until creamy. Alternatively, you can transfer to a stand-alone blender or food processor and blend it in batches if necessary.

Serve hot and season with additional salt and pepper if necessary.

NUTRITION FACTS, per one serving (recipe makes one serving):
373 cal, 22 g protein, 27 g carbohydrate, 7 g fiber, 18 g fat

Oven-Baked Chicken with Sweet Potato

Phase 1 or Phase 2 Diet

This is a simple chicken dish that's perfect when you don't have time for a lot of prep. I use black cumin for its healing properties and peppery flavor, but also add a pinch of black pepper to boost the absorption of turmeric.

For convenience, use an entire sweet potato, which takes about the same amount of time to cook as the chicken.

Makes two servings

4 chicken drumsticks or thighs, bone-in (around 1 pound or so raw)—skin on or off depending on your preference

3 tablespoons olive oil

2 cloves garlic, minced

1 teaspoon onion powder

1 teaspoon turmeric powder

½ teaspoon black cumin powder

1 teaspoon salt, or to taste

A pinch of black pepper

1 large sweet potato

1 large red onion, sliced

Preheat your oven to 400°F. Rinse and dry the chicken with a paper towel to remove any residual moisture. This helps ensure a crispy exterior after baking.

In a mixing bowl, combine the olive oil, garlic, turmeric, black cumin, black pepper, and salt to make a paste. Include the onion powder but not the sliced onions.

Coat the chicken well with the paste on both sides. Place in a single layer on an oven-safe tray.

Wash the sweet potato and poke a few holes in it with a knife. Place the potato whole on a separate oven-safe dish.

Bake for 20 minutes, then remove the chicken from the oven and turn the meat over. Spread the sliced onion all around the pan and over the chicken.

Return to oven and bake for another 10–15 minutes or until chicken is cooked through. The sweet potato should be ready around the same time. Allow to cool for a few minutes before serving.

NUTRITION FACTS, per one serving: (recipe makes two servings)
576 cal, 30 g protein, 35 g carbohydrate, 5 g fiber, 35 g fat

Salmon Fish Curry

Phase I or Phase 2 Diet

This recipe originated in South India, where my family hails from, and it has been passed down through generations. We typically make it with salmon, but you can substitute other types of fish.

Makes two servings

2 teaspoons olive oil, divided

¼ teaspoon turmeric powder

½ teaspoon coriander powder

⅛ teaspoon black pepper

½ teaspoon salt

1 tablespoon lemon juice

8 oz salmon fillet, cut into 2-inch pieces

1 medium onion, white or yellow, thinly sliced

1 clove garlic, minced

½ inch ginger, chopped

1 tomato, medium sized, chopped

8 oz full-fat coconut milk (about half a can)

I tablespoon cilantro, finely chopped

I cup quinoa (measured dry), cooked according to package instructions

In a bowl, mix 1 teaspoon of olive oil with turmeric, coriander, black pepper, salt, and lemon juice to form a paste. Add the salmon to the bowl and mix to coat evenly. Cover and allow to marinate for at least 30 minutes (or up to 2 hours).

In a skillet, add the remaining oil and sauté the onions for about a minute. Add the garlic and ginger and cook on medium heat until the onions become translucent. Add the chopped tomato, stir well, and cook covered for about a minute until the tomatoes blend well with the rest of the mixture.

Add 2 tablespoons of water to the pan and mix well on medium heat. When the sauce simmers, transfer the fish and any remaining marinade from the bowl to the pan. Stir gently without breaking up the fish. Cook on medium heat for around 2 minutes.

Add the coconut milk and stir gently. Cover and cook for another 2 minutes or until fish is done. Check on the salt level and add salt to taste. Transfer to a serving dish and garnish with the cilantro. Serve over cooked quinoa.

NUTRITION FACTS, per one serving (recipe makes two servings): 552 cal, 27 g protein, 15 g carbohydrate, 4 g fiber, 45 g fat

Pumpkin Soup

Phase I or Phase 2 Diet

Pumpkin is an underutilized ingredient; we rarely see it outside of special holidays. This is a shame because pumpkin is an outstanding source of vitamin A, which is critical for optimal immune function. It is also a good source of vitamin C, potassium, copper, manganese, antioxidants, and fiber.

This delectable pumpkin soup pairs well with roasted green beans (recipe immediately following this one).

Makes two servings

2 tablespoons olive oil

I onion, chopped

2 cloves garlic, crushed

¼ teaspoon ground cinnamon

¼ teaspoon ground nutmeg

⅛ teaspoon clove powder

½ teaspoon salt

4 cups raw pumpkin, peeled and chopped into 1-inch pieces (or, substitute 2 cups of canned sugar-free pumpkin purée)

2 cups vegetable or chicken broth

½ cup coconut milk

1 pinch black pepper

Heat the olive oil in a skillet, add onion and sauté until translucent. Add garlic, spices, and salt, and sauté for another minute.

Add the pumpkin along with the broth. Bring to a boil, cover and reduce heat. Simmer until the pumpkin is fully cooked and soft, around 20 minutes or so, stirring occasionally.

When the pumpkin is soft, add the coconut milk and cook for another 2 minutes. It works better to add the coconut milk after the pumpkin has finished cooking.

Blend in the pot with an immersion blender until creamy. Alternatively, you can transfer to a stand-alone blender or food processor and blend it in batches.

When ready, transfer to a bowl and garnish with a sprinkle of black pepper before serving.

NUTRITION FACTS, per one serving (recipe makes two servings):
363 cal, 5 g protein, 27 g carbohydrate, 4 g fiber, 29 g fat

Roasted Green Beans with Black Cumin

Phase 1 or Phase 2 Diet

Green beans are an excellent source of fiber, potassium, and vitamins, including folate. This dish features black cumin, which is not widely known but is an incredibly powerful spice with high levels of antioxidants, anticancer properties, anti-inflammatory effects, and beneficial effects for the gut microbiome, blood sugar regulation, and cholesterol levels. This is an easy way to incorporate black cumin into a healthy vegetable dish.

Makes two servings

½ pound green beans

1 tablespoon olive oil

½ teaspoon sea salt

½ teaspoon black cumin seeds

Preheat an oven to 400°F.

Trim the edges of the green beans and wash well. Pat dry with paper towels until they are completely dry (any residual moisture on the beans will lead to soggy beans in the final dish).

Line a baking tray with aluminum foil or parchment paper.

Spread the olive oil around the beans and toss or mix by hand until the oil is evenly spread. Spread the green beans out on a single layer without overlapping if possible. You might need more than one baking tray depending on size.

Sprinkle the salt and black cumin seeds on top of the beans. Place the baking tray in the oven for about 12–14 minutes.

Check for a few brown caramelized spots on the beans—that's when you know they are done. Do not continue to cook at that point because the beans will become excessively caramelized.

Remove from oven and allow to cool for a couple of minutes before serving.

NUTRITION FACTS, per one serving (recipe makes two servings):
98 cal, 2 g protein, 8 g carbohydrate, 3 g fiber, 7 g fat

Stir-Fried Ground Beef and Kale over Quinoa

Phase 1 or Phase 2 Diet

Ground beef is easy to find and relatively inexpensive. It is an excellent source of protein and important vitamins and minerals. Combine it with kale and you get an incredibly nutrient-dense meal that tastes amazing. Green onions are featured here because they are close to the way wild onions used to be, and therefore an outstanding source of phytochemicals (140 times more than white onions). As

I discussed in my first book, wild plants have been bred to be larger and sweeter but have lost many of their nutrients, so selecting plants that are close to their wild ancestors is a good way to boost the nutrient density of your diet.

Makes two servings

  1 tablespoon olive oil
  ½ onion, chopped
  2 garlic cloves, crushed
  2 tablespoons green onions, chopped
  8 ounces ground beef
  ½ teaspoon salt, or to taste
  ¼ teaspoon turmeric
  ¼ teaspoon ginger powder, or half-inch chopped ginger
  pinch of black pepper
  3 cups kale (measured raw), chopped and roughly separated into stems and
    leaves
  1 cup quinoa (measured dry), cooked according to package instructions

In a skillet over medium heat, add the oil, onion, garlic, and green onions and cook until the onions start to become opaque. Add the ground beef and all the spices, and mix well. Stir and cook for about 5 minutes until the meat is browned, breaking up the meat with a spoon frequently.

Add in the kale stems. Cover and simmer for 2–3 minutes until the stems begin to soften. Then add the kale leaves, cover, and cook for another 2 minutes until done. Serve over the quinoa immediately while the kale is still somewhat crunchy.

NUTRITION FACTS, per one serving (recipe makes two servings): 729 cal, 36 g protein, 67 g carbohydrate, 10 g fiber, 36 g fat

Spiced Salmon Burgers in Lettuce Wrap

Phase 1 or Phase 2 Diet

The beneficial omega-3 fats in salmon, along with generous amounts of vitamin A, B vitamins, magnesium, selenium, and vitamin D, make it one of the most powerful healing foods. Ajwain is a spice that strengthens the digestive system and the microbiome, and ginger adds anti-inflammatory properties to the dish.

In Phase 1, because we are avoiding eggs, use the gelatin powder to help the salmon patties stick together. If you are making this during Phase 2, you can substitute one whisked egg for the gelatin powder as a binder.

Makes two servings

1 tablespoon unflavored gelatin powder

½ pound salmon fillet, cut into half-inch pieces

1-inch piece ginger, finely diced

¼ teaspoon black cumin

2 teaspoons ajwain seeds

¼ cup chopped cilantro

½ teaspoon sea salt

2 tablespoons olive oil, divided

4 leaves romaine lettuce

Mix the gelatin with 3 tablespoons of warm water and stir for a few seconds until the gelatin is dissolved.

Add the gelatin, salmon, and all the remaining ingredients except for the olive oil and lettuce, to a bowl. Mix well and divide into approximately 4 patties. Set aside on a plate or pan.

Heat 1 tablespoon of olive oil in a skillet. When hot, sauté 2 salmon patties at a time until golden brown. It will take approximately 2 minutes on each side. Then add the remaining 1 tablespoon of olive oil to cook the remaining 2 patties.

Wrap each patty in one leaf of romaine lettuce and enjoy as a lettuce wrap. Alternatively, this pairs well with the Coconut Flatbread (recipe under Side Dishes below). If you like you can add lettuce, tomato, and onion to make salmon sandwiches using the flatbread or other bun substitute.

NUTRITION FACTS, per one serving of 2 patties using romaine lettuce wrap (recipe makes two servings):
396 cal, 33 g protein, 3 g carbohydrate, 1 g fiber, 28 g fat

Ginger-Lime Scallops and Quinoa

Phase 1 or Phase 2 Diet

This dish is a nutritional powerhouse, with the essential omega-3 fats from the scallops and the anti-inflammatory compounds from the ginger and turmeric. The briny taste of the scallops pairs well with the sharpness of ginger and lime.

This recipe includes plain quinoa, but if you have a little extra time, I recommend pairing it with the Basil Pesto Quinoa (see recipe on p. 313).

Makes two servings

12 sea scallops (frozen or fresh)

½ teaspoon sea salt

1 teaspoon turmeric powder

2 tablespoons coconut oil

2 teaspoons minced fresh ginger

1 tablespoon lime juice, freshly squeezed

1 cup quinoa (measured dry), cooked per package directions

Preparation of the scallops is key for this recipe. Whether they are frozen or fresh, rinse them with water and make sure they are completely dry. Too much moisture means the scallops will steam while cooking instead of searing.

Sprinkle the sea salt over the scallops and then rub turmeric powder on both sides, coating the scallops evenly.

Heat the coconut oil in a skillet over high heat until the oil in the pan is hot. Add the ginger and cook for 20 seconds. Then arrange the scallops on the pan in a single layer.

Cook for about 2 minutes until they are browned on the bottom, then flip over and cook the other side for another 2 minutes. The scallops should be firm but not tough and rubbery. They should start to release from the pan when they are ready. Turn off heat, pour the lime juice over the scallops, and mix well with the minced ginger in the pan.

Transfer to a plate and serve immediately with the quinoa on the side.

NUTRITION FACTS, per one serving (recipe makes two servings):
564 cal, 34 g protein, 62 g carbohydrate, 6 g fiber, 20 g fat

Oregano-Thyme Roasted Black Cod over Spinach and Rice

Phase 1 or Phase 2 Diet

Black cod, also known as sablefish or butterfish, is a nutrient-dense and sustainable option that is low in mercury. It contains as much beneficial omega-3 fatty acids as wild salmon.

If you cannot find black cod, you can substitute with Pacific cod, which is leaner and has a milder flavor, and is technically a different species (but it will work for this recipe). Pacific cod is not as rich in omega-3s, but it is easier to find and less expensive. This recipe calls for fresh fish but you can substitute with frozen cod fillets—no need to thaw before baking, but add about 10 minutes to the cooking time.

The thyme provides a sharp, peppery flavor which pairs well with the buttery taste of the black cod, and oregano adds a polyphenol and phytochemical boost.

Makes one serving

2 cloves garlic, chopped

4 ounces black cod

½ teaspoon salt, or to your taste

1 tablespoon olive oil

1 tablespoon fresh oregano leaves

1 tablespoon fresh thyme, leaves and stalks

3 cups raw spinach, with salad dressing of your choice

1 cup white rice (measured dry), cooked according to package instructions

Chop the garlic and set aside.

Preheat the oven to 375°F. Dry the cod with a paper towel and then season on both sides with salt.

In a baking dish, combine the olive oil, garlic, oregano, and thyme. Mix well and coat the fish on both sides. Bake until the fish is opaque (not translucent) and flakes easily with a fork, about 10–15 minutes.

Serve over the cooked rice with the spinach salad on the side.

NUTRITION FACTS, per one serving (recipe makes one serving):
596 cal, 17 g protein, 81 g carbohydrate, 6 g fiber, 23 g fat

Romaine Lettuce-Artichoke Salad with Black Beans

Phase 2 Diet

Romaine lettuce contains four times the phytochemicals of iceberg lettuce and is an excellent nutrient-dense option. I've included a recipe for making homemade lemon vinaigrette, although you can use any other salad dressing of your choice.

If you prefer, you can use canned beans instead of dry (substitute 1 cup of canned beans). Your microbiome will be thrilled with the prebiotics from the artichokes, mushrooms, and black beans—contributing to a massive 30 g of total dietary fiber.

Makes one serving

For the salad:

½ cup black beans (measured dry)

3 cups romaine lettuce (from around one head of romaine lettuce)

½ cup artichoke hearts (drained from water-packed container or thawed from frozen)

2 medium-sized tomatoes

I cup white button mushrooms, thinly sliced

For the dressing:

2 tablespoons lemon juice, ideally freshly squeezed from I lemon

I teaspoon salt

2 cloves of garlic, minced

2 teaspoons Dijon mustard

2 tablespoons olive oil

For garnish:

I tablespoon pumpkin seeds

Soak the black beans overnight in water that covers them by at least 2–3 inches, as they will expand. In the morning, discard the water. Rinse well and add the beans to a pot with enough water to cover the beans by 2–3 inches. Bring to a boil and then simmer over medium heat until tender, which may take 30–40 minutes or so. Drain and set aside the beans.

Separate the leaves from your head of romaine lettuce. Rinse them with water and then dry very well using paper towels. Removing as much water from the lettuce as possible will help it to remain crisp and prevent a soggy salad. You can use a salad spinner as well if you have one.

Chop the romaine lettuce into 1-inch pieces and set aside. Rinse the artichoke hearts and dry well. Cut the tomatoes into bite-size pieces and set aside.

In a small bowl, combine the lemon juice, salt, garlic, and Dijon mustard and mix well. Making sure your dressing has enough salt is a pro tip for a delicious salad, because ensuring adequate salt levels is key to any salad.

Use a fork to continuously whisk the mixture while slowly adding in the olive oil. Our goal is to make an emulsion, which is a mixture of 2 liquids that do not dissolve in each other. This will not last long (the elements will separate) so make the dressing just before you are ready to eat.

In a large bowl, toss the lettuce, artichoke hearts, tomatoes, mushrooms, and black beans with about three quarters of the salad dressing. Don't be afraid to use your hands to mix thoroughly and evenly, and "fluff up" the salad.

Drizzle with the remaining dressing and sprinkle the seeds on top before serving.

NUTRITION FACTS, per one serving (recipe makes one serving):
779 cal, 33 g protein, 94 g carbohydrate, 30 g fiber, 35 g fat

Chicken Tikka Masala over Rice

Phase 2 Diet

This is a famous dish and most popular at Indian restaurants. Traditionally, the chicken is roasted separately and added to the sauce later, but I have simplified it in this one-pan recipe. Restaurants usually add dairy in the form of yogurt and heavy cream. This version works equally well with nondairy substitutions. Here, the red bell pepper offers additional phytochemicals and fiber.

I suggest using chicken thighs because they are juicier and work better in this dish; if you are using chicken breast, simply marinate it longer to compensate.

This is a complex recipe, but it is truly rewarding. On a day that you have some extra time or motivation, try this out—the taste is worth it!

Makes three servings

1 cup nondairy yogurt (e.g., coconut or almond), divided

3 tablespoons olive oil, divided

2 teaspoons lemon juice

1 teaspoon cumin powder

1 teaspoon onion powder

½ teaspoon turmeric powder

½ teaspoon fenugreek powder

½ inch ginger, finely chopped

pinch of black pepper

2 cloves garlic, chopped

3 tablespoons tomato paste

1 teaspoon salt

8 ounces boneless, skinless chicken thigh or chicken breast, cut into 1-inch cubes

1 onion, peeled and chopped

1 red bell pepper, seeded and finely diced

6 ounces coconut milk, full fat

2 tablespoons chopped cilantro

1 cup rice (measured dry), cooked according to package instructions

Set aside ¼ cup of the nondairy yogurt and 1 tablespoon of the olive oil for later. In a mixing bowl combine ¾ cup of the nondairy yogurt, 2 tablespoons of olive oil, lemon juice, cumin, onion, turmeric, fenugreek, ginger, black pepper, garlic, tomato paste, salt, and chicken. Mix well to coat. Cover the bowl and refrigerate for at least one hour, or overnight if possible.

Heat the remaining 1 tablespoon of olive oil in a large skillet over medium until hot. Add onions and red bell pepper and cook until the onions become translucent.

Add the marinated chicken, spreading it around evenly throughout the pan in a single layer. Cook for about 3–4 minutes, without stirring much, browning one side. Flip the pieces and cook for another 3–4 minutes. The goal is not to fully cook the chicken but to sear the surface—it will finish cooking in the sauce.

Add the remaining ¼ cup of nondairy yogurt as well as the coconut milk and stir well. Bring the curry to a boil on high heat, then reduce to medium heat.

Cover and cook for 5–6 minutes more, stirring occasionally, or until the chicken is fully cooked. Garnish with the chopped cilantro and serve immediately over rice.

NUTRITION FACTS, per one serving (recipe makes three servings):
651 cal, 23 g protein, 70 g carbohydrate, 5 g fiber, 32 g fat

Macadamia-Encrusted Wild Salmon with Buckwheat

Phase 2 Diet

Salmon has unparalleled health benefits largely due to its high omega-3 content. This dish includes macadamia nuts, which are extremely low in omega-6 fats and therefore help improve your balance of omega-3 and omega-6 fats, which aid with reducing inflammation in the body.

Buckwheat is a gluten-free grain substitute that is not widely known but versatile and delicious. Like quinoa it is technically a seed and therefore low-glycemic and high in protein.

Makes two servings

½ teaspoon ground black pepper

1 teaspoon lemon juice

½ teaspoon sea salt

8 ounces wild salmon fillets

1 whole egg

¼ cup chopped Macadamia nuts

1 tablespoon extra-virgin olive oil

1 cup buckwheat (measured dry), cooked according to package instructions

Preheat oven to 400°F.

Mix together the black pepper, lemon juice, and salt and rub into the salmon flesh.

In a shallow bowl, whisk egg until it is well mixed. Dip the fish in the egg mixture and then coat with the nuts on one side. Spread any remaining nuts over the fish and gently pat down.

Brush a baking sheet with the olive oil. Place the fish nut-side up and bake for 6–8 minutes, depending upon the thickness of the fillets, or until they are easily flaked with a fork.

Serve with the buckwheat on the side.

Nutrition Facts, per one serving (recipe makes two servings): 639 cal, 27 g protein, 63 g carbohydrate, 10 g fiber, 31 g fat

Dover Sole with Red Pesto and Sweet Potato

Phase 2 Diet

Dover sole is a type of whitefish. It is mild yet delicious, while being an excellent source of minerals such as selenium, magnesium, potassium, and iodine. The wild-caught version is relatively low in mercury and fairly easy to find. This is a one-pot dish that is simple to make in the oven.

Red pesto is a common condiment typically made from sun-dried tomatoes, basil, and garlic; it is a lesser-known product that I consider one of my kitchen hacks, because it's a convenient way to add excellent flavor to any dish using just a single product. If you prefer to make this yourself at home, I have included the ingredients below.

Makes one serving

- 1 pound sweet potato or yam, sliced into quarter-inch thick circles
- 1 tablespoon extra-virgin olive oil
- ½ teaspoon salt, or to your taste
- 4 ounces wild-caught Dover sole fillet
- 1 tablespoon red pesto (if you prefer not to use store-bought, you can substitute by mixing together 2 teaspoons tomato sauce, 1 teaspoon dried basil, 1 teaspoon lemon juice, one chopped garlic clove, and 1 teaspoon olive oil)
- 1 tablespoon chopped cilantro, for garnish

Coat both sides of the sweet potato slices with the olive oil. Place the sweet potato slices flat on a single layer in a baking pan.

Sprinkle the salt over both sides of the Dover sole fillet. Place the fish on top of the sweet potato slices. Spread the red pesto evenly on top of the fillet.

Bake in a 400°F oven for 10–15 minutes, until the fish is opaque. Be sure not to overcook. The flesh should be white all the way through and slightly flake with a fork.

Remove the tray from the oven and transfer to a plate, garnishing with the chopped cilantro.

NUTRITION FACTS, per one serving (recipe makes one serving):
589 cal, 30 g protein, 74 g carbohydrate, 6 g fiber, 20 g fat

Black Cumin Shrimp Curry

Phase 2 Diet

This is yet another delicious recipe that incorporates black cumin. The shrimp are a good source of B12 and the fenugreek and cumin provide support for healthy blood sugar and metabolism.

This pairs well with quinoa but feel free to substitute rice if you prefer. This recipe includes regular quinoa but for a flavor boost I suggest having it with the Basil Pesto Quinoa (see recipe on p. 313).

Makes two servings

1 tablespoon coconut oil, divided

¼ teaspoon fenugreek seeds

¼ teaspoon ajwain seeds

½ teaspoon nigella sativa seeds

2 medium cloves of garlic, chopped

½ medium-sized onion, chopped

1 medium tomato, diced

½ teaspoon turmeric

1 teaspoon cumin powder

½ cup coconut milk

½ teaspoon salt

½ pound shrimp, peeled and deveined

1 cup of quinoa (measured dry), cooked according to package instructions

In a medium-sized pot, heat 1 teaspoon of coconut oil. When the oil is hot, add fenugreek, ajwain, nigella sativa, and the garlic. Stir and sauté for about 30 seconds.

Add chopped onion and sauté for 2–3 minutes over medium heat until onions are opaque. Then add tomatoes, turmeric, cumin powder, coconut milk, and salt and cook over medium heat for about 10 minutes or until the sauce begins to thicken slightly. At this time, the sauce is ready and can be removed from the stove and set aside.

In a skillet or cast-iron pan, heat the remaining 2 teaspoons of coconut oil. When the oil is hot add the shrimp and stir fry for about 2 minutes. Add the sauce, mix well and cook for another 2 minutes, or until the shrimp are fully cooked.

Serve immediately over the quinoa.

NUTRITION FACTS, per one serving (recipe makes two servings): 623 cal, 40 g protein, 63 g carbohydrate, 8 g fiber, 24 g fat

Beef Curry over Rice

Phase 2 Diet

This beef curry is loaded with aromatic spices that make it taste amazing and add therapeutic properties to the dish. The raisins provide a lightness and sweet flavor that pairs well with the heartiness of the beef.

The first step is to sear the beef. This preserves the juices inside while caramelizing the outside. Although this takes additional time, it adds a great deal of flavor to the final dish. I recommend bone broth to add richness to this dish, but you can substitute vegetable broth or water for a lighter version.

Makes two servings

1 tablespoon olive oil
1 medium onion, chopped (any color onion is fine)
¼ teaspoon turmeric powder
¼ teaspoon cumin powder
8 ounces lean beef stew meat, cut into 1-inch pieces

I clove garlic, minced

½ teaspoon ginger paste or fresh ginger, finely chopped

¼ teaspoon fenugreek powder

I medium carrot, chopped into circles

2 tablespoons raisins

I cup beef bone broth (or chicken bone broth)

I tablespoon tomato paste

8 ounces full-fat coconut milk (about half a can)

½ teaspoon salt, or to taste

I tablespoon chopped parsley

½ cup rice (measured dry), cooked according to package instructions

Heat the oil in a large saucepan and add the onion, turmeric, and cumin powder. Sauté for 2–3 minutes until the onions turn translucent.

Mix in the beef, garlic, ginger, and fenugreek and sear the beef for 10–12 minutes, stirring occasionally to brown the meat as evenly as possible.

Add the carrot, raisins, bone broth, tomato paste, coconut milk, and salt and bring to a boil after stirring well. Reduce to a simmer and cook partially covered for another 20 minutes or until the beef is tender. Garnish with the chopped parsley and serve over the rice.

NUTRITION FACTS, per one serving (recipe makes two servings):
755 cal, 36 g protein, 68 g carbohydrate, 6 g fiber, 40 g fat

Spiced Turkey Meatloaf with Sweet Potatoes

Phase 2 Diet

This is a dish that we make all the time at home, since it is easy, nutritious, and tastes great. We usually keep ginger in the freezer because it is easy to grate when frozen. Cremini mushrooms have an earthy flavor that pairs well with turkey.

Cast-iron pans can go from stovetop to oven, but if you do not have one, any other pan would work too.

Makes four servings

I teaspoon coconut oil

I medium-sized white onion, diced

4 small cloves garlic

1 tablespoon ginger, grated or finely chopped

½ teaspoon turmeric powder

½ teaspoon fennel powder

¼ teaspoon cumin powder

¼ teaspoon black pepper

¼ teaspoon black cumin powder

1 teaspoon salt, or to taste

1 pound ground turkey

2 eggs, beaten

1 tablespoon cilantro, chopped

juice of ½ lemon, squeezed

1 cup cremini mushrooms, thinly sliced

4 sweet potatoes

Preheat oven to 375°F.

Note: You could simply mix and bake all the ingredients and skip this first step, but I find that roasting the spices makes the overall dish more savory and piquant.

In a cast-iron pan heat the coconut oil. When hot, add the onion and sauté until translucent. Then add the garlic, ginger, spices, and salt and roast on medium heat for another minute or so. Allow to cool for a minute.

In the meantime, add the ground meat to a mixing bowl. Break it up with your hands and add the eggs and mix well. Transfer the sautéed mixture from the pan to the bowl, add the cilantro, lemon juice, and mushrooms and mix well. Once ready, transfer the mixture back to the cast-iron pan (or other well-greased oven safe dish) and place in the oven.

Wash the sweet potatoes. Ideally, leave the skin on because most of the phyto-chemicals are in the skin and close to the external surface. Place them whole on a different pan and place them in the oven.

Bake for 38–40 minutes or until the turkey is well-cooked internally. For a crispy top, broil for the final few minutes of baking.

NUTRITION FACTS, per one serving (recipe makes four servings):
465 cal, 21 g protein, 43 g carbohydrate, 6 g fiber, 24 g fat

SIDE DISHES & LIGHTER FARE

Oven Roasted Artichoke

Phase 1 or Phase 2 Diet

The artichoke is an outstanding source of prebiotic inulin fiber. Although it can have an intimidating appearance, you can work with it without a lot of fuss. The reward is a delicious dish that is nearly unmatched in benefits for your microbiome.

When choosing an artichoke, find one that has tightly packed leaves and does not have too many brown areas. To cook, a baking pan with a lid is your best option. You can also cover the artichokes with aluminum foil while baking.

Makes one serving

2 fresh globe artichokes
1 tablespoon lemon juice
1 tablespoon olive oil

Preheat your oven to 400°F.

Chop off about a half-inch piece at the base of the artichoke, and 1 inch off of the top, and discard both. Pull off any small, fibrous leaves at the base and discard. You'll notice that the leaves have a small spike at the end. Use scissors to trim off a tiny strip at the end of each leaf (along with the spike) and discard.

Slice the artichoke down the middle vertically so you have 2 symmetric halves. At the center, you'll find an area with fuzzy hairs called the "choke." Use a spoon to scoop this area out completely and discard, because these fine hairs can get caught in your throat (hence the name).

Rub the lemon juice all over the cut surfaces of the artichoke to counteract oxidation. Line a baking pan with the olive oil, and place the 4 artichoke halves, cut surface up, on the tray in a single layer.

Roast in the oven for about 10 minutes, to brown the edges. Then, cover the pan tightly with a lid or aluminum foil. This is an important step to ensure that the flesh does not dry out. Return to the oven and bake for another 30–40 minutes, or until the artichoke is tender and the leaves can be pulled off easily.

Artichoke pairs well with Avocado Hummus (see recipe on p. 315), or any other sauce you prefer. In case this is your first time cooking a fresh artichoke, to eat it: pull off each leaf one by one and dip in the sauce. Place in your mouth and scrape off the tender flesh at the end of the leaf along with the dipping sauce, and discard/compost the remainder. Repeat until the leaves are done, and do the same with the heart and base of the artichoke.

NUTRITION FACTS, per one serving (recipe makes one serving):
187 cal, 4 g protein, 14 g carbohydrate, 7 g fiber, 14 g fat

Garlicky Shiitake Mushrooms

Phase 1 or Phase 2 Diet

Asian mushrooms, such as shiitake and maitake, have a tremendous amount of umami, the fifth basic taste that provides depth and richness of flavor. Mushrooms also contain unique prebiotics that feed the microbiome and immune-enhancing compounds like beta-glucans, which have cancer-fighting properties.

This recipe calls for fresh shiitake mushrooms, which are widely available in Asian markets and most grocery stores. As an alternative, you can use dehydrated shiitake mushrooms and rehydrate them with water before cooking. These mushrooms are very hardy and it is nearly impossible to overcook them, so don't be afraid to use high heat.

Makes two servings

16 ounces shiitake mushrooms, trimmed to bite-sized pieces (try to make them approximately the same size)

2 teaspoons coconut oil

½ onion, diced

2 small garlic cloves, minced

¼ teaspoon salt

Remove and discard the mushroom stems. Wash the mushroom caps after removing and pat dry with a paper towel to remove as much moisture as you can.

Heat the coconut oil in a large saucepan and add the onion when the oil is hot. Sauté for 2 minutes until the onions start to turn translucent.

Add the mushrooms and spread them apart in a single layer. Cook on high heat for 3–4 minutes, stirring occasionally.

At this point, adjust the heat based on how much liquid has been released from the mushrooms (this can vary). If there's not much liquid in the pan, reduce to medium heat. If a lot of water has come out from the mushrooms, maintain high heat to evaporate as much of the water as possible. This will enrich the taste of the mushrooms and provide a more seared flavor.

Add the minced garlic and salt and continue to sauté for another 3 minutes, stirring occasionally. You can tell they are done when they become soft and golden brown; they will have reduced in size as well.

NUTRITION FACTS, per one serving (recipe makes two servings):
128 cal, 5 g protein, 18 g carbohydrate, 6 g fiber, 6 g fat

Gluten-Free Coconut Flatbread

Phase 1 or Phase 2 Diet

This flatbread made with coconut flour is soft and delicious, like regular flatbread but with the advantage of being gluten-free. Psyllium husk gives it an outstanding fiber content of 15 g for each flatbread.

Makes four servings

1 cup coconut flour
4 tablespoons psyllium husk
2 tablespoons extra-virgin olive oil, divided
½ teaspoon baking soda
½ teaspoon salt

In a bowl, mix together the coconut flour and psyllium husk. Add 1 tablespoon of the olive oil and the remaining ingredients. Mix well and then use your hands to knead the dough. If the dough is too moist or sticking to your hands, you may add another ¼ teaspoon of psyllium husk until it is soft but not sticky. Then allow the dough to set for about 5 minutes.

Divide the dough into 4 parts. Place an individual piece of dough between two sheets of parchment paper and roll it flat with your hands or a rolling pin. Any shape will work—it doesn't need to be circular.

To a saucepan or cast-iron pan, add the remaining 1 tablespoon of olive oil and heat on medium. Place each piece of dough on the pan and immediately cover the pan with a lid. Cook for 2 minutes on one side, then remove the lid, flip, cover again and cook for one more minute. Repeat until all the dough has been used up.

This flatbread pairs well with the Chicken Tikka Masala or any other curry, and can be used as a bun substitute with the Spiced Salmon Burgers. It will last for up to 2 days in an airtight container stored in the refrigerator.

NUTRITION FACTS, per one serving (recipe makes four servings): 195 cal, 4 g protein, 21 g carbohydrate, 15 g fiber, 11 g fat

Basil Pesto Quinoa

Phase 2 Diet

Some find quinoa boring but preparing it in the right way can make it a delicious and even exciting part of your meal. I think you will not be disappointed with this version. It leads to a flavorful dish that can accompany any vegetable or meat curry but can also stand alone.

Makes two servings

½ cup quinoa (measured dry), cooked according to package instructions

1 cup fresh basil leaves, stems removed

½ cup pine nuts (may substitute with pumpkin seeds if pine nuts are not available, or in case of allergies)

1 tablespoon lemon juice, freshly squeezed from half a lemon

1 tablespoon olive oil

½ teaspoon salt

Cook the quinoa according to package instructions. While it is cooking, prepare the pesto.

In a blender or food processor, combine the basil leaves with the pine nuts, lemon juice, olive oil, and salt. Blend until smooth.

Combine the cooked quinoa with the pesto in a bowl and mix well. Serve immediately.

NUTRITION FACTS, per one serving (recipe makes two servings): 435 cal, 10 g protein, 35 g carbohydrate, 7 g fiber, 30 g fat

Sunflower Seed Hummus with Cumin

Phase 2 Diet

Sunflower seeds are an excellent source of magnesium and zinc, and tahini is one of the richest nondairy food sources of calcium. You can substitute premade sunflower butter if you prefer not having to grind the sunflower seeds.

Chickpeas are a good source of resistant starch, B vitamins, fiber, potassium, and selenium. The cumin provides a toasted flavor that complements the other ingredients well.

Makes four servings

2 tablespoons roasted sunflower seeds (or 1 tablespoon of sunflower butter)

2 ½ cups cooked chickpeas (equivalent of one 15-ounce can)

2 tablespoons tahini

2 tablespoons lemon juice

2 cloves of garlic

⅛ teaspoon cumin powder

2 tablespoons water

½ teaspoon sea salt, or to taste

In a blender or food processor, add sunflower seeds and pulse until they become a paste, adding tablespoons of water as necessary; the texture should be smooth and creamy. If you opt to use sunflower seed butter, you can skip this step and add it directly to the blender.

Add all of the remaining ingredients and blend until smooth. If necessary, add more water to get the consistency to your liking. Spread on the Toasted Rosemary Crackers (see recipe on p. 315) or use as a dipping sauce for raw celery or carrots as a snack.

NUTRITION FACTS, per one serving (recipe makes four servings):
274 cal, 13 g protein, 38 g carbohydrate, 11 g fiber, 9 g fat

Avocado Hummus

Phase 2 Diet

Makes four servings

2 ½ cups cooked chickpeas (equivalent of one 15-ounce can)

2 tablespoons water

2 tablespoons tahini

2 tablespoons lemon juice

2 cloves of garlic

2 medium-sized avocados, peeled and pitted

½ teaspoon sea salt

⅛ teaspoon black pepper

Add the chickpeas to a food processor or blender and blend for about 3–4 minutes until it becomes a paste, adding water by the tablespoon to thin the mixture if necessary. Add in the tahini, lemon juice, and garlic and blend for another minute. Scoop in the avocados, salt, and pepper, and blend for another minute or until smooth.

NUTRITION FACTS, per one serving (recipe makes four servings): 341 cal, 14 g protein, 42 g carbohydrate, 14 g fiber, 15 g fat

Toasted Rosemary Crackers

Phase 2 Diet

These gluten-free crackers made with almond flour are an excellent substitute for saltines or traditional crackers. The rosemary provides an additional antioxidant boost and a savory flavor. The psyllium makes these crackers an excellent source of fiber. They are delicious on their own or with traditional hummus or the Sunflower Seed Hummus.

Makes four servings (8 crackers)

1 cup almond flour

4 tablespoons psyllium husk

2 tablespoons extra-virgin olive oil, divided

1 teaspoon rosemary leaves (fresh or dried)

½ teaspoon baking soda

½ teaspoon salt

In a bowl, mix together the almond flour and psyllium husk. Add 1 table-spoon of olive oil and the remaining ingredients. Mix well and then use your hands to knead the dough. If the dough is too moist or sticking to your hands, add another ¼ teaspoon of psyllium husk until it is soft but not sticky. Set aside for 5 minutes.

Divide the dough into 4 parts. Break each part into two roughly equal pieces. Place each piece of dough between two sheets of parchment paper and roll it flat with your hands or a rolling pin. Cut out a circular shape using the lid of a glass bottle or the top of a can. Save any remaining dough for another cracker.

On a griddle or cast-iron pan, add the remaining 1 tablespoon of olive oil and heat on medium. Place each piece of dough on the pan and cook uncovered for 2 minutes on one side, then flip and cook for 1 minute more. Repeat until all the dough has been used up. These crackers can be stored in an airtight container for up to 7 days.

NUTRITION FACTS, per one serving (recipe makes four servings): 214 cal, 5 g protein, 10 g carbohydrate, 7 g fiber, 19 g fat

FERMENTED FOODS

Cooling Cucumber Raita

Phase 1 or Phase 2 Diet

Raita is a traditional Indian fermented food traditionally made with yogurt. This version is modified to use nondairy yogurt. The cilantro, cucumber, and mint make a cooling side dish that pairs very well with spice-heavy curries and entrees.

In the Phase 1 Diet I suggest using coconut yogurt, and if you are in Phase 2 you can use almond yogurt or other acceptable nondairy yogurts.

Makes two servings

½ medium cucumber, cut into 4 pieces

¼ cup cilantro

¼ cup mint leaves

1 cup plain unsweetened nondairy yogurt (e.g., coconut or almond)

pinch of cumin powder

In a food processor or blender, combine cucumber, cilantro, mint, and yogurt. Pulse until the cucumber is chopped and a chunky mixture is formed.

Top with a pinch of cumin powder. Serve immediately or store in the refrigerator for up to 48 hours.

NUTRITION FACTS, per one serving (recipe makes two servings): 81 cal, 3 g protein, 13 g carbohydrate, 1 g fiber, 2 g fat

Homemade Sauerkraut

Phase 1 or Phase 2 Diet

Sauerkraut is a staple fermented food in many different cultures. Even a tablespoon as a condiment to accompany your meals will provide a significant number of beneficial bacteria. If you are interested in making a more nutrient-dense sauerkraut you can purchase red cabbage, which will work just as well and has higher levels of antioxidants.

Makes eight servings

1 head of cabbage, green or red

1 teaspoon sea salt

Filtered water

Coarsely chop the cabbage and place it in a mixing bowl. Start to use your hands to mash and mix the cabbage as vigorously as you can. It should start to release water into the bowl as cabbage has a fairly high water content.

Add a teaspoon of sea salt to the cabbage and then mash it with the back of a wooden spoon or other solid kitchen utensil to break it down further.

Spoon the cabbage into a mason jar and, using the back of the wooden spoon or other utensil, pack it down as tightly as you can into the bottom of the jar.

When you are done, if there was adequate fluid released from the cabbage, the water should cover the very top of the cabbage, i.e., there should not be any cabbage sticking out above the water. If some of the cabbage is above the water, add some filtered water until all of the cabbage is completely submerged. Cover the jar loosely with a kitchen towel or cheesecloth.

Set the jar in a cool, dry place away from sunlight and check it every couple of days to make sure that all the cabbage is submerged. If not, add more filtered water until all the cabbage is below the water line.

After 5 days, start to taste the cabbage. It should have a tart, tangy taste but still retain some of its crunch. If it's not ready, check again every 1 or 2 days until ready. Depending on the temperature and local climate, it can take anywhere from 7–14 days to be ready.

When it is done, cover tightly and refrigerate the sauerkraut. It should last for at least a couple of months in the fridge.

NUTRITION FACTS, per one serving (recipe makes eight servings):
22 cal, 5 g carbohydrate, 2 g fiber, not a significant source of protein or fat

Pickled Ginger

Phase 1 or Phase 2 Diet

Pickled ginger combines the anti-inflammatory effects of ginger with the microbiome benefits of a fermented food. It's an excellent condiment that adds flavor to any cooked meat or vegetable dish. I often drop a spoonful in the corner of my dinner plates to boost the probiotic capacity of the meal.

Makes eight servings

¼ pound fresh ginger

Filtered water

¼ teaspoon sea salt

Start by peeling the ginger and slicing it into thin half-inch pieces. If it's easier you can grate the ginger—it just depends what consistency you prefer for the final product.

Fill a glass Mason jar about halfway with filtered water and add the salt. Stir well.

Add the ginger and then, if necessary, add more water until the top of the ginger is completely submerged. Do not seal the jar but cover loosely with a cheesecloth, paper towel, or kitchen towel.

Check it every 24 hours. If the water level drops and any ginger comes up above the water, add more water until all the ginger is completely submerged. After 3 days, begin tasting. Once the ginger tastes tangy or tart, it's ready. Seal tightly and store in the fridge where it will last for up to a month.

NUTRITION FACTS, per one serving (recipe makes eight servings):
10 cal, 2 g carbohydrate, not a significant source of protein, fiber, or fat

Acknowledgments

After publishing my first book several years ago, I made a silent vow not to do this again because of the amount of work involved. Of course, as time went on, I forgot that vow. More importantly, a new dream developed—to share my knowledge and understanding about autoimmune conditions with as many people as possible. It has taken a small army of people to make this dream a reality. There are far more people than I can mention individually here, but I hope that you know who you are and that you have my sincere gratitude.

To my agent, Jud Laghi, your belief in this project from the beginning was unwavering. What you have accomplished exceeded all my expectations. I thank you for the sage advice, acumen, and wisdom you brought to every step of the process.

To my editor, Nana Twumasi, and the team at Grand Central Balance, I thank you for your masterful shepherding of the process, insightful editing, and skillful transformation of my rough ideas into the polished final version.

I would like to thank everyone at my clinic, the Sutter Health Institute for Health and Healing, especially my director, Judith Tolson, for the unflagging support and encouragement.

I owe a debt of gratitude to many teachers, but I want to especially thank Dr. Andrew Weil for giving me a solid foundation in integrative medicine. I also want to thank my patients who have been and continue to be my teachers.

My friends and family have been the biggest blessings in my life. I would like to extend a deep bow and my heartfelt gratitude to each and every one of you. To my wife, Aiswarya, and my daughter, Alisha—thank you for being on this fantastic journey with me. I am so lucky to have you both in my life. Everything I do and strive for—is for you.

Notes

Introduction

1. DeLis Fairweather, Sylvia Frisancho-Kiss, and Noel R. Rose, "Sex Differences in Autoimmune Disease from a Pathological Perspective," *The American Journal of Pathology* 173, no. 3 (September 2008): 600–609, doi: 10.2353/ajpath.2008.071008.
2. Gregg E. Dinse et al., "Increasing Prevalence of Antinuclear Antibodies in the United States," *Arthritis Rheumatology* 72, no. 6 (June 2020): 1026–1035, doi: 10.1002/art.41214.
3. Manuel J. Amador-Patarroyo, Alberto Rodriguez-Rodriguez, and Gladis Montoya-Ortiz, "How Does Age at Onset Influence the Outcome of Autoimmune Diseases?", *Autoimmune Diseases* 2012 (December 13, 2011): 251730, doi: 10.1155/2012/251730.
4. "Disease List," Autoimmune Association, accessed June 23, 2021, https://www.aarda.org /diseaselist/.
5. Dinse, "Increasing Prevalence," 1026–1035.
6. Miriam E. Tucker, "Autoimmune Disease," *Autoimmune Association* (October 4, 2018), accessed April 10, 2022, https://www.aarda.org/closing-care-gap-autoimmune-disease.
7. Yehuda Shoenfeld et al., "The Mosaic of Autoimmunity: Prediction, Autoantibodies, and Therapy in Autoimmune Diseases—2008," *Israel Medical Association Journal* 10, no. 1 (January 2008): 13–19, https://pubmed.ncbi.nlm.nih.gov/18300564/.
8. In Young Choi et al., "Diet Mimicking Fasting Promotes Regeneration and Reduces Autoimmunity and Multiple Sclerosis Symptoms," *Cell Reports* 15, no. 10 (June 7, 2016): 2136–2146, doi: 10.1016/j.celrep.2016.05.009.
9. Bruce Stevens et al., "Increased Human Intestinal Barrier Permeability Plasma Biomarkers Zonulin and FABP2 Correlated with Plasma LPS and Altered Gut Microbiome in Anxiety or Depression," *Gut* 67, no. 8 (2018): 1555–1557, doi: 10.1136/gutjnl-2017-314759.
10. Sun Kwang Kim and Hyunsu Bae, "Acupuncture and Immune Modulation," *Autonomic Neuroscience: Basic and Clinical* 157, nos. 1–2 (October 28, 2010): 38–41, doi: 10.1016/j .autneu.2010.03.010.

Chapter 1

1. Vlma Harjutsalo, Reijo Sund, and Mikael Knip, "Incidence of Type 1 Diabetes in Finland," *Jama Network* (July 24/31, 2013): 427–428, doi: 10.1001/jama.2013.8399.
2. James A. King et al., "Incidence of Celiac Disease Is Increasing Over Time: A Systematic Review and Meta-analysis," *American Journal of Gastroenterology* 115, no. 4 (April 2020): 507–525, doi: 10.14309/ajg.0000000000000523.
3. Christina Ong et al., "Rapid Rise in the Incidence and Clinical Characteristics of Pediatric Inflammatory Bowel Disease in a South-East Asian Cohort in Singapore, 1994–2015," *Journal of Digestive Diseases* 19, no. 7 (July 2018): 395–403, doi: 10.1111/1751-2980.12641.
4. Aaron Lerner, Patricia Jeremias, and Torsten Matthias, "The World Incidence and Prevalence of Autoimmune Diseases is Increasing," *International Journal of Celiac Disease* 3, no. 4 (2015): 151–155, doi: 10.12691/ijcd-3-4-8.

5. Jacqueline Parkin and Bryony Cohen, "An Overview of the Immune System," *Immunology* 357, no. 9270 (June 2, 2001): 1777–1789, accessed January 18, 2022, doi: 10.1016 /S0140-6736(00)04904-7.

6. Parkin, "An Overview," 1777–1789.

7. Maria K. Smatti et al., "Viruses and Autoimmunity: A Review on the Potential Interaction and Molecular Mechanisms," *Viruses* 11, no. 8 (August 19, 2019): 762, accessed January 18, 2022, doi: 10.3390/v11080762.

8. Richard A.C. Hughes and Jeremy H. Rees, "Clinical and Epidemiologic Features of Guillain-Barré Syndrome," *The Journal of Infectious Diseases* 176, no. 2 (December 1997): S92–S98, accessed January 18, 2022, doi: 10.1086/513793.

9. Kai W. Wucherpfennig, "Mechanisms for the Induction of Autoimmunity by Infectious Agents," *The Journal of Clinical Investigation* 108, no. 8 (2001): 1097–1104, accessed January 18, 2022, doi: 10.1172/JCI14235.

10. Robert S. Fujinami, "Molecular Mimicry, Bystander Activation, or Viral Persistence: Infections and Autoimmune Disease," *Clinical Microbiology Review* 19, no. 1 (January 2006): 80–94, accessed January 18, 2022, 10.1128/CMR.19.1.80-94.2006.

11. Gilbert J. Fournié et al., "Induction of Autoimmunity through Bystander Effects: Lessons from Immunological Disorders Induced by Heavy Metals," *Journal of Autoimmunity* 16, no. 3 (May 2001): 319–326, doi: 10.1006/jaut.2000.0482.

12. Margarita Dominguez-Villar and David A. Hafler, "Regulatory T Cells in Autoimmune Disease," *Nature Immunology* 19 (June 20, 2018): 665–673, doi: 10.1038/s41590-018-0120-4.

13. R.D.G. Leslie and M. Hawa, "Twin Studies in Auto-immune Disease," *ACTA Geneticae Medicae et Gemellologiae: Twin Research* 43, nos. 1–2 (1994): 71–81, doi: 10.1017/s000156600000297x.

14. Zachary H. Harvey, Yiwen Chen, and Daniel F. Jarosz, "Protein-Based Inheritance: Epigenetics beyond the Chromosome," *Molecular Cell* 69, no. 2 (January 2018): 195–202, doi: 10.1016/j .molcel.2017.10.030.

15. Dhinoth K. Bangarusamy et al., "Nutri-epigenetics: The Effect of Maternal Diet and Early Nutrition on the Pathogenesis of Autoimmune Diseases," *Minerva Pediatrics* 73, no. 2 (April 2021): 98–110, doi: 10.23736/S2724-5276.20.06166-6.

16. Aristo Vojdani et al., "The Role of Exposomes in the Pathophysiology of Autoimmune Diseases I: Toxic Chemicals and Food," *Pathophysiology* 28, no. 4 (2021): 513–543, doi: 10.3390 /pathophysiology28040034.

17. Christina E. West et al., "The Gut Microbes and Inflammatory Noncommunicable Diseases: Associations and Potentials for Gut Microbes Therapies," *The Journal of Allergy and Clinical Immunology* 135, no. 1 (January 1, 2015): 3–13, doi: 10.1016/j.jaci.2014.11.012.

18. Ron Sender, Shai Fuchs, and Ron Milo, "Revised Estimates for the Number of Human and Bacteria Cells in the Body," *PLoS Biology* 14, no. 8 (August 2016): e1002533, doi: 10.1371 /journal.pbio.1002533.

19. Jack A. Gilbert et al., "Current Understanding of the Human Microbiome," *Nature Medicine* 24 (April 1, 2018): 392–400, accessed January 18, 2022, doi: 10.1038/nm.4517.

20. Edoardo Pasolli et al., "Extensive Unexplored Human Microbiome Diversity Revealed by Over 150,000 Genomes from Metagenomes Spanning Age, Geography, and Lifestyle," *Cell* 178, no. 3 (January 17, 2019): 649–662, doi: 10.1016/j.cell.2019.01.001.

21. C. Manichanh et al., "Reduced Diversity of Faecal Microbiota in Crohn's Disease Revealed by a Metagenomic Approach," *Gut* 55, no. 2 (February 2006): 205–211, doi: 10.1136 /gut.2005.073817.

22. Marsha C. Wibowo et al., "Reconstruction of Ancient Microbial Genomes from the Human Gut," *Nature* 594 (May 12, 2021): 234–239, doi: 10.1038/s41586-021-03532-0.

23. Martin J. Blaser, "The Theory of Disappearing Microbiota and the Epidemics of Chronic Diseases," *Nature Reviews Immunology* 17 (July 27, 2017): 461–463, doi: 10.1038/nri.2017.77.

24. Christian Milani et al., "The First Microbial Colonizers of the Human Gut: Composition, Activities, and Health Implications of the Infant Gut Microbes," *Microbiology and Molecular Biology Reviews* 81, no. 4 (November 8, 2017): e00036-17, doi: 10.1128/MMBR.00036-17.

25. Lieke W. J. van den Elsen et al., "Shaping the Gut Microbes by Breastfeeding: The Gateway to Allergy Prevention?", *Frontiers in Pediatrics* (February 27, 2019), doi: 10.3389/fped.2019.00047.

26. Philip Bowler, Christine Murphy, and Randall Woolcott, "Biofilm Exacerbates Antibiotic Resistance: Is This a Current Oversight in Antimicrobial Stewardship?", *Antimicrobial Resistance and Infection Control* 9, no. 1 (October 20, 2020), doi: 10.1186/s13756-020-00830-6.

27. Kelly S. Swanson et al., "The International Scientific Association for Probiotics and Prebiotics (ISAPP) Consensus Statement on the Definition and Scope of Synbiotics," *Nature Reviews Gastroenterology & Hepatology* 17, no. 11 (November 2020): 687–701, accessed January 18, 2011, doi: 10.1038/s41575-020-0344-2.

28. Jakub Żółkiewicz et al., "Postbiotics—A Step Beyond Pre- and Probiotics," *Nutrients* 12, no. 8 (July 23, 2020): 2189, doi: 10.3390/nu12082189.

29. Jeff D. Leach and Kristin D. Sobolik, "High Dietary Intake of Prebiotic Inulin-Type Fructans in the Prehistoric Chihuahuan Desert," *British Journal of Nutrition* 13, no. 11 (April 26, 2010): 1558–1561, doi: 10.1017/S0007114510000966.

30. Stephanie L. Schnorr et al., "Gut Microbiome of the Hadza Hunter-gatherers," *Nature Communications* 5, no. 3654 (April 15, 2014), doi: 10.1038/ncomms4654.

31. Bjoern O. Schroeder, "Fight Them or Feed Them: How the Intestinal Mucus Layer Manages the Gut Microbiota," *Gastrenterology Report* 7, no. 1 (February 2019): 3–12, doi: 10.1093/gastro/goy052.

32. Mahesh S. Desai, "A Dietary Fiber-Deprived Gut Microbe Degrades the Colonic Mucus Barrier and Enhances Pathogen Susceptibility," *Cell* 167, no. 5 (November 17, 2016): 1339–1353, doi: 10.1016/j.cell.2016.10.043.

33. Bjoern O. Schroeder et al., "Bifidobacteria or Fiber Protect Against Diet-Induced Microbiota-Mediated Colonic Mucus Deterioration," *Cell Host & Microbe* 23, no. 1 (January 10, 2018): 27–40, doi: 10.1016/j.chom.2017.11.004.

34. Pascal Juillerat et al., "Prevalence of Inflammatory Bowel Disease in the Canton of Vaud (Switzerland): A Population-based Cohort Study," *Journal of Crohn's and Colitis* 2, no. 2 (June 2008): 131–141, doi: 10.1016/j.crohns.2007.10.006.

35. Moises Velasquez-Manoff, *An Epidemic of Absence: A New Way of Understanding Allergies and Autoimmune Diseases* (New York: Simon and Schuster, 2012), 110.

36. Velasquez-Manoff, *An Epidemic of Absence*, 113.

37. John W. Frew, "The Hygiene Hypothesis, Old Friends, and New Genes," *Frontiers in Immunology* 10 (March 6, 2019): 388, doi: 10.3389/fimmu.2019.00388.

38. Martin Blaser, *Missing Microbes* (New York: Henry Holt and Company, 2014), 138–139.

39. Sergio Castañeda et al., "Microbiota Characterization in Blastocystis-colonized and Blastocystis-free School-age Children from Colombia," *Parasites & Vectors* 13 (October 16, 2020): 521, accessed January 18, 2022, doi: 10.1186/s13071-020-04392-9.

40. Helle Gotfred-Rasmussen et al., "Impact of Metronidazole Treatment and Dientamoeba Fragilis Colonization on Gut Microbes Diversity," *Journal of Pediatric Gastroenterology and Nutrition* 73, no. 1 (July 1, 2021): 23–29, doi: 10.1097/MPG.0000000000003096.

41. Bethany M. Henrick et al., "Elevated Fecal pH Indicates a Profound Change in the Breastfed Infant Gut Microbiome Due to Reduction of *Bifidobacterium* over the Past Century," *mSphere* (March 7, 2018), doi: 10.1128/mSphere.00041-18.

42. Tommi Vatanen et al., "Variation in Microbiome LPS Immunogenicity Contribute to Autoimmunity in Humans," *Cell* 165, no. 4 (May 5, 2016): 842–853, doi: 10.1016/j.cell.2016.04.007.

43. Mikael Knip and Heli Siljander, "The Role of the Intestinal Microbiota in Type 1 Diabetes Mellitus," *Nature Reviews Endocrinology* 12 (January 4, 2016): 154–167, doi: 10.1038/nrendo.2015.218.

44. Henrick, "Elevated."

45. Knip, "The Role of the Intestinal Microbiota," 154–167.

46. Sarah Esther Chang et al., "New-Onset IgG Autoantibodies in Hospitalized Patients with COVID-19," *medRxiv* (January 29, 2021), doi: 10.1101/2021.01.27.21250559.

47. Mariam Ahmed Saad et al., "COVID-19 and Autoimmune Diseases: A Systematic Review of Reported Cases," *Current Rheumatology Reviews* 17, no. 2 (2021): 193–204, doi: 10.2174/15733 97116666201029155856.

48. Nahid Bhadelia et al., "Distinct Autoimmune Antibody Signatures Between Hospitalized Acute COVID-19 Patients, SARS-CoV-2 Convalescent Individuals, and Unexposed Pre-Pandemic Controls," *medRxiv* (January 25, 2021), doi: 10.1101/2021.01.21.21249176.

49. Shin Jie Yong et al., "Long COVID or Post-COVID-19 Syndrome: Putative Pathophysiology, Risk Factors, and Treatments," *Infectious Diseases* 53, no. 10 (October 2021): 737–754, doi: 10.1080/23744235.2021.1924397.

50. Aristo Vojdani and Datis Kharrazian, "Potential Antigenic Cross-Reactivity between SARS-COV-2 and Human Tissue with a Possible Link to an Increase in Autoimmune Diseases," *Journal of Clinical Immunology* 217 (August 2020): 108480, doi: 10.1016/j.clim.2020.108480.

Chapter 2

1. Bruce P. Lanphear, "The Impact of Toxins on the Developing Brain," *Annu Rev Public Health* 36 (2015): 211–30, doi: 10.1146/annurev-publhealth-031912-114413.

2. Emily C. Somers et al., "Mercury Exposure and Antinuclear Antibodies among Females of Reproductive Age in the United States: NHANES," *Environmental Health Perspectives* 123, no. 8 (August 2015): 792–798, doi: 10.1289/ehp.1408751.

3. EPA Press Office, "EPA Releases First Major Update to Chemicals List in 40 Years," Environmental Protection Agency (February 19, 2019), accessed April 5, 2022, https://archive.epa.gov/epa/newsreleases/epa-releases-first-major-update-chemicals-list-40-years.html.

4. Vladimir N. Uversky et al., "Synergistic Effects of Pesticides and Metals on the Fibrillation of Alpha-Synuclein: Implications for Parkinson's Disease," *Neurotoxicology* 23, nos. 4–5 (October 2002): 527–536, doi: 10.1016/s0161-813x(02)00067-0.

5. "National Report on Human Exposure to Environmental Chemicals: Updated Tables, March 2021," Centers for Disease Control and Prevention, https://www.cdc.gov/exposurereport/.

6. "Group: EWG/Commonweal Study #1, Industrial Chemicals and Pesticides in Adults Found 155–171 of 214 Tested Chemicals (9 Participants)," Human Toxome Project, accessed April 10, 2022, https://www.ewg.org/sites/humantoxome/participants/participant-group.php?group=bb1.

7. "Body Burden: The Pollution in Newborns," EWG (July 14, 2005), accessed January 19, 2022, https://www.ewg.org/research/body-burden-pollution-newborns.

8. Rachel Morello-Frosch et al., "Environmental Chemicals in an Urban Population of Pregnant Women and Their Newborns from San Francisco," *Environmental Science & Technology* 50, no. 22 (October 4, 2016): 12464–12472, doi: 10.1021/acs.est.6b03492.

9. Guomao Zheng et al., "Per- and Polyfluoroalkyl Substances (PFAS) in Breast Milk: Concerning Trends for Current-Use PFAS," *Environmental Science & Technology* 55, no. 11 (May 13, 2021): 7510–7520, https://doi.org/10.1021/acs.est.0c06978.

10. Bevin E. Blake and Suzanne E. Fenton, "Early Life Exposure to Per- and Polyfluoroalkyl Substances (PFAS) and Latent Health Outcomes: A Review Including the Placenta as a Target Tissue and Possible Driver of Peri- and Postnatal Effects," *Toxicology* 443 (October 2020): 152, doi: 10.1016/j.tox.2020.152565.

11. Fabrizia Bamonti et al., "Metal Chelation Therapy in Rheumatoid Arthritis: A Case Report. Successful Management of Rheumatoid Arthritis by Metal Chelation Therapy," *BioMetals* 24, no. 6 (December 2011): 1093–1098, doi: 10.1007/s10534-011-9467-9.

12. Alessandro Fulgenzi et al., "A Case of Multiple Sclerosis Improvement Following Removal of Heavy Metal Intoxication: Lessons Learnt from Matteo's Case," *BioMetals* 25, no. 3 (March 2012): 569–576, doi: 10.1007/s10534-012-9537-7.

13. M.P. Webber et al., "Nested Case-Control Study of Selected Systemic Autoimmune Diseases in World Trade Center Rescue/Recovery Workers," *Arthritis & Rheumatology* 67, no. 5 (May 2015): 1369–1376, doi: 10.1002/art.39059.

14. Edith M. Williams et al., "A Geographic Information Assessment of Exposure to a Toxic Waste Site and Development of Systemic Lupus Erythematosus (SLE): Findings from the Buffalo Lupus Project," *Journal of Toxicology and Environmental Health Sciences* 3, no. 3 (March 2011): 52–64, https://scholarcommons.sc.edu/cgi/viewcontent.cgi?article=1004&context=sph_epidemiology_biostatistics_facpub.

15. Edith M. Williams et al., "A Case Study of Community Involvement Influence on Policy Decisions: Victories of a Community-Based Participatory Research Partnership," *International Journal of Environmental Research and Public Health* 13, no. 5 (May 20, 2016): 515, doi: 10.3390/ijerph13050515

16. Yanpei Gu et al., "Biomarkers, Oxidative Stress and Autophagy in Skin Aging," *Ageing Research Reviews* 59 (February 24, 2020): 101036, doi: 10.1016/j.arr.2020.101036.

17. Sheetal Ramani et al., "Oxidative Stress in Autoimmune Diseases: An Under Dealt Malice," *Current Protein & Peptide Science* 21, no. 6 (2020): 611–621, doi: 10.2174/138920372166620 0214111816; Shunichi Kumagai, Takumi Jikimoto, and Jun Saegusa, "Pathological Roles of Oxidative Stress in Autoimmune Diseases," *Rinsho Byori (Japanese Journal of Clinical Pathology)* 51, no. 2 (February 2003): 126–132, https://pubmed.ncbi.nlm.nih.gov/12690629/.

18. Dorothy J. Pattison et al., "Dietary Beta-Cryptoxanthin and Inflammatory Polyarthritis: Results from a Population-based Prospective Study," *The American Journal of Clinical Nutrition* 82, no. 2 (August 2005): 451–455, doi: 10.1093/ajcn.82.2.451.

19. Lindsey A. Criswell et al., "Smoking Interacts with Genetic Risk Factors in the Development of Rheumatoid Arthritis among Older Caucasian Women," *Annals of the Rheumatic Diseases* 65, no. 9 (September 2006): 1163–1167, doi: 10.1136/ard.2005.049676.

20. Eyal Zifman et al., "Antioxidants and Smoking in Autoimmune Disease—Opposing Sides of the Seesaw?", *Autoimmunity Reviews* 8, no. 2 (December 2008): 165–169, doi: 10.1016/j.autrev.2008.06.011.

21. Jian-Hua Wang et al., "Acupuncture for Smoking Cessation: A Systematic Review and Meta-Analysis of 24 Randomized Controlled Trials," *Tobacco Induced Diseases* 17 (June 4, 2019): 48, doi: 10.18332/tid/109195.

22. Margaret Sears E et al. "Arsenic, Cadmium, Lead, and Mercury in Sweat: A Systematic Review," *Journal of Environmental and Public Health* Vol. 2012 (February 2012): 184745, doi: 10.1155/2012/184745.

23. Sears, "Arsenic," 184745.

24. Stephen J. Genuis et al., "Blood, Urine, and Sweat (BUS) Study: Monitoring and Elimination of Bioaccumulated Toxic Elements," *Archives of Environmental Contamination and Toxicology* 61, no. 2 (August 2011): 344–357, doi: 10.1007/s00244-010-9611-5.

25. Geary W. Olsen et al., "Half-Life of Serum Elimination of Perfluorooctanesulfonate, Perfluorohexanesulfonate, and Perfluorooctanoate in Retired Fluorochemical Production Workers," *Environmental Health Perspectives* 115, no. 9 (September 2007): 1298–1305, doi: 10.1289/ehp.10009.

26. US Food and Drug Administration, "Recommendations About the Use of Dental Amalgam in Certain High-Risk Populations: FDA Safety Communication," September 2020, https://www.fda.gov/medical-devices/safety-communications/recommendations-about-use-dental-amalgam-certain-high-risk-populations-fda-safety-communication, accessed on June 1, 2022.

27. US Food and Drug Administration, "Recommendations," accessed on April 6, 2022.

28. "Basic Information about Mercury," United States Environmental Protection Agency, https://www.epa.gov/mercury/basic-information-about-mercury.

29. Monisha Jaishankar et al., "Toxicity, Mechanism and Health Effects of Some Heavy Metals," *Interdisciplinary Toxicology* 7, no. 2 (June 2014): 60–72, doi: 10.2478/intox-2014-0009.

30. Somers, "Mercury Exposure," 792–798.

31. Ahmad Movahedian Attar et al., "Serum Mercury Level and Multiple Sclerosis," *Biological Trace Element Research* 146 (2012): 150–153, doi: 10.1007/s12011-011-9239-y.

32. Benjamin Rowley and Marc Monestier, "Mechanisms of Heavy Metal-induced Autoimmunity," *Molecular Immunology* 42, no. 7 (May 2005): 833–838, doi: 10.1016/j.molimm.2004.07.050.

33. Glinda S. Cooper et al., "Occupational Risk Factors for the Development of Systemic Lupus Erythematosus," *The Journal of Rheumatology* 31, no. 10 (October 2004): 1928–1933, https://pubmed.ncbi.nlm.nih.gov/15468355/.

34. Frank C. Arnett et al., "Urinary Mercury Levels in Patients with Autoantibodies to U3-RNP (Fibrillarin)," *The Journal of Rheumatology* 27, no. 2 (February 2000): 405–410, https://pubmed.ncbi.nlm.nih.gov/10685806/.

35. Jennifer F. Nyland et al., "Biomarkers of Methylmercury Exposure Immunotoxicity among Fish Consumers in Amazonian Brazil," *Environmental Health Perspectives* 119, no. 12 (December 2011): 1733–1738, doi: 10.1289/ehp.1103741.

36. Carolyn M. Gallagher and Jaymie R. Meliker, "Mercury and Thyroid Autoantibodies in U.S. Women, NHANES 2007–2008," *Environment International* 40 (April 2012): 39–43, doi: 10.1016/j.envint.2011.11.014.

37. Jaishankar, "Toxicity," 60–72.

38. "Regulations for Lead Emissions from Aircraft," United States Environmental Protection Agency, https://www.epa.gov/regulations-emissions-vehicles-and-engines/regulations-lead-emissions-aircraft.

39. "Lead in Food, Foodwares, and Dietary Supplements," U.S. Food & Drug Administration (February 27, 2020), https://www.fda.gov/food/metals-and-your-food/lead-food-foodwares-and-dietary-supplements.

40. Monika Rusin et al., "Concentration of Cadmium and Lead in Vegetables and Fruits," *Scientific Reports* 11 (June 7, 2021): 11913, doi: 10.1038/s41598-021-91554-z.

41. Kaushala Prasad Mishra et al., "Lead Exposure and Its Impact on Immune System: A Review," *Toxicology in Vitro* 23, no. 6 (September 2009): 969–972, doi: 10.1016/j.tiv.2009.06.014.

42. Geir Bjørklund et al., "Metals, Autoimmunity, and Neuroendocrinology: Is There a Connection?", *Environmental Research* 187 (August 2020): 109541, doi: 10.1016/j.envres.2020.109541.

43. Jaishankar, "Toxicity," 60–72.

44. Andy Menke et al., "Blood Lead Below 0.48 Micromol/L (10 Microg/Dl) and Mortality among US Adults," *Circulation* 114, no. 13 (September 26, 2006): 1388–1394, doi: 10.1161/CIRCULATIONAHA.106.628321.

45. Richard L. Canfield et al., "Intellectual Impairment in Children with Blood Lead Concentrations below 10 μg per Deciliter," *The New England Journal of Medicine* 348 (April 17, 2003): 1517–1526, doi: 10.1056/NEJMoa022848.

46. "Lead in Food," U.S. Food & Drug Administration.

47. Wolfgang Maret, "The Bioinorganic Chemistry of Lead in the Context of Its Toxicity," *Metal Ions in Life Sciences* 17 (April 10, 2017), doi: 10.1515/9783110434330-001.

48. Kelley Herring, "The Hidden Danger in Your Slow Cooker," The Wellness Blog (February 26, 2014), accessed on April 10, 2022, https://discover.grasslandbeef.com/blog/the-hidden-danger-in-your-slow-cooker/.

49. Anne E. Nigra et al., "Poultry Consumption and Arsenic Exposure in the US Population," *Environmental Health Perspectives* 125, no. 3 (March 2017): 370–377, doi: 10.1289/EHP351.

50. Rizwanul Haque, Archana Chaudhary, and Nadra Sadaf, "Immunomodulatory Role of Arsenic in Regulatory T Cells," *Endocrine, Metabolic & Immune Disorders—Drug Targets* 17, no. 3 (2017): 176–181, doi: 10.2174/1871530317666170818114454.

51. Daniele Ferrario, Laura Gribaldo, and Thomas Hartung, "Arsenic Exposure and Immunotoxicity: a Review Including the Possible Influence of Age and Sex," *Current Environmental Health Reports* 3 (2016): 1–12, doi: 10.1007/s40572-016-0082-3.

52. Maria Grau-Pérez et al., "The Association of Arsenic Exposure and Metabolism with Type 1 and Type 2 Diabetes in Youth: The SEARCH Case-Control Study," *Diabetes Care* 40, no. 1 (January 2017): 46–53, doi: 10.2337/dc16-0810.

53. Jonas Ludvigsson, P. Andersson-White, and Carlos Guerrero-Bosagna, "Toxic Metals in Cord Blood and Later Development of Type 1 Diabetes," *Pediatric Dimensions* 4, no. 2 (June 2019), doi: 10.15761/PD.1000186.

54. Chun Fa Huang et al., "Arsenic and Diabetes: Current Perspectives," *The Kaohsiung Journal of Medical Sciences* 27, no. 9 (September 2011): 402–410, doi: 10.1016/j.kjms.2011.05.008.

55. Kobra Bahrampour Juybari et al., "Evaluation of Serum Arsenic and Its Effects on Antioxidant Alterations in Relapsing-Remitting Multiple Sclerosis Patients," *Multiple Sclerosis and Related Disorders* 19 (January 2018): 79–84, doi: 10.1016/j.msard.2017.11.010.

56. Rusin, "Concentration of Cadmium," 11913.

57. Sandra Mounicou et al., "Concentrations and Bioavailability of Cadmium and Lead in Cocoa Powder and Related Products," *Food Additives & Contaminants* 20, no. 4 (April 2003): 343–352, https://pubmed.ncbi.nlm.nih.gov/12775476/.

58. Theoharris Frangos and Wolfgang Maret, "Zinc and Cadmium in the Aetiology and Pathogenesis of Osteoarthritis and Rheumatoid Arthritis," *Nutrients* 13, no. 1 (December 26, 2020): 53, doi: 10.1080/0265203031000077888.

59. Motoyasu Ohsawa, "Heavy Metal-induced Immunotoxicity and Its Mechanisms," *Yakugaku Zasshi* 129, no. 3 (March 2009): 305–319, doi: 10.1248/yakushi.129.305.

60. Marta Wacewicz-Muczyńska et al., "Cadmium, Lead and Mercury in the Blood of Psoriatic and Vitiligo Patients and their Possible Associations with Dietary Habits," *Science of the Total Environment* 757 (February 25, 2021): 143967, doi: 10.1016/j.scitotenv.2020.143967.

61. Aleksandra Popov Aleksandrov et al., "Immunomodulation by Heavy Metals as a Contributing Factor to Inflammatory Diseases and Autoimmune Reactions: Cadmium as an Example," *Immunology Letters* 240 (December 2021): 106–122, doi: 10.1016/j.imlet.2021.10.003.

62. Andrea Hartwig, "Cadmium and Cancer," *Metal Ions in Life Sciences* 11 (2013): 491–507, doi: 10.1007/978-94-007-5179-8_15.

63. Ernie Hood, "Measuring Autoimmunity in America," *Environmental Factor* (April 2018), https://factor.niehs.nih.gov/2018/4/science-highlights/autoimmunity/index.htm.

64. Jürgen Angerer et al., *Opinion on Triclosan Antimicrobial Resistance* (Brussels: European Commission Directorate-General for Health & Consumers, June 22, 2010), accessed January 22, 2022, https://ec.europa.eu/health/scientific_committees/consumer_safety/docs/sccs_o_023.pdf.

65. Juliette Legler et al., "Obesity, Diabetes, and Associated Costs of Exposure to Endocrine-Disrupting Chemicals in the European Union," *The Journal of Clinical Endocrinology & Metabolism* 100, no. 4 (April 2015): 1278–1288, doi: 10.1210/jc.2014-4326.

66. Barbara Predieri et al., "Endocrine Disrupting Chemicals and Type 1 Diabetes," *International Journal of Molecular Sciences* 21, no. 8 (April 2020): 2937, doi: 10.3390/ijms21082937.

67. Guomao Zheng et al., "Per- and Polyfluoroalkyl Substances (PFAS) in Breast Milk: Concerning Trends for Current-Use PFAS," *Environmental Science & Technology* 55, no. 11 (May 13, 2021): 7510–7520, doi: 10.1021/acs.est.0c06978

68. Joseph Braun et al., *NTP Monograph on Immunotoxicity Associated with Exposure to Perfluorooctanoic Acid (PFOA) or Perfluorooctane Sulfonate (PFOS)* (Washington, DC: Office of Health Assessment and Translation Division of the National Toxicology Program, National Institute of Environmental Health Sciences, National Institutes of Health, U.S. Department of Health and Human Services, September, 2016), accessed December 14, 2021, https://ntp.niehs.nih.gov/ntp/ohat/pfoa_pfos/pfoa_pfosmonograph_508.pdf.

69. Abigail Gaylord et al., "Persistent Organic Pollutant Exposure and Celiac Disease: A Pilot Study," *Environmental Research* 186 (July 2020): 109439, doi: 10.1016/j.envres.2020.109439.

70. Glenys M. Webster et al., "Associations Between Perfluoroalkyl Acids (PFASs) and Maternal Thyroid Hormones in Early Pregnancy: A Population-based Cohort Study," *Environmental Research* 133 (August 2014): 338–347, doi: 10.1016/j.envres.2014.06.012.

71. "Learn about Polychlorinated Biphenyls (PCBs)," United States Environmental Protection Agency, https://www.epa.gov/pcbs/learn-about-polychlorinated-biphenyls-pcbs.

72. Salvatore Benvenga, "Endocrine Disruptors and Thyroid Autoimmunity," *Best Practice & Research: Clinical Endocrinology & Metabolism* 34, no. 1 (January 2020): 101377, doi: 10.1016/j .beem.2020.101377.

73. Predieri, "Endocrine Disrupting Chemicals," 2937.

74. "PCBs in Farmed Salmon," Environmental Working Group (July 31, 2003), https://www.ewg .org/research/pcbs-farmed-salmon.

75. Walter J. Crinnion, "Polychlorinated Biphenyls: Persistent Pollutants with Immunological, Neurological, and Endocrinological Consequences," *Alternative Medicine Review* 16, no. 1 (March 2011): 5013, https://pubmed.ncbi.nlm.nih.gov/21438643/.

76. Michael C.R. Alavanja, "Pesticides Use and Exposure Extensive Worldwide," *Reviews on Environmental Health* 24, no. 4 (October–December 2009): 303–309, doi: 10.1515 /reveh.2009.24.4.303.

77. "National Report on Human Exposure to Environmental Chemicals: Updated Tables, March 2021," Centers for Disease Control and Prevention, https://www.cdc.gov/exposurereport/.

78. Doaa A. El-Morsi, Rania H. Abdel Rahman, and Assem A.K. Abou-Arab, "Pesticides Residues in Egyptian Diabetic Children: A Preliminary Study," *Journal of Clinical Toxicology* (2012): 2–6, accessed January 22, 2022, doi: 10.4172/2161-0495.1000138.

79. Navdep Kaur et al., "Longitudinal Association of Biomarkers of Pesticide Exposure with Cardiovascular Disease Risk Factors in Youth with Diabetes," *Environmental Research* 181 (February 2020): 108916, doi: 10.1016/j.envres.2019.108916.

80. Gaylord, "Persistent Organic Pollutant Exposure," 109439.

81. Christine G. Parks et al., "Insecticide Use and Risk of Rheumatoid Arthritis and Systemic Lupus Erythematosus in the Women's Health Initiative Observational Study," *Arthritis Care and Research* 63, no. 2 (February 2011): 184–194, doi: 10.1002/acr.20335.

82. Parks, "Insecticide Use," 184–194.

83. L.S. Gold et al., "Systemic Autoimmune Disease Mortality and Occupational Exposures," *Arthritis & Rheumatology* 56, no. 10 (October 2007): 3189–3201, doi: 10.1002/art.22880.

84. Armando Meyer et al., "Pesticide Exposure and Risk of Rheumatoid Arthritis among Licensed Male Pesticide Applicators in the Agricultural Health Study," *Environmental Health Perspectives* 125, no. 7 (July 14, 2017): 077010, doi: 10.1289/EHP1013.

85. Marcin Baranski et al., "Higher Antioxidant and Lower Cadmium Concentrations and Lower Incidence of Pesticide Residues in Organically Grown Crops: A Systematic Literature Review and Meta-analyses," *British Journal of Nutrition* 112, no. 5 (Sept. 14, 2014): 794–811, doi: 10.1017/S0007114514001366.

86. Baranski, "Higher Antioxidant and Lower Cadmium Concentrations," 794–811.

87. Antonio Suppa et al., "Roundup Causes Embryonic Development Failure and Alters Metabolic Pathways and Gut Microbes Functionality in Non-Target Species," *Microbiome* 8, no. 170 (December 15, 2020), doi: 10.1186/s40168-020-00943-5.

88. Anthony Samsel and Stephanie Seneff, "Glyphosate, Pathways to Modern Diseases II: Celiac Sprue and Gluten Intolerance," *Interdisciplinary Toxicology* 6, no. 4 (December 2013): 159–184, accessed January 22, 2022, doi: 10.2478/intox-2013-0026.

89. "IARC Monographs Volume 112: Evaluation of Five Organophosphate Insecticides and Herbicides," International Agency for Research on Cancer / World Health Organization (March 20, 2015), accessed January 22, 2022, https://www.iarc.who.int/wp-content/uploads/2018/07 /MonographVolume112-1.pdf.

90. Anthony Samsel and Stephanie Seneff, "Glyphosate's Suppression of Cytochrome P450 Enzymes and Amino Acid Biosynthesis by the Gut Microbiome: Pathways to Modern Diseases," *Entropy* 15, no. 4 (April 18, 2013): 1416–1463, doi: 10.3390/e15041416.

91. Samsel, "Glyphosate," 159–184.

92. Samsel, "Glyphosate's Suppression," 1416–1463.

93. Christine G. Parks et al., "Rheumatoid Arthritis in Agricultural Health Study Spouses: Associations with Pesticides and Other Farm Exposures," *Environmental Health Perspectives* 124, no. 11 (November 1, 2016): 1728–1734, accessed January 22, 2022, doi: 10.1289/EHP129.

94. Gary M. Williams, Robert Kroes, and Ian C. Munro, "Safety Evaluation and Risk Assessment of the Herbicide Roundup and Its Active Ingredient, Glyphosate, for Humans," *Regulatory Toxicology and Pharmacology* 31, no. 2 (2000): 117–165, accessed January 22, 2022, doi: 10.1006/rtph.1999.1371.

95. Joël Spiroux de Vendômois et al., "Debate on GMOs Health Risks after Statistical Findings in Regulatory Tests," *International Journal of Biological Sciences* 6, no. 6 (2010): 590–598, accessed January 22, 2022, doi: 10.7150/ijbs.6.590.

96. Centers for Disease Control and Prevention, *Fourth National Report on Human Exposure to Environmental Chemicals* (Washington, DC: U.S. Department of Health and Human Services, 2009), accessed April 10, 2022, http://www.cdc.gov/exposurereport/pdf/FourthReport.pdf.

97. Antonia M. Calafat et al., "Exposure of the U.S. Population to Bisphenol A and 4-Tertiary-Octylphenol: 2003–2004," *Environmental Health Perspectives* 116, no. 1 (January 2008): 39–44, accessed January 22, 2022, doi: 10.1289/ehp.10753.

98. Datis Kharrazian, "The Potential Roles of Bisphenol A (BPA) Pathogenesis in Autoimmunity," *Environmental Triggers and Autoimmunity* (April 7, 2014), doi: 10.1155/2014/743616.

99. Yanshan Lv, "Higher Dermal Exposure of Cashiers to BPA and its Association with DNA Oxidative Damage," *Environment International* 98 (January 2017): 69–74, doi: 0.1016/j.envint.2016.10.001.

100. Predieri, "Endocrine Disrupting Chemicals," 2937.

101. Tolga Ince et al., "Urinary Bisphenol-A Levels in Children with Type 1 Diabetes Mellitus," *Journal of Pediatric Endocrinology and Metabolism* 31, no. 8 (August 28, 2018): 829–836, https://pubmed.ncbi.nlm.nih.gov/29975667/.

102. Iain A. Lang et al., "Association of Urinary Bisphenol A Concentration with Medical Disorders and Laboratory Abnormalities in Adults," *Journal of the American Medical Association* 300, no. 11 (September 17, 2008): 1303–1310, doi: 10.1001/jama.300.11.1303.

103. Xiaoqian Gao et al., "Rapid Responses and Mechanism of Action for Low-Dose Bisphenol S on *ex Vivo* Rat Hearts and Isolated Myocytes: Evidence of Female-Specific Proarrhythmic Effects," *Environmental Health Perspectives*, Advance Publication (February 26, 2015), doi: 10.1289/ehp.1408679.

104. Yanshan, "Higher Dermal Exposure," 69–74.

105. Glinda S. Cooper et al., "Evidence of Autoimmune-Related Effects of Trichloroethylene Exposure from Studies in Mice and Humans," *Environmental Health Perspectives* 117, no. 5 (May 1, 2009): 696–702, accessed January 22, 2022, https://ehp.niehs.nih.gov/doi/pdf/10.1289/ehp.11782.

106. Alavanja, "Pesticides Use," 303–309.

107. Xindi C. Hu et al., "Detection of Poly- and Perfluoroalkyl Substances (PFASs) in U.S. Drinking Water Linked to Industrial Sites, Military Fire Training Areas, and Wastewater Treatment Plants," *Environmental Science & Technology Letters* 3, no. 10 (August 9, 2016): 344–350, doi: 10.1021/acs.estlett.6b00260.

108. Rob Smith, "Study Finds Drugs Seeping into Drinking Water," interview by Joan Rose, *Talk of the Nation*, NPR, March 10, 2008, audio, 16:33, accessed December 15, 2021, https://www.npr.org/templates/story/story.php?storyId=88062858.

109. Donna Jackson Nakazawa, *The Autoimmune Epidemic* (New York: Touchstone/Simon & Schuster, 2008), xvii.

110. Joseph Pizzorno, *The Toxin Solution* (New York: HarperCollins, 2017), 1, 32.

111. EcoWatch, "84,000 Chemicals on the Market, Only 1% Have Been Tested for Safety," July 2015, https://www.ecowatch.com/84-000-chemicals-on-the-market-only-1-have-been-tested-for-safety-1882062458.html, accessed on April 20, 2022.

112. Rubén D. Arias-Pérez et al., "Inflammatory Effects of Particulate Matter Air Pollution," *Environmental Science and Pollution Research International* 27, no. 34 (December 27, 2020): 2390–2404, doi: 10.1007/s11356-020-10574-w.

113. Cha-Na Zhao et al., "Emerging Role of Air Pollution in Autoimmune Diseases," *Autoimmunity Reviews* 18, no. 6 (June 2019): 607–614, https://doi.org/10.1016/j.autrev.2018.12.010.

114. Zhao, "Emerging Role of Air Pollution," 607–614.

115. Susanna D. Mitro et al., "Consumer Product Chemicals in Indoor Dust: A Quantitative Meta-analysis of U.S. Studies," *Environmental Science & Technology* 50, no. 19 (September 14, 2016): 10661–10672, doi: 10.1021/acs.est.6b02023.

116. Gaylord, "Persistent Organic Pollutant Exposure," 109439.

117. Lacey Robinson and Rachel Miller, "The Impact of Bisphenol A and Phthalates on Allergy, Asthma, and Immune Function: A Review of Latest Findings," *Current Environmental Health Reports* 2, no. 4 (December 2015): 379–387, doi: 10.1007/s40572-015-0066-8.

118. Robert M. Gogal Jr. and S.D. Holladay, "Perinatal TCDD Exposure and the Adult Onset of Autoimmune Disease," *Journal of Immunotoxicology* 5, no. 4 (October 2008): 413–418, doi: 10.1080/10408360802483201.

119. Zehua Yan et al., "Analysis of Microplastics in Human Feces Reveals a Correlation between Fecal Microplastics and Inflammatory Bowel Disease Status," *Environmental Science & Technology* 56, no. 1 (December 22, 2021): 414–421, doi: 10.1021/acs.est.1c03924.

120. Junjie Zhang et al., "Occurrence of Polyethylene Terephthalate and Polycarbonate Microplastics in Infant and Adult Feces," *Environmental Science & Technology Letters* 8, no. 11 (September 22, 2021): 989–994, doi: 10.1021/acs.estlett.1c00559.

121. Greg Seaman, "The Top 10 Plants for Removing Indoor Toxins," Eartheasy (September 6, 2020), accessed January 3, 2022, https://learn.eartheasy.com/articles/the-top-10-plants-for-removing-indoor-toxins/.

122. Jonathan Wilson et al., "An Investigation into Porch Dust Lead Levels," *Environmental Research* 137 (February 2015): 129–135, doi: 10.1016/j.envres.2014.11.013.

123. Marcia G. Nishioka, "Distribution of 2,4-Dichlorophenoxyacetic Acid in Floor Dust throughout Homes Following Homeowner and Commercial Lawn Applications: Quantitative Effects of Children, Pets, and Shoes," *Environmental Science & Technology* 33, no. 9 (March 31, 1999): 1359–1365, doi: 10.1021/es980580o.

124. M. Jahangir Alam et al., "Investigation of Potentially Pathogenic *Clostridium Difficile* Contamination in Household Environs," *Anaerobe* 27 (June 2014): 31–33, doi: 10.1016/j.anaerobe.2014.03.002.

125. Alison K. Cohen, Sarah Janssen, and Gina Solomon, "Clearing the Air: Hidden Hazards of Air Fresheners," Natural Resources Defense Council (2007), https://www.researchgate.net/publication/262872839_Clearing_the_Air_Hidden_Hazards_of_Air_Fresheners.

126. "Wood Smoke and Your Health," United States Environmental Protection Agency (April 26, 2021), accessed January 3, 2022, https://www.epa.gov/burnwise/wood-smoke-and-your-health.

127. "Use of Lead-Free Pipes, Fittings, Fixtures, Solder, and Flux for Drinking Water," United States Environmental Protection Agency (March 11, 2021), accessed January 5, 2022, https://www.epa.gov/sdwa/use-lead-free-pipes-fittings-fixtures-solder-and-flux-drinking-water.

128. Amine Kassouf et al., "Migration of Iron, Lead, Cadmium and Tin from Tinplate-coated Cans into Chickpeas," *Food Additives & Contaminants: Part A: Chemistry, Analysis, Control, Exposure & Risk Assessment* 30, no. 11 (2013): 1987–1992, doi: 10.1080/19440049.2013.832399.

129. Kunlun Liu, Jiabao Zheng, and Fusheing Chen, "Effects of Washing, Soaking and Domestic Cooking on Cadmium, Arsenic and Lead Bioaccessibilities in Rice," *Journal of the Science of Food and Agriculture* 98, no. 10 (August 2018): 3829–3835, doi: 10.1002/jsfa.8897.

130. Lisa L. Gill, "Your Herbs and Spices Might Contain Arsenic, Cadmium, and Lead," *Consumer Reports* (November 9, 2021), accessed January 15, 2022, https://www.consumerreports.org/food-safety/your-herbs-and-spices-might-contain-arsenic-cadmium-and-lead/.

131. Meredith Schneider, "Taking Psyllium to Aid Digestion Could be Dangerous," The Swell Score (March 24, 2021), https://theswellscore.com/taking-psyllium-to-aid-digestion-could-be-dangerous/.

132. Sa Liu, S. Katharine Hammond, and Ann Rojas-Cheatham, "Concentrations and Potential Health Risks of Metals in Lip Products," *Environmental Health Perspectives* 121, no. 6 (June 1, 2013), doi: 10.1289/ehp.1205518.

133. "PCBs in Farmed Salmon," Environmental Working Group (July 31, 2003), https://www.ewg.org/research/pcbs-farmed-salmon.

134. "Dirty Dozen: EWG's 2022 Shopper's Guide to Pesticides in Produce," Environmental Working Group, accessed April 9, 2022, https://www.ewg.org/foodnews/dirty-dozen.php.

135. Afrooz Saadatzadeh et al., "Determination of Heavy Metals (Lead, Cadmium, Arsenic, and Mercury) in Authorized and Unauthorized Cosmetics," *Cutaneous and Ocular Toxicology* 38, no. 3 (September 2019): 207–211, doi: 10.1080/15569527.2019.1590389.

136. "UL GREENGUARD Certification Program Fact Sheet," https://www.ul.com/resources/ul-greenguard-certification-program, accessed on April 3, 2022.

137. Deborah J. Watkins et al., "Exposure to PBDEs in the Office Environment: Evaluating the Relationships between Dust, Handwipes, and Serum," *Environmental Health Perspectives* 119, no. 9 (September 2011): 1247–1252, accessed January 24, 2022, doi: 10.1289/ehp.1003271.

138. Craig M. Butt et al., "Metabolites of Organophosphate Flame Retardants and 2-ethylhexyl Tetrabromobenzoate in Urine from Paired Mothers and Toddlers," *Environmental Science and Technology* 48, no. 17 (August 4, 2014): 10432–10438, accessed January 24, 2022, doi: 10.1021/es5025299.

Chapter 3

1. Mariana Karamanou et al., "From Miasmas to Germs: A Historical Approach to Theories of Infectious Disease Transmission," *Le Infezioni in Medicina* 20, no. 1 (March 2012): 58–62, https://pubmed.ncbi.nlm.nih.gov/22475662/.

2. Seun Ayoade, "Thalassemias Validate Germ Terrain Duality of Malaria," *Health Science Journal* (2017), doi: 10.21767/1791-809X.1000512.

3. Ashutosh K. Mangalam, Meeta Yadav, and Rajwardhan Yadav, "The Emerging World of Microbiome in Autoimmune Disorders: Opportunities and Challenges," *Indian Journal of Rheumatology* 16, no. 1 (March 2021): 57–72, doi: 10.4103/injr.injr_210_20.

4. Chiara Bellocchi and Elizabeth R. Volkmann, "Update on the Gastrointestinal Microbiome in Systemic Sclerosis," *Current Rheumatology Reports* 20, no. 8 (June 25, 2018): 49, doi: 10.4103/injr.injr_210_20.

5. Mangalam, "The Emerging World," 57–72.

6. Bilal Ahmad Paray et al., "Leaky Gut and Autoimmunity: An Intricate Balance in Individuals Health and the Diseased State," *International Journal of Molecular Sciences* 21, no. 24 (December 2020): 9770, doi: 10.3390/ijms21249770.

7. Alexandr Parlesak et al., "Increased Intestinal Permeability to Macromolecules and Endotoxemia in Patients with Chronic Alcohol Abuse in Different Stages of Alcohol-Induced Liver Disease," *Journal of Hepatology* 32, no. 5 (May 2000): 742–747, doi: 10.1016/s0168 -8278(00)80242-1.

8. Peter C. Konturek, Tomasz Brzozowski, and Stanislaw J. Konturek, "Stress and the Gut: Pathophysiology, Clinical Consequences, Diagnostic Approach and Treatment Options," *Journal of Physiology and Pharmacology* 62, no. 6 (December 2011): 591–599, https://pubmed.ncbi.nlm .nih.gov/22314561/.

9. Qinghui Mu et al., "Leaky Gut as a Danger Signal for Autoimmune Diseases," *Frontiers in Immunology* 8 (2017): 598, doi: 10.3389/fimmu.2017.00598.

10. Maisa C. Takenaka and Francisco J. Quintana, "Tolerogenic Dendritic Cells," *Seminars in Immunopathology* 39, no. 2 (February 2017): 113–120, doi: 10.1007/s00281-016-0587-8.

11. Andrew T. Gewirtz and James L. Madara, "Periscope, Up! Monitoring Microbes in the Intestine," *Nature Immunology* 2 (April 2001): 288–290, doi: 10.1038/86292.

12. Guy C. Brown, "The Endotoxin Hypothesis of Neurodegeneration," *Journal of Neuroinflammation* 16, no. 180 (September 13, 2019), doi: 10.1186/s12974-019-1564-7.

13. Brown, "The Endotoxin Hypothesis."

14. Marie-Caroline Michalski et al., "Dietary Lipid Emulsions and Endotoxemia," *Lipid Consumption and Functionality: New Perspectives* 23, no. 3 (October 2016): D306, doi: 10.1051 /OCL/2016009.

15. Rui Lin et al., "Abnormal Intestinal Permeability and Microbiota in Patients with Autoimmune Hepatitis," *International Journal of Clinical and Experimental Pathology* 8, no. 5 (May 1, 2015): 5153–5160, https://pubmed.ncbi.nlm.nih.gov/26191211/.

16. Nobuo Fuke et al., "Regulation of Gut Microbes and Metabolic Endotoxemia with Dietary Factors," *Nutrients* 11, no. 10 (September 23, 2019): 2277, doi: 10.3390/nu11102277.

17. Jill A. Parnell, Teja Klancic, and Raylene A. Reimer, "Oligofructose Decreases Serum Lipopolysaccharide and Plasminogen Activator Inhibitor-1 in Adults with Overweight/Obesity," *Obesity* 25, no. 3 (March 2017): 510–513, doi: 10.1002/oby.21763.

18. Bruce R. Stevens et al., "Increased Human Intestinal Barrier Permeability Plasma Biomarkers Zonulin and FABP2 Correlated with Plasma LPS and Altered Gut Microbiome in Anxiety or Depression," 1555–1557, doi: 10.1136/gutjnl-2017-314759.

19. Michael Berk et al., "So Depression Is an Inflammatory Disease, But Where Does the Inflammation Come From?", *BMC Medicine* 11, no. 200 (September 12, 2013), https://bmcmedicine .biomedcentral.com/articles/10.1186/1741-7015-11-200.

20. Alison C. Bested, Alan C. Logan, and Eva M. Selhub, "Intestinal Microbiota, Probiotics and Mental Health: From Metchnikoff to Modern Advances: Part II—Contemporary Contextual Research," *Gut Pathogens* 5, no. 1 (March 14, 2013): 3, doi: 10.1186/1741-7015-11-200.

21. Michalski, "Dietary Lipid Emulsions," D306.

22. Patty W. Siri-Tarino et al., "Meta-Analysis of Prospective Cohort Studies Evaluating the Association of Saturated Fat with Cardiovascular Disease," *American Journal of Clinical Nutrition* 91, no. 3 (March 2010): 535–546, doi: 10.3945/ajcn.2009.27725.

23. Rajiv Chowdhury et al., "Association of Dietary, Circulating, and Supplement Fatty Acids with Coronary Risk: A Systematic Review and Meta-analysis," *Annals of Internal Medicine* 160, no. 6 (March 18, 2014): 398–406, doi: 10.7326/M13-1788.

24. L.A. Waddell et al., "The Zoonotic Potential of Mycobacterium Avium Ssp. Paratuberculosis: A Systematic Review and Meta-Analyses of the Evidence," *Epidemiol Infect* 143, no. 15, (2015): 3135–57, doi: 10.1017/S095026881500076X.

25. S. Masala et al., "Antibodies Recognizing Mycobacterium Avium Paratuberculosis Epitopes Cross-react with the Beta-cell Antigen Znt8 in Sardinian Type 1 Diabetic Patients," *PLoS One* 6(10), (2011): e26931, doi: 10.1371/journal.pone.0026931.

26. Raja Atreya et al., "Facts, Myths and Hypotheses on the Zoonotic Nature of Mycobacterium Avium Subspecies Paratuberculosis," *International Journal of Medical Microbiology* 304, (2014): 858–867, doi: 10.1016/j.ijmm.2014.07.006.

27. Atreya et al., "Facts, Myths and Hypotheses," 858–867.

28. Martin Feller et al., "Mycobacterium Avium Subspecies Paratuberculosis and Crohn's Disease: A Systematic Review and Meta-analysis," *Lancet Infect Dis* 7, no. 9 (2007): 607–13, doi: 10.1016/S1473-3099(07)70211-6.

29. John Aitken et al., "A Mycobacterium Species for Crohn's Disease?", *Pathology* 53, no. 7 (2021): 818–823, doi: 10.1016/j.pathol.2021.03.003.

30. Waddell et al., "The Zoonotic Potential," 3135–3157.

31. Guanxiang Liang and Frederic D. Bushman, "The Human Virome: Assembly, Composition and Host Interactions," *Nature Reviews Microbiology* 19 (March 30, 2021): 514–527, doi: 10.1038/s41579-021-00536-5.

32. Andrey N. Shkoporov and Colin Hill, "Bacteriophages of the Human Gut: The 'Known Unknown' of the Microbiome," *Cell Host & Microbe* 25, no. 2 (February 13, 2019): 195–209, doi: 10.1016/j.chom.2019.01.017.

33. Guoyan Zhao et al., "Intestinal Virome Changes Precede Autoimmunity in Type I Diabetes-Susceptible Children," *Proceedings of the National Academy of Sciences of the United States of America* 114, no. 30 (July 25, 2017): E6166–E6175, doi: 10.1073/pnas.1706359114.

34. Katri Lindfors et al., "Metagenomics of the Faecal Virome Indicate a Cumulative Effect of Enterovirus and Gluten Amount on the Risk of Coeliac Disease Autoimmunity in Genetically At-Risk Children: The TEDDY Study," *Gut* 69, no. 8 (August 2020): 1416–1422, doi: 10.1136/gutjnl-2019-319809.

35. Melissa A. Fernandes et al., "Enteric Virome and Bacterial Microbiota in Children with Ulcerative Colitis and Crohn's Disease," *Journal of Pediatric Gastroenterology and Nutrition* 68, no. 1 (January 2019): 30–36, doi: 10.1097/MPG.0000000000002140.

36. Adam G. Clooney et al., "Whole-Virome Analysis Sheds Light on Viral Dark Matter in Inflammatory Bowel Disease," *Cell Host & Microbe* 26, no. 6 (December 11, 2019): 764–778.e5, doi: 10.1016/j.chom.2019.10.009.

37. Tao Zuo et al., "Gut Mucosal Virome Alterations in Ulcerative Colitis," *Gut* 68, no. 7 (July 2019): 1169–1179, doi: 10.1136/gutjnl-2018-318131.

38. John B. Harley et al., "Transcription Factors Operate across Disease Loci, with EBNA2 Implicated in Autoimmunity," *Nature Genetics* 50, no. 5 (May 2018): 699–707, doi: 10.1038/s41588-018-0102-3.

39. Anette Holck Draborg, Karen Duus, and Gunnar Houen, "Epstein-Barr Virus in Systemic Autoimmune Diseases," *Systemic Autoimmune Diseases* 535738 (August 24, 2013), doi: 10.1155/2013/535738.

40. Draborg, "Epstein-Barr Virus."

41. Draborg, "Epstein-Barr Virus."

42. Shotaro Masuoka et al., "Epstein-Barr Virus Infection and Variants of Epstein-Barr Nuclear Antigen-1 in Synovial Tissues of Rheumatoid Arthritis," *PLoS One* 13, no. 12 (December 11, 2018): e0208957, doi: 10.1371/journal.pone.0208957.

43. Amit Bar-Or et al., "Epstein-Barr Virus in Multiple Sclerosis: Theory and Emerging Immunotherapies," *Trends in Molecular Medicine* 26, no. 3 (March 2020): 296–310, doi: 10.1016/j.molmed.2019.11.003.

44. Bar-Or, "Epstein-Barr Virus," 296–310.

45. Alexander G. Gabibov, "Combinatorial Antibody Library from Multiple Sclerosis Patients Reveals Antibodies that Cross-React with Myelin Basic Protein and EBV Antigen," *The FASEB Journal* 25, no. 12 (December 2011): 4211–4221, doi: 10.1096/fj.11-190769.

46. "Epstein-Barr Virus and Infectious Mononucleosis: Laboratory Testing," Centers for Disease Control and Prevention, https://www.cdc.gov/epstein-barr/laboratory-testing.html.

47. Lin Zhang et al., "The Role of Gut Mycobiome in Health and Diseases," *Therapeutic Advances in Gastroenterology* 2021, no. 14 (September 23, 2021), doi: 10.1177/17562848211047130.

48. Zhang, "The Role of Gut Mycobiome."

49. Yu Gu et al., "The Potential Role of Gut Mycobiome in Irritable Bowel Syndrome," *Frontiers in Microbiology* 10 (August 21, 2019): 1894, doi: 10.3389/fmicb.2019.01894.

50. Helen Tremlett et al., "The Gut Microbiome in Human Neurological Disease: A Review," *Annals of Neurology* 81, no. 3 (March 2017): 369–382, doi: 10.1002/ana.24901.

51. Julián Benito-León, "Association Between Multiple Sclerosis and Candida Species: Evidence from a Case-Control Study," *European Journal of Clinical Microbiology & Infectious Diseases* 29, no. 9 (September 2010): 1139–1145, doi: 10.1007/s10096-010-0979-y.

52. Shahla Amri Saroukolaei et al., "The Role of Candida Albicans in the Severity of Multiple Sclerosis," *Mycoses* 59, no. 11 (November 2016): 697–704, doi: 10.1111/myc.12489.

53. Romain Gerard et al., "An Immunological Link Between Candida Albicans Colonization and Crohn's Disease," *Critical Reviews in Microbiology* 41, no. 2 (June 2015): 135–139, doi: 10.3109/1040841X.2013.810587.

54. Lerner Aaron and Matthias Torsten, "Candida Albicans in Celiac Disease: A Wolf in Sheep's Clothing," *Autoimmunity Reviews* 19, no. 9 (September 2020): 102621, doi: 10.1016/j.autrev.2020.102621.

55. Matthew L. Wheeler et al., "Immunological Consequences of Intestinal Fungal Dysbiosis," *Cell Host & Microbe* 19, no. 6 (June 8, 2016): 865–873, doi: 10.1016/j.chom.2016.05.003.

56. Mafalda Cavalheiro and Miguel Cacho Teixeira, "*Candida* Biofilms: Threats, Challenges, and Promising Strategies," *Frontiers in Medicine* 5 (2018): 28, doi: 10.3389/fmed.2018.00028.

57. Hans-Curt Flemming et al., "Biofilms: An Emergent Form of Bacterial Life," *Nature Reviews Microbiology* 14, no. 9 (August 11, 2016): 563–575, doi: 10.1038/nrmicro.2016.94.

58. Lindsay Kalan et al., "Redefining the Chronic-Wound Microbiome: Fungal Communities Are Prevalent, Dynamic, and Associated with Delayed Healing," *mBio* 7, no. 5 (September–October 2016): e01058–16, doi: 10.1128/mBio.01058-16.

59. Voon Kin Chin et al., "Mycobiome in the Gut: A Multiperspective Review," *Mediators of Inflammation* 2020 (April 4, 2020), doi: 10.1155/2020/9560684.

60. Pedro H. Gazzinelli-Guimaraes and Thomas B. Nutman, "Helminth Parasites and Immune Regulation," *F1000Research* 7 (October 23, 2018): F1000 Faculty Rev-1685, doi: 10.12688/f1000research.15596.1.

61. Anne M. Ercolini and Stephen D. Miller, "The Role of Infections in Autoimmune Disease," *Clinical & Experimental Immunology* 155, no. 1 (January 2009): 1–15, doi: 10.1111/j.1365-2249.2008.03834.x.

62. Laura Eme and W. Ford Doolittle, "Archaea," *Current Biology* 25, no. 19 (October 5, 2015): R851–855, doi: 10.1016/j.cub.2015.05.025.

63. Katelyn E. Madigan, Richa Bundy, and Richard B. Weinberg, "Distinctive Clinical Correlates of Small Intestinal Bacterial Overgrowth with Methanogens," *Clinical Gastroenterology and Hepatology* (September 29, 2021), doi: 10.1016/j.cgh.2021.09.035.

64. Erika Ruback Bertges and Júlio Maria Fonseca Chebli, "Prevalence and Factors Associated with Small Intestinal Bacterial Overgrowth in Patients with Crohn's Disease: A Retrospective Study at a Referral Center," *Arquivos de Gastroenterologia* 57, no. 3 (July–September 2020): 283–288, doi: 10.1590/S0004-2803.202000000-64.

65. Jeremy Liu Chen Kiow et al., "High Occurrence of Small Intestinal Bacterial Overgrowth in Primary Biliary Cholangitis," *Neurogastroenterology & Motility* 31, no. 11 (November 2019): e13691, doi: 10.1111/nmo.13691.

Chapter 4

1. Arun Parashar and Malairaman Udayabanu, "Gut Microbiota Regulates Key Modulators of Social Behavior," *European Neuropsychopharmacology* 26, no. 1 (January 2016): 78–91, doi: 10.1016/j.euroneuro.2015.11.002.

2. Zachary Blount, "The Unexhausted Potential of E. Coli," *eLife* 4 (2015): e05826, doi: 10.7554/eLife.05826.

3. Jack Gilbert et al., "Current Understanding of the Human Microbiome," *Nature Medicine* 24, no. 4 (April 10, 2018): 392–400, doi: 10.1038/nm.4517.

4. Sylvie Miquel, "*Faecalibacterium prausnitzii* and Human Intestinal Health," *Current Opinion in Microbiology* 16, no. 3 (June 2013): 255–261, doi: 10.1016/j.mib.2013.06.003.

5. Yun Kit Yeoh et al., "Gut Microbiota Composition Reflects Disease Severity and Dysfunctional Immune Responses in Patients with COVID-19," *Gut* 70, no. 4 (April 2021): 698–706, doi; 10.1136/gutjnl-2020-323020.

6. Tao Zuo et al., "Alterations in Gut Microbes of Patients with COVID-19 During Time of Hospitalization," *Gastroenterology* 159, no. 3 (September 2020): 944–955, doi: 10.1053/j.gastro.2020.05.048.

7. Alison N. Thorburn, Laurence Macia, and Charles R. Mackay, "Diet, Metabolites, and 'Western-Lifestyle' Inflammatory Diseases," *Immunity* 40, no. 6 (June 19, 2014): 833–842, doi: 10.1016/j.immuni.2014.05.014.

8. Omaida C. Velázquez, Howard M. Lederer, John L. Rombeau, "Butyrate and the Colonocyte. Production, Absorption, Metabolism, and Therapeutic Implications," *Advances in Experimental Medicine and Biology* 427 (1997): 123–134, https://pubmed.ncbi.nlm.nih.gov/9361838/.

9. Hu Liu et al., "Butyrate: A Double-Edged Sword for Health?", *Advances in Nutrition* 9, no. 1 (January 2018): 21–29, doi: 10.1093/advances/nmx009.

10. Petra Louis and Harry J. Flint, "Formation of Propionate and Butyrate by the Human Colonic Microbiota," *Environmental Microbiology* 19, no. 1 (January 2017): 29–41, doi: 10.1111/1462-2920.13589.

11. Jindong Zhang et al., "Beneficial Effect of Butyrate-Producing Lachnospiraceae on Stress-Induced Visceral Hypersensitivity in Rats," *Journal of Gastroenterology and Hepatology* 34, no. 8 (August 2019): 1368–1376, doi: 10.1111/jgh.14536.

12. Roman M. Stilling et al., "The Neuropharmacology of Butyrate: The Bread and Butter of the Microbiota-Gut-Brain Axis?", *Neurochemistry International* 99 (October 2016): 110–132, doi: 10.1016/j.neuint.2016.06.011.

13. Tennekoon B. Karunaratne et al., "Niacin and Butyrate: Nutraceuticals Targeting Dysbiosis and Intestinal Permeability in Parkinson's Disease," *Nutrients* 13, no. 1 (January 2021): 28, doi: 10.3390/nu13010028.

14. Miquel, "*Faecalibacterium prausnitzii*," 255–261.

15. Harry Sokol et al., "*Faecalibacterium prausnitzii* is an Anti-Inflammatory Commensal Bacterium Identified by Gut Microbes Analysis of Crohn Disease Patients," *Proceedings of the National Academy of Sciences of the United States of America* 105, no. 43 (October 28, 2008): 16731–16736, doi: 10.1073/pnas.0804812105.

16. Mireia Lopez-Siles et al., "*Faecalibacterium prausnitzii*: From Microbiology to Diagnostics and Prognostics," *The ISME Journal* 11, no. 4 (April 2017): 841–852, doi: 10.1038/ismej.2016.176.

17. Patrice D. Cani and William M. de Vos, "Next-Generation Beneficial Microbes: The Case of *Akkermansia muciniphila*," *Frontiers in Microbiology* 8 (2017): 1765, doi: 10.3389/fmicb.2017.01765.

18. Muriel Derrien et al., "*Akkermansia*," in *Bergey's Manual of Systematics of Archaea and Bacteria*, ed. William B. Whitman (Hoboken, NJ: John Wiley & Sons, Inc., 2015), doi: 10.1002/9781118960608.gbm01282.

19. Kequan Zhou, "Strategies to Promote Abundance of *Akkermansia muciniphila*, an Emerging Probiotics in the Gut, Evidence from Dietary Intervention Studies," *Journal of Functional Foods* 33 (June 2017): 194–201, doi: 10.1016/j.jff.2017.03.045.

20. Hubert Plovier et al., "A Purified Membrane Protein from *Akkermansia muciniphila* or the Pasteurized Bacterium Improves Metabolism in Obese and Diabetic Mice," *Nature Medicine* 23, no. 1 (January 2017): 107–113, doi: 10.1038/nm.4236.

21. Yuji Naito, Kazuhiko Uchiyama, and Tomohisa Takagi, "A Next-generation Beneficial Microbe: *Akkermansia muciniphila,*" *Journal of Clinical Biochemistry and Nutrition* 63, no. 1 (July 2018): 33–35, doi: 10.3164/jcbn.18-57.

22. Cani, "Next-Generation Beneficial Microbes," 1765.

23. Kouichi Miura and Hirohide Ohnishi, "Role of Gut Microbes and Toll-like Receptors in Non-alcoholic Fatty Liver Disease," *World Journal of Gastroenterology* 20, no. 23 (June 21, 2014): 7381–7391, accessed January 9, 2022, doi: 10.3748/wjg.v20.i23.7381.

24. Maria Carlota Dao et al., "*Akkermansia muciniphila* and Improved Metabolic Health during a Dietary Intervention in Obesity: Relationship with Gut Microbiome Richness and Ecology," *Gut* 65, no. 3 (March 2016): 426–436, doi: 10.1136/gutjnl-2014-308778.

25. Arun P. Lakshmanan et al., "Akkermansia, a Possible Microbial Marker for Poor Glycemic Control in Qataris Children Consuming Arabic Diet—A Pilot Study on Pediatric T1DM in Qatar." *Nutrients* vol. 13, no. 3 (2021): 836, doi: 10.3390/nu13030836.

26. Rapat Pittayanon et al., "Differences in Gut Microbiota in Patients With vs Without Inflammatory Bowel Diseases: A Systematic Review," *Gastroenterology* 158 (2020): 930–946.e1, doi: 10.1053/j.gastro.2019.11.294.

27. Huajun Zheng et al., "Altered Gut Microbiota Composition Associated with Eczema in Infants," *PLoS One* 11, no. 11 (2016): e0166026, doi: 10.1371/journal.pone.0166026.

28. Y Wu et al., "Breast Milk Flora Plays an Important Role in Infantile Eczema: Cohort Study in Northeast China," *Journal of Applied Microbiology* 131 (2021): 2981–2993, doi: 10.1111/jam.15076.

29. Angelina Volkova et al., "Predictive Metagenomic Analysis of Autoimmune Disease Identifies Robust Autoimmunity and Disease-Specific Microbial Signatures," *Frontiers in Microbiology* 12 (2021): 621310, doi: 10.3389/fmicb.2021.621310.

30. Ali Mirza et al., "The Multiple Sclerosis Gut Microbiota: A Systematic Review," *Mult Scler Relat Disord* 37 (2020): 101427, doi: 10.1016/j.msard.2019.101427.

31. Zhou, "Strategies," 194–201.

32. Pittayanon et al., "Differences," 930–946.e1.

33. Cani, "Next-Generation Beneficial Microbes," 1765.

34. Claire Depommier et al., "Supplementation with *Akkermansia muciniphila* in Overweight and Obese Human Volunteers: A Proof-of-Concept Exploratory Study," *Nature Medicine* 25, no. 7 (July 2019): 1096–1103, doi: 10.1038/s41591-019-0495-2.

35. Depommier, "Supplementation," 1096–1103.

36. Zhou, "Strategies," 194–201.

37. Robert Caesar et al., "Crosstalk between Gut Microbes and Dietary Lipids Aggravates WAT Inflammation through TLR Signaling," *Cell Metabolism* 22, no. 4 (October 6, 2015): 658–668, doi: 10.1016/j.cmet.2015.07.026.

38. Ceren Özkul, Meltem Yalınay, and Tarkan Karakan, "Islamic Fasting Leads to an Increased Abundance of *Akkermansia muciniphila* and *Bacteroides fragilis* Group: A Preliminary Study on Intermittent Fasting," *Turkish Journal of Gastroenterology* 30, no. 12 (December 2019): 1030–1035, doi: 10.5152/tjg.2019.19185.

39. Naito, "A Next-generation Beneficial Microbe," 33-35.

40. Olusegun V. Oyetayo, "Medicinal Uses of Mushrooms in Nigeria: Towards Full and Sustainable Exploitation," *African Journal of Traditional, Complementary and Alternative Medicines* 8, no. 3 (2011): 267–274, doi: 10.4314/ajtcam.v8i3.65289.

41. Amy O'Callaghan and Douwe van Sinderen, "Bifidobacteria and Their Role as Members of the Human Gut Microbes," *Frontiers in Microbiology* 7 (2016): 925, doi: 10.3389/fmicb.2016.00925.

42. Audrey Rivière et al., "Bifidobacteria and Butyrate-Producing Colon Bacteria: Importance and Strategies for Their Stimulation in the Human Gut," *Frontiers in Microbiology* 7 (June 28, 2016): 979, doi: 10.3389/fmicb.2016.00979.

43. Sabrina Duranti et al., "Exploring the Ecology of Bifidobacteria and Their Genetic Adaptation to the Mammalian Gut," *Microorganisms* 9, no. 1 (January 2021): 8, doi: 10.3390/microorganisms9010008.

44. Rivière, "Bifidobacteria," 979.

45. O'Callaghan, "Bifidobacteria," 925.

46. Timur Liwinski et al., "A Disease-Specific Decline of the Relative Abundance of Bifidobacterium in Patients with Autoimmune Hepatitis," *Alimentary Pharmacology & Therapeutics* 51, no. 12 (June 2020): 1417–1428, doi: 10.1111/apt.15754.

47. Flávia Martinello, Camila Fontana Roman, and Paula Alves de Souza, "Effects of Probiotic Intake on Intestinal Bifidobacteria of Celiac Patients," *Arquivos de Gastroenterologia* 54, no. 2 (April–June 2017): 85–90, https://pubmed.ncbi.nlm.nih.gov/28273274/.

48. Helioswilton Sales-Campos, Siomar Castro Soares, and Carlo José Freire Oliveira, "An Introduction of the Role of Probiotics in Human Infections and Autoimmune Diseases," *Critical Reviews in Microbiology* 45, no. 4 (August 2019): 423–432, doi: 10.1590/S0004-2803.201700000-07.

49. Li-Hao Cheng et al., "Psychobiotics in Mental Health, Neurodegenerative and Neurodevelopmental Disorders," *Journal of Food and Drug Analysis* 27, no. 3 (July 2019): 632–648, doi: 10.1016/j.jfda.2019.01.002.

50. O'Callaghan, "Bifidobacteria," 925.

51. Hend Elsaghir and Anil Reddivari, "Bacteroides Fragilis," in *StatPearls* [Internet] (Treasure Island, FL: StatPearls Publishing, 2022), https://pubmed.ncbi.nlm.nih.gov/31971708/.

52. Ezequiel Valguarnera and Juliane Wardenburg, "Good Gone Bad: One Toxin Away from Disease for Bacteroides fragilis," *Journal of Molecular Biology* 432, no. 4 (February 14, 2020): 765–785, doi: 10.1016/j.jmb.2019.12.003.

53. Hannah M. Wexler, "*Bacteroides*: The Good, the Bad, and the Nitty-Gritty," *Clinical Microbiology Reviews* 20, no. 4 (October 2007): 593–621, doi: 10.1128/CMR.00008-07.

54. Amanda Jacobson et al., "A Gut Commensal-Produced Metabolite Mediates Colonization Resistance to Salmonella Infection," *Cell Host & Microbe* 24, no. 2 (August 2018): 296–307.e7, doi: 10.1016/j.chom.2018.07.002.

55. Helle Krogh Pedersen, "Human Gut Microbes Impact Host Serum Metabolome and Insulin Sensitivity," *Nature* 535, no. 7612 (June 21, 2016): 376–381, doi: 10.1038/nature18646.

56. Alf A. Lindberg et al., "Structure-activity Relationships in Lipopolysaccharides of Bacteroides Fragilis," *Research and Reviews of Infectious Diseases* 12, suppl. 2 (January-February 1990): 133–141, doi: 10.1093/clinids/12.supplement_2.s133.

57. Diogo Costa et al., "Human Microbiota and Breast Cancer—Is There Any Relevant Link?—A Literature Review and New Horizons Toward Personalized Medicine," *Frontiers in Microbiology* 12 (February 25, 2021): 584332, doi: 10.3389/fmicb.2021.584332.

58. D.H Kim and Y.H. Jin, "Intestinal Bacterial Beta-glucuronidase Activity of Patients with Colon Cancer," *Archives of Pharmacal Research* 24, no. 6 (December 2001): 564–567, doi: 10.1007/BF02975166.

59. Knip, "The Role of the Intestinal Microbiota," 154–167.

60. R.T. Krawczyk and A. Banaszkiewicz, "Dr. Józef Brudziński—the True 'Father of Probiotics'," *Beneficial Microbes* 12, no. 3 (June 15, 2021): 211–213, doi: 10.3920/BM2020.0201.

61. Laura Marin et al., "Bioavailability of Dietary Polyphenols and Gut Microbes Metabolism: Antimicrobial Properties," *BioMed Research International* 2015, no. 905215 (February 23, 2015), doi: 10.1155/2015/905215.

62. Rebecca L. Fine, Derek L. Mubiru, and Martin A. Kriegel, *Advances in Immunology* 146 (2020): 29–56, doi: 10.1016/bs.ai.2020.02.002.

63. V. Buchta, "Vaginal Microbiome," *Ceska Gynekologie* 83, no. 5 (2018 Winter): 371–379, https://pubmed.ncbi.nlm.nih.gov/30848142/.

64. José Matos et al., "Insights from *Bacteroides* Species in Children with Type 1 Diabetes," *Microorganisms* 9, no. 7 (July 2, 2021): 1436, 10.3390/microorganisms9071436.

65. Lin, "Abnormal Intestinal Permeability," 5153–5160.

66. Alok K. Paul et al., "Probiotics and Amelioration of Rheumatoid Arthritis: Significant Roles of *Lactobacillus casei* and *Lactobacillus acidophilus,*" *Microorganisms* 9, no. 5 (May 16, 2021): 1070, doi: 10.3390/microorganisms9051070.

67. Douglas J. Morrison and Tom Preston, "Formation of Short-Chain Fatty Acids by the Gut Microbes and Their Impact on Human Metabolism," *Gut* 7, no. 3 (2016): 189–200, doi: 10.1080/19490976.2015.1134082.

68. Eva C. Soto-Martin et al., "Vitamin Biosynthesis by Human Gut Butyrate-Producing Bacteria and Cross-Feeding in Synthetic Microbial Communities," *mBio* 11, no. 4 (July-August 2020): e00886-20, doi: 10.1128/mBio.00886-20.

69. Alison M. Stephen and J.H. Cummings, "The Microbial Contribution to Human Faecal Mass," *Journal of Medical Microbiology* 13, no. 1 (February 1, 1980), doi: 10.1099/00222615-13-1-45.

70. Maria Sanchez and Premysl Bercik, "Epidemiology and Burden of Chronic Constipation," *Canadian Journal of Gastroenterology* 25, suppl. B (October 2011): 11B–15B, doi: 10.1155/2011/974573.

71. Francesco Asnicar et al., "Blue Poo: Impact of Gut Transit Time on the Gut Microbiome Using a Novel Marker," *Gut* 70 (2021): 1665–1674, doi: 10.1136/gutjnl-2020-323877.

72. Tuwilika P.T. Keendjele et al., "Corn? When Did I Eat Corn? Gastrointestinal Transit Time in Health Science Students," *Advances in Physiology Education* 45, no. 1 (March 1, 2021): 103–108, doi: 10.1152/advan.00192.2020.

73. Satish S.C. Rao et al., "Evaluation of Gastrointestinal Transit in Clinical Practice: Position Paper of the American and European Neurogastroenterology and Motility Societies," *Neurogastroenterology & Motility* 23, no. 1 (December 7, 2010): 8–23, doi: 10.1111/j.1365-2982.2010.01612.x.

74. Stephen J. Lewis and Ken W. Heaton, "Stool Form Scale as a Useful Guide to Intestinal Transit Time," *Scandinavian Journal of Gastroenterology* 32, no. 9 (1997): 920–924, doi: 10.3109/00365529709011203.

75. Jan Bures et al., "Small Intestinal Bacterial Overgrowth Syndrome," *World Journal of Gastroenterology* 16, no. 24 (June 28, 2010): 2978–2990, doi: 10.3748/wjg.v16.i24.2978.

76. Asnicar, "Blue Poo," 1665–1674.

77. Asnicar, "Blue Poo," 1665–1674.

78. Chin Wai Ho, "Varieties, Production, Composition and Health Benefits of Vinegars: A Review," *Food Chemistry* 221 (April 15, 2017): 1621–1630, doi: 10.1016/j.foodchem.2016.10.128.

79. Darshna Yagnik, Vlad Serafin, and Ajit J. Shah, "Antimicrobial Activity of Apple Cider Vinegar against *Escherichia coli*, *Staphylococcus aureus* and *Candida albicans*; Downregulating Cytokine and Microbial Protein Expression," *Scientific Reports* 8 (2018): 1732, doi: 10.1038/s41598-017-18618-x.

80. Keng-Liang Wu et al., "Effects of Ginger on Gastric Emptying and Motility in Healthy Humans," *European Journal of Gastroenterology and Hepatology* 20, no. 5 (May 2008): 436–440, doi: 10.1097/MEG.0b013e3282f4b224.

81. Edzard Ernst and Max H. Pittler, "Efficacy of Ginger for Nausea and Vomiting: A Systematic Review of Randomized Clinical Trials," *British Journal of Anaesthesia* 84, no. 3 (2000): 367–371, https://www.ncbi.nlm.nih.gov/books/NBK68168/.

82. Fumiko Higashikawa, "Improvement of Constipation and Liver Function by Plant-derived Lactic Acid Bacteria: A Double-blind, Randomized Trial," *Nutrition* 26, no. 4 (April 2010): 367–374, doi: 10.1016/j.nut.2009.05.008.

83. Angela Saviano et al., "Lactobacillus Reuteri DSM 17938 *(Limosilactobacillus reuteri)* in Diarrhea and Constipation: Two Sides of the Same Coin?", *Medicina* 57, no. 7 (June 23, 2021): 643, doi: 10.3390/medicina57070643.

Chapter 5

1. Francis Coucke, "Food Intolerance in Patients with Manifest Autoimmunity: Observational Study," *Autoimmunity Reviews* Volume 17, Issue 11, (2018): 1078–1080, doi: 10.1016/j.autrev.2018.05.011.

2. M. Hvatum et al., "The Gut-Joint Axis: Cross Reactive Food Antibodies in Rheumatoid Arthritis," *Gut* 55, no. 9 (September 2006), http://dx.doi.org/10.1136/gut.2005.076901.

3. Giuseppe Losurdo et al., "Extra-intestinal Manifestations of Non-Celiac Gluten Sensitivity: An Expanding Paradigm," *World Journal of Gastroenterology* 24, no. 14 (April 14, 2018): 1521–1530, doi: 10.3748/wjg.v24.i14.1521.

4. Widjaja Lukito, "From 'Lactose Intolerance' to 'Lactose Nutrition'," *Asia Pacific Journal of Clinical Nutrition* 24, suppl. 1 (2015): S1–S8, doi: 10.6133/apjcn.2015.24.s1.01.

5. Chaysavanh Manichanh, "Reduced Diversity of Faecal Microbiota in Crohn's Disease Revealed by a Metagenomic Approach," *Gut* 55, no. 2 (February 2006): 205–211, doi: 10.1136/gut.2005.073817.

6. Schnorr, "Gut Microbiome of the Hadza Hunter-gatherers."

7. Monica Barone et al., "Gut Microbiome Response to a Modern Paleolithic Diet in a Western Lifestyle Context," *PLoS One* 14, no. 8 (August 8, 2019): e0220619, doi: 10.1371/journal.pone.0220619.

8. Barone, "Gut Microbiome Response," e0220619.

9. Natália Ellen Castilho de Almeida et al., "Digestion of Intact Gluten Proteins by *Bifidobacterium* Species: Reduction of Cytotoxicity and Proinflammatory Responses," *Journal of Agricultural and Food Chemistry* 68, no. 15 (April 15, 2020): 4485–4492, doi: 10.1021/acs.jafc.0c01421.

10. Alberto Caminero et al., "Duodenal Bacterial Proteolytic Activity Determines Sensitivity to Dietary Antigen through Protease-Activated Receptor-2," *Sedici* 10, no. 1 (2019), doi: 10.1038/s41467-019-09037-9.

11. Karl Mårild et al., "Antibiotic Exposure and the Development of Coeliac Disease: A Nationwide Case-control Study," *BMC Gastroenterology* 13 (2013): 109, doi: 10.1186/1471-230X-13-109.

12. Mårild, "Antibiotic Exposure," 109.

13. James A. King et al., "Incidence of Celiac Disease Is Increasing Over Time: A Systematic Review and Meta-analysis," *The American Journal of Gastroenterology* 115, no. 4 (April 2020): 507–525, doi: 10.14309/ajg.0000000000000523.

14. Ángel Ferrero-Serrano, Christian Cantos, and Sarah M. Assmann, "The Role of Dwarfing Traits in Historical and Modern Agriculture with a Focus on Rice," *Cold Spring Harbor Perspectives in Biology* 11, no. 11 (November 2019): a034645, doi: 10.1101/cshperspect.a034645.

15. Alyssa Hidalgo and Andrea Brandolini, "Nutritional Properties of Einkorn Wheat (*Triticum monococcum L.*)," *Journal of the Science of Food and Agriculture* 94, no. 4 (March 15, 2014): 601–612, doi: 10.1002/jsfa.6382.

16. Jun He et al., "A High-Amylopectin Diet Caused Hepatic Steatosis Associated with More Lipogenic Enzymes and Increased Serum Insulin Concentration," *British Journal of Nutrition* 106, no. 10 (November 2011): 1470–1475, doi: 10.1017/S0007114511001966.

17. David Perlmutter, *Grain Brain* (New York: Little, Brown and Company, 2013), 63.

18. Hetty C. van den Broeck et al., "Presence of Celiac Disease Epitopes in Modern and Old Hexaploid Wheat Varieties: Wheat Breeding May Have Contributed to Increased Prevalence of Celiac Disease," *Theoretical and Applied Genetics* 121, no. 8 (2010): 1527–1539, accessed January 26, 2022, doi: 10.1007/s00122-010-1408-4.

19. Daniela Pizzuti et al., "Lack of Intestinal Mucosal Toxicity of Triticum Monococcum in Celiac Disease Patients," *Scandinavian Journal of Gastroenterology* 41, no. 11 (November 2006): 1305–1311, accessed January 26, 2022, doi: 10.1080/00365520600699983.

20. Rittika Chunder et al., "Antibody Cross-Reactivity Between Casein and Myelin-Associated Glycoprotein Results in Central Nervous System Demyelination," *Proceedings of the National Academy of Sciences of the United States of America* 119, no. 10 (March 2, 2022): e2117034119, doi: 10.1073/pnas.2117034119.

21. Jorge E. Chavarro et al., "A Prospective Study of Dairy Foods Intake and Anovulatory Infertility," *Human Reproduction* 22, no. 5 (May 2007): 1340–1347, accessed January 26, 2022, doi: 10.1093/humrep/dem019.

22. Katayoun Khoshbin and Michael Camilleri, "Neurogastroenterology and Motility: Effects of Dietary Components on Intestinal Permeability in Health and Disease," *The American Journal of Physiology-Gastrointestinal and Liver Physiology* 319, no. 5 (November 1, 2020): G589–G608, doi: 10.1152/ajpgi.00245.2020.

23. "Polysorbate 80," Bell Chem (May 18, 2014), https://www.bellchem.com/news/polysorbate-80.

24. D. Partridge et al., "Food Additives: Assessing the Impact of Exposure to Permitted Emulsifiers on Bowel and Metabolic Health—Introducing the FADiets Study," *Nutrition Bulletin* 44, no. 4 (December 2019): 329–349, doi: 10.1111/nbu.12408.

25. Robert D. Abbott, Adam Sadowski, and Angela G. Alt, "Efficacy of the Autoimmune Protocol Diet as Part of a Multi-disciplinary, Supported Lifestyle Intervention for Hashimoto's Thyroiditis," *Cureus* 11, no. 4 (April 2019): e4556, doi: 10.7759/cureus.4556.

26. Gauree G. Konijeti et al., "Efficacy of the Autoimmune Protocol Diet for Inflammatory Bowel Disease," *Inflammatory Bowel Diseases* 23, no. 11 (November 2017): 2054–2060, doi: 10.1097/MIB.0000000000001221.

27. Anita Chandrasekaran et al., "The Autoimmune Protocol Diet Modifies Intestinal RNA Expression in Inflammatory Bowel Disease," *Crohn's & Colitis 360* 1, no. 3 (October 2019): otz016, doi: 10.1093/crocol/otz016.

28. Jotham Suez et al., "Artificial Sweeteners Induce Glucose Intolerance by Altering the Gut Microbiota," *Nature* 514 (2014): 181–186, doi: 10.1038/nature13793.

29. Carol Johnston et al., "Examination of the Antiglycemic Properties of Vinegar in Healthy Adults," *Annals of Nutrition & Metabolism* 56, no. 1 (2010): 74–79, doi: 10.1159/000272133.

30. E. Östman et al., "Vinegar Supplementation Lowers Glucose and Insulin Responses and Increases Satiety After a Bread Meal in Healthy Subjects," *European Journal of Clinical Nutrition* 59 (2005): 983–988, doi: 10.1038/sj.ejcn.1602197.

31. Carol Johnston et al., "Vinegar Ingestion at Mealtime Reduced Fasting Blood Glucose Concentrations in Healthy Adults at Risk for Type 2 Diabetes," *Journal of Functional Foods* 5, no. 4 (2013): 2007–2011, doi: 10.1016/j.jff.2013.08.003.

32. Tomoo Kondo et al., "Vinegar Intake Reduces Body Weight, Body Fat Mass, and Serum Triglyceride Levels in Obese Japanese Subjects," *Bioscience, Biotechnology, and Biochemistry* 73, no. 8, (2009): 1837–1843, doi: 10.1271/bbb.90231.

33. QiQi Zhou et al., "Randomised Placebo-controlled Trial of Dietary Glutamine Supplements for Postinfectious Irritable Bowel Syndrome," *Gut* 68, no. 6 (2019), doi: 10.1136/gutjnl-2017-315136.

34. Michael Gleeson, "Dosing and Efficacy of Glutamine Supplementation in Human Exercise and Sport Training," *Journal of Nutrition* 138, no. 10 (October 2008): 2045S–2049S, doi: 10.1093/jn/138.10.2045S.

35. Lara Costantini et al., "Impact of Omega-3 Fatty Acids on the Gut Microbiota," *International Journal of Molecular Sciences* 18, no. 12 (December 2017): 2645, doi: 10.3390/ijms18122645.

36. Ines Barkia, Nazamid Saari, and Schonna R. Manning, "Microalgae for High-Value Products Towards Human Health and Nutrition," *Marine Drugs* 17, no. 5 (May 24, 2019): 304, doi: 10.3390/md17050304.

37. Losurdo, "Extra-intestinal Manifestations," 1521–1530.

38. K. de Punder, and L. Pruimboom, "The Dietary Intake of Wheat and Other Cereal Grains and Their Role in Inflammation," *Nutrients* 5(3) (2013): 771–787, doi: 10.3390/nu5030771.

39. Pizzuti, "Lack of Intestinal Mucosal Toxicity," 1305–1311.

40. Carlo G. Rizzello et al., "Highly Efficient Gluten Degradation by Lactobacilli and Fungal Proteases during Food Processing: New Perspectives for Celiac Disease," *Applied and Environmental Microbiology* 73, no. 14 (July 2007): 4499–4507, accessed January 26, 2022, doi: 10.1128/AEM.00260-07.

41. Luigi Greco et al., "Safety for Patients with Celiac Disease of Baked Goods Made of Wheat Flour Hydrolyzed during Food Processing," *Clinical Gastroenterology and Hepatology* 9, no. 1 (January 2011): 24–29, accessed January 26, 2022, doi: 10.1016/j.cgh.2010.09.025.

Chapter 6

1. Susan L. Worley, "The Extraordinary Importance of Sleep," *P & T: A Peer-Reviewed Journal for Formulary Management* 43, no. 12 (2018): 758–763, https://www.ncbi.nlm.nih.gov/pmc/articles/PMC6281147/.

2. Tracey J. Smith et al., "Impact of Sleep Restriction on Local Immune Response and Skin Barrier Restoration with and without 'Multi-Nutrient' Nutrition Intervention," *Journal of Applied Physiology* Vol. 124, (2018): 190, doi: 10.1152/japplphysiol.00547.2017.

3. Séverine Lamon et al., "The Effect of Acute Sleep Deprivation on Skeletal Muscle Protein Synthesis and the Hormonal Environment," *Physiological Reports* 9, no. 1 (2021): e14660, doi: 10.14814/phy2.14660.

4. Fatin Atrooz and Samina Salim, "Sleep Deprivation, Oxidative Stress and Inflammation," *Advances in Protein Chemistry and Structural Biology* 119, (2020): 309–336 doi: 10.1016/bs.apcsb.2019.03.001.

5. Luciana Besedovsky et al., "The Sleep-Immune Crosstalk in Health and Disease," *Physiological Reviews* 99, no. 3 (2019): 1325–1380, doi: 10.1152/physrev.00010.2018.

6. Taylor A. James, Dara James, and Linda K. Larkey, "Heart-focused Breathing and Perceptions of Burden in Alzheimer's Caregivers: An Online Randomized Controlled Pilot Study," *Geriatric Nursing* 42, no. 2 (March–April 2021): 397–404, doi: 10.1016/j.gerinurse.2021.02.006.

7. Savita Srivastava and James L. Boyer, "Psychological Stress Is Associated with Relapse in Type 1 Autoimmune Hepatitis," *Liver International* 30, no. 10 (September 16, 2010): 1439–1447, accessed January 26, 2022, doi: 10.1111/j.1478-3231.2010.02333.x.

8. Elizabeth K. Pradhan et al., "Effect of Mindfulness-based Stress Reduction in Rheumatoid Arthritis Patients," *Arthritis & Rheumatology* 57, no. 7 (October 2007): 1134–1142, doi: 10.1002/art.23010.

9. Andrew Octavian Sasmita, Joshua Kuruvilla, and Anna Pick Kiong Ling, "Harnessing Neuroplasticity: Modern Approaches and Clinical Future," *International Journal of Neuroscience* 128, no. 11 (November 2018): 1061–1077, doi: 10.1080/00207454.2018.1466781.

10. Neeraj S. Limaye, Lilian Braighi Carvalho, and Sharon Kramer, "Effects of Aerobic Exercise on Serum Biomarkers of Neuroplasticity and Brain Repair in Stroke: A Systematic Review," *Archives of Physical Medicine and Rehabilitation* 102, no. 8 (August 2021): 1633–1634, doi: 10.1016/j.apmr.2021.04.010.

11. Julie Tseng and Jordan Poppenk, "Brain Meta-state Transitions Demarcate Thoughts across Task Contexts Exposing the Mental Noise of Trait Neuroticism," *Nature Communications* 11, no. 3480 (July 13, 2020), doi: 10.1038/s41467-020-17255-9.

12. Kristen A. Lindquist et al., "The Brain Basis of Emotion: A Meta-analytic Review," *Behavioral and Brain Sciences* 35, no. 3 (June 2012): 121–143, doi: 10.1017/S0140525X11000446.

13. Estela M. Pardos-Gascón et al., "Differential Efficacy between Cognitive-Behavioral Therapy and Mindfulness-based Therapies for Chronic Pain: Systematic Review," *International Journal of Clinical and Health Psychology* 21, no. 1 (January-April 2021): 100197, doi: 10.1016/j.ijchp.2020.08.001.

14. Nicholas A. Coles, Jeff T. Larsen, and Heather C. Lench, "A Meta-analysis of the Facial Feedback Literature: Effects of Facial Feedback on Emotional Experience are Small and Variable," *Psychological Bulletin* 145, no. 6 (2019): 610–651, doi: 10.1037/bul0000194.

15. Fernando Marmolejo-Ramos et al., "Your Face and Moves Seem Happier When I Smile: Facial Action Influences the Perception of Emotional Faces and Biological Motion Stimuli," *Experimental Psychology* 67, no. 1 (January 2020): 14–22, doi: 10.1027/1618-3169/a000470.

16. Michael B. Lewis and Patrick J. Bowler, "Botulinum Toxin Cosmetic Therapy Correlates with a More Positive Mood," *Journal of Cosmetic Dermatology* 8 (2009): 24–26, https://onlinelibrary.wiley.com/doi/pdf/10.1111/j.1473-2165.2009.00419.x.

17. Suzanne C. Segerstrom and Gregory E. Miller, "Psychological Stress and the Human Immune System: A Meta-analytic Study of 30 Years of Inquiry," *Psychological Bulletin* 130, no. 4 (July 2004): 601–630, doi: 10.1037/0033-2909.130.4.601.

18. Soroor Behbahani and Farhad Shahram, "Electrocardiogram and Heart Rate Variability Assessment in Patients with Common Autoimmune Diseases: A Methodological Review," *Turk Kardiyoloji Dernegi Arsivi* 48, no. 3 (April 2020): 312–327, doi: 10.5543/tkda.2019.21112.

19. Harun Evrengül et al., "Heart Rate Variability in Patients with Rheumatoid Arthritis," *Rheumatology International* 24, no. 4 (July 2004): 198–202, doi: 10.1007/s00296-003-0357-5.

20. Marco A. Perrone et al., "Heart Rate Variability Modifications in Response to Different Types of Exercise Training in Athletes," *The Journal of Sports Medicine and Physical Fitness* 61, no. 10 (October 2021): 1411–1415, doi: 10.23736/S0022-4707.21.12480-6.

21. Hayley A. Young and David Benton, "Heart-rate Variability: A Biomarker to Study the Influence of Nutrition on Physiological and Psychological Health?", *Behavioral Pharmacology* 29, 2 and 3-Spec Issue (April 2018): 140–151, doi: 10.1097/FBP.0000000000000383.

22. Julian F. Thayer, Shelby S. Yamamoto, and Jos F. Brosschot, "The Relationship of Autonomic Imbalance, Heart Rate Variability and Cardiovascular Disease Risk Factors," *International Journal of Cardiology* 141, no. 2 (May 28, 2010): 122–131, doi: 10.1016/j.ijcard.2009.09.543.

23. Wei Xin, Wei Wei, and Xiao-Ying Li, "Short-Term Effects of Fish-Oil Supplementation on Heart Rate Variability in Humans: A Meta-analysis of Randomized Controlled Trials," *The American Journal of Clinical Nutrition* 97, no. 5 (May 2013): 926–935, doi: 10.3945/ajcn.112.049833.

24. Cecilie Rovsing et al., "Deep Breathing Increases Heart Rate Variability in Patients with Rheumatoid Arthritis and Systemic Lupus Erythematosus," *Journal of Clinical Rheumatology* 27, no. 7 (October 1, 2021): 261–266, doi: 10.1097/RHU.0000000000001300.

25. Tim Vanuytsel et al., "Psychological Stress and Corticotropin-Releasing Hormone Increase Intestinal Permeability in Humans by a Mast Cell-dependent Mechanism," *Gut* 63, no. 8 (August 2014): 1293–1299, doi: 10.1136/gutjnl-2013-305690.

26. Rosa M. Arin et al., "Adenosine: Direct and Indirect Actions on Gastric Acid Secretion," *Frontiers in Physiology* 8, no. 737 (September 22, 2017), doi: 10.3389/fphys.2017.00737

27. Aitor Lanas-Gimeno, Gonzalo Hijos, and Ángel Lanas, "Proton Pump Inhibitors, Adverse Events and Increased Risk of Mortality," *Expert Opinion on Drug Safety* 18, no. 11 (November 2019): 1043–1053, doi: 10.1080/14740338.2019.1664470.

28. Rashmi Chandra and Rodger A. Liddle, "Neural and Hormonal Regulation of Pancreatic Secretion," *Current Opinion in Gastroenterology* 25, no. 5 (September 2009): 441–446, doi: 10.1097/MOG.0b013e32832e9c41.

29. Shanta R. Dube et al., "Cumulative Childhood Stress and Autoimmune Diseases in Adults," *Psychosomatic Medicine* 71, no. 2 (February 2009): 243–250, doi: 10.1097/PSY.0b013e3181907888.

30. Mario F. Juruena et al., "The Role of Early Life Stress in HPA Axis and Anxiety," *Advances in Experimental Medicine and Biology* 1191 (2020): 141–153, doi: 10.1007/978-981-32-9705-0_9.

31. Martin H. Teicher, Carl M. Anderson, and Ann Pocari, "Childhood Maltreatment Is Associated with Reduced Volume in the Hippocampal Subfields CA3, Dentate Gyrus, and Subiculum," *Proceedings of the National Academy of Sciences of the United States of America* 109, no. 9 (February 28, 2012): E563–572, doi: 10.1073/pnas.1115396109.

32. Shanta R. Dube et al., "Cumulative Childhood Stress and Autoimmune Diseases in Adults," *Psychosomatic Medicine* 71, no. 2 (February 2009): 243–350, doi: 10.1097/PSY.0b013e3181907888.

33. Sanne L. Nijhof et al., "Healthy Play, Better Coping: The Importance of Play for the Development of Children in Health and Disease," *Neuroscience and Biobehavioral Reviews* 95 (December 2018): 421–429, doi: 10.1016/j.neubiorev.2018.09.024.

34. Michael Yogman et al., "The Power of Play: A Pediatric Role in Enhancing Development in Young Children," *Pediatrics* 142, no. 3 (September 2018): e20182058, doi: 10.1542/peds.2018-2058.

35. Suzanne D.E. Held and Marek Spinka, "Animal Play and Animal Welfare," *Animal Behaviour* 81, no. 5 (May 2011): 891–899, doi: 10.1016/j.anbehav.2011.01.007.

36. Thomas E. Gorman, Douglas E. Gentile, and C. Shawn Green, "Problem Gaming: A Short Primer," *American Journal of Play* 10, no. 3 (Spring 2018): 309–327, https://pubmed.ncbi.nlm.nih.gov/34721754/.

37. "George Bernard Shaw >Quotes >Quotable Quote," GoodReads, accessed January 8, 2022, https://www.goodreads.com/quotes/413462-we-don-t-stop-playing-because-we-grow-old-we-grow.

Chapter 7

1. Fabrizia Bamonte et al., "Metal Chelation Therapy in Rheumatoid Arthritis: A Case Report. Successful Management of Rheumatoid Arthritis by Metal Chelation Therapy," *BioMetals* 24, no. 6 (December 2011): 1093–1098, doi: 10.1007/s10534-011-9467-9.

2. Allesandro Fulghenzi et al., "A Case of Multiple Sclerosis Improvement Following Removal of Heavy Metal Intoxication Lessons Learnt from Matteo's Case," *BioMetals* 25, no. 3 (March 2012): 569–576, doi: 10.1007/s10534-012-9537-7.

3. Jonna Jalanka et al., "The Effect of Psyllium Husk on Intestinal Microbiota in Constipated Patients and Healthy Controls," *International Journal of Molecular Sciences* 20, no. 2 (January 20, 2019): 433, doi: 10.3390/ijms20020433.

4. Mayara Belaorio and Manuel Gómez, "Psyllium: A Useful Functional Ingredient in Food Systems," *Critical Reviews in Food Science and Nutrition* 62, no. 2 (September 1, 2020): 527–538, doi: 10.1080/10408398.2020.1822276.

5. G. Quartarone, "Role of PHGG as a Dietary Fiber: A Review Article," *Minerva Gastroenterologica e Dietologica* 59, no. 4 (December 2013): 329–340, https://pubmed.ncbi.nlm.nih.gov/24212352/.

6. Simon J. Reider et al., "Prebiotic Effects of Partially Hydrolyzed Guar Gum on the Composition and Function of the Human Microbiota—Results from the PAGODA Trial," *Nutrients* 12, no. 5 (May 2020): 1257, doi: 10.3390/nu12051257.

7. Zenta Yasukawa et al., "Effect of Repeated Consumption of Partially Hydrolyzed Guar Gum on Fecal Characteristics and Gut Microbiota: A Randomized, Double-Blind, Placebo-Controlled, and Parallel-Group Clinical Trial," *Nutrients* 11, no. 9 (September 10, 2019): 2170, doi: 10.3390/nu11092170.

8. Rosemary Waring, "Cytochrome P450: Genotype to Phenotype," *Xenobiotica* 50 (January 2020): 9–18, doi: 10.1080/00498254.2019.1648911.

9. Robin P. Peeters and Theo J. Visser, "Metabolism of Thyroid Hormone," *Endotext* [Internet] (January 1, 2017), https://www.ncbi.nlm.nih.gov/books/NBK285545/.

10. Genjiro Kimura, "Sodium, Kidney, and Circadian Rhythm of Blood Pressure," *Clinical and Experimental Nephrology* 5 (2001): 13–18, doi: 10.1007/PL00012172.

11. Karen Schmitt et al., "Circadian Control of DRP1 Activity Regulates Mitochondrial Dynamics and Bioenergetics," *Cell Metabolism* 27, no. 3 (March 6, 2018): 657–666, doi: 10.1016/j.cmet.2018.01.011.

12. Robin M. Voigt et al., "Circadian Rhythm and the Gut Microbiome," *International Review of Neurobiology* 131 (September 6, 2016): 193–205, doi: 10.1016/bs.irn.2016.07.002.

13. Jiffin K. Paulose and Vincent M. Cassone, "The Melatonin-Sensitive Circadian Clock of the Enteric Bacterium *Enterobacter Aerogenes,*" *Gut Microbes* 7, no. 5 (July 7, 2016): 424–427, doi: 10.1080/19490976.2016.1208892.

14. Margaret E. Sears, Kathleen J. Kerr, and Riina I. Bray, "Arsenic, Cadmium, Lead, and Mercury in Sweat: A Systematic Review," *Journal of Environmental and Public Health* 2012 (February 22, 2012): 184745, doi: 10.1155/2012/184745.

15. Genuis, "Blood, Urine, and Sweat," 344–357.

16. Masaki Iguchi et al., "Heat Stress and Cardiovascular, Hormonal, and Heat Shock Proteins in Humans," *Journal of Athletic Training* 47, no. 2 (March–April 2012): 184–190, doi: 10.4085/1062-6050-47.2.184.

17. K. Kukkonen-Harjula and K. Kauppinen, "How the Sauna Affects the Endocrine System," *Annals of Clinical Research* 20, no. 4 (1988): 262–266, https://pubmed.ncbi.nlm.nih.gov/3218898/.

18. Rhonda P. Patrick and Teresa L. Johnson, "Sauna Use as a Lifestyle Practice to Extend Healthspan," *Experimental Gerontology* 154 (October 15, 2021): 111509, doi: 10.1016/j.exger.2021.111509.

19. Tanjaniina Laukkanen et al., "Association Between Sauna Bathing and Fatal Cardiovascular and All-Cause Mortality Events," *JAMA Internal Medicine* 175, no. 4 (April 2015): 542–548, doi: 10.1001/jamainternmed.2014.8187.

20. Shan Liao, Pierre-Yves von der Weid, and Inflammation Research Network, Snyder Institute for Chronic Diseases, "Lymphatic System: An Active Pathway for Immune Protection," *Seminars in Cell and Developmental Biology* 38 (February 2015): 83–89, doi: 10.1016/j.semcdb.2014.11.012.

21. Weston Petroski and Deanna M. Minich, "Is There Such a Thing as 'Anti-Nutrients'? A Narrative Review of Perceived Problematic Plant Compounds," *Nutrients* 12, no. 10 (October 2020): doi: 10.3390/nu12102929.

22. Takuya Uchikawa et al., "Chlorella Suppresses Methylmercury Transfer to the Fetus in Pregnant Mice," *Journal of Toxicological Sciences* 36, no. 5 (2011): 675–680, doi: 10.2131/jts.36.675.

23. Carlo Perricone, Caterina De Carolis, and Roberto Perricone, "Glutathione: A Key Player in Autoimmunity," *Autoimmunity Reviews* 8, no. 8 (July 2009): 697–701, doi: 10.1016/j.autrev.2009.02.020.

24. Raghu Sinha et al., "Oral Supplementation with Liposomal Glutathione Elevates Body Stores of Glutathione and Markers of Immune Function," *European Journal of Clinical Nutrition* 72, no. 1 (January 2018): 105–111, doi: 10.1038/ejcn.2017.132.

25. John P. Richie Jr. et al., "Randomized Controlled Trial of Oral Glutathione Supplementation on Body Stores of Glutathione," *European Journal of Nutrition* 54, no. 2 (March 2015): 251–263, doi: 10.1007/s00394-014-0706-z.

26. Yasushi Honda et al., "Efficacy of Glutathione for the Treatment of Nonalcoholic Fatty Liver Disease: An Open-Label, Single-Arm, Multicenter, Pilot Study," *BMC Gastroenterology* 17 (August 8, 2017): 96, doi: 10.1186/s12876-017-0652-3.

Chapter 8

1. S.B. Naaeder, D.F. Evans, and E.Q. Archampong, "Effect of Chronic Dietary Fibre Supplementation on Colonic pH on Healthy Volunteers," *West African Journal of Medicine* 17, no. 3 (July–September 1998): 165–167, https://pubmed.ncbi.nlm.nih.gov/9814085/.

2. Shadi Lal Malhotra, "Faecal Urobilinogen Levels and pH of Stools in Population Groups with Different Incidence of Cancer of the Colon, and their Possible Role in its Aetiology," *Journal of the Royal Society of Medicine* 75, no. 9 (September 1982): 709–714, doi: 10.1177/014107688207500907.

3. CK Yao et al., "Review Article: Insights into Colonic Protein Fermentation, Its Modulation and Potential Health Implications," *Alimentary Pharmacology & Therapeutics*, 43 no. 2 (2016): 181–196, doi: 10.1111/apt.13456.

4. Jane G. Muir et al., "Measurement of Short-Chain Carbohydrates in Common Australian Vegetables and Fruits by High-Performance Liquid Chromatography (HPLC)," *Journal of Agricultural and Food Chemistry* 57, no. 2 (February 2009): 554–565, doi: 10.1021/jf802700e.

5. Mohammad Hossein Boskabady, Saeed Alitaneh, and Azam Alavinezhad, "Carum Copticum L.: An Herbal Medicine with Various Pharmacological Effects," *BioMed Research International* 2014 (June 25, 2014): 569087, doi: 10.1155/2014/569087.

6. Jason A. Hawrelak et al., "Essential Oils in the Treatment of Intestinal Dysbiosis: A Preliminary In Vitro Study," *Alternative Medicine Review* 14, no. 4 (2009): 380–384, https://www.researchgate.net/publication/40765979_Essential_Oils_in_the_Treatment_of_Intestinal_Dysbiosis_A_Preliminary_in_vitro_Study.

7. Boskabady, "Carum Copticum L.," 569087.

8. Prasanthi Karna et al., "Benefits of Whole Ginger Extract in Prostate Cancer," *British Journal of Nutrition* 107, no. 4 (August 18, 2011): 473–484, doi: 10.1017/S0007114511003308.

9. Jung San Chang et al., "Fresh Ginger (Zingiber Officinale) Has Anti-Viral Activity against Human Respiratory Syncytial Virus in Human Respiratory Tract Cell Lines," *Journal of Ethnopharmacology* 145, no. 1 (January 9, 2013): 146–151, doi: 10.1016/j.jep.2012.10.043.

10. Ponmurugan Karuppiah and Shyamkumar Rajaram, "Antibacterial Effect of *Allium Sativum* Cloves and *Zingiber Officinale* Rhizomes against Multiple-Drug Resistant Clinical Pathogens," *Asian Pacific Journal of Tropical Biomedicine* 2, no. 8 (August 2012): 597–601, doi: 10.1016/S2221-1691(12)60104-X.

11. Gill Paramdeep, "Efficacy and Tolerability of Ginger (Zingiber Officinale) in Patients of Osteoarthritis of Knee," *Indian Journal of Physiology and Pharmacology* 57, no. 2 (April–June 2013): 177–183, https://pubmed.ncbi.nlm.nih.gov/24617168/.

12. R.D. Altman and K.C. Marcussen, "Effects of a Ginger Extract on Knee Pain in Patients with Osteoarthritis," *Arthritis and Rheumatology* 44, no. 11 (2001): 2531–2538, doi: 10.1002/1529-0131.

13. Jerry O. Ciocon, Daisy G. Ciocon, and Diana Galindo, "Dietary Supplements in Primary Care: Botanicals Can Affect Surgical Outcomes and Follow-up," *Geriatrics* 59, no. 9 (October 2004): 20–24, https://pubmed.ncbi.nlm.nih.gov/15461234/.

14. Ao Shang et al., "Bioactive Compounds and Biological Functions of Garlic (*Allium sativum* L.)," *Foods* 8, no. 7 (July 5, 2019): 246, doi: 10.3390/foods8070246.

15. Rodrigo Arreola et al., "Immunomodulation and Anti-Inflammatory Effects of Garlic Compounds," *Journal of Immunology Research* 2015 (April 19, 2015): 401630, doi: 10.1155/2015/401630.

16. Kun Song and John A. Milner, "The Influence of Heating on the Anticancer Properties of Garlic," *The Journal of Nutrition* 131, no. 3 (March 2001): 1054S–1057S, doi: 10.1093/jn/131.3.1054S.

17. Bharat B. Aggarwal with Debra Yost, *Healing Spices* (New York: Sterling Publishing, 2011), 47–48.

18. B.H. Ali and Gerald Blunden, "Pharmacological and Toxicological Properties of Nigella Sativa," *Phytotherapy Research* 17, no. 4 (April 2003): 299–305, doi: 10.1002/ptr.1309.

19. H. Mahmoudvand et al., "Evaluation of Antifungal Activities of the Essential Oil and Various Extracts of *Nigella Sativa* and its Main Component, Thymoquinone against Pathogenic Dermatophyte Strains," *Journal de Mycologie Médicale* 24, no. 4 (December 2014): e155–e161, doi: 10.1016/j.mycmed.2014.06.048.

20. Huda Kaatabi et al., "Nigella Sativa Improves Glycemic Control and Ameliorates Oxidative Stress in Patients with Type 2 Diabetes Mellitus: Placebo Controlled Participant Blinded Clinical Trial," *PLoS One* 10, no. 2 (February 23, 2015): e0113486, doi: 10.1371/journal.pone.0113486.

21. Tamer A. Gheita and Sanaa A. Kenawy, "Effectiveness of Nigella Sativa Oil in the Management of Rheumatoid Arthritis Patients: A Placebo Controlled Study," *Phytotherapy Research* 26, no. 8 (August 2012): 1246–1248, doi: 10.1002/ptr.3679.

22. Ali, "Pharmacological and Toxicological Properties of Nigella Sativa," 299–305.

23. Mahmoud Aqel and Rola Shaheen, "Effects of the Volatile Oil of Nigella Sativa Seeds on the Uterine Smooth Muscle of Rat and Guinea Pig," *Journal of Ethnopharmacology* 52, no. 1 (May 1, 1996): 23–26, doi: 10.1016/0378-8741(95)01330-x.

24. Subash Chandra Gupta et al., "Neem (*Azadirachta indica*): An Indian Traditional Panacea with Modern Molecular Basis," *Phytomedicine* 34 (October 15, 2017): 14–20, doi: 10.1016/j.phymed.2017.07.001.

25. Usharani Pingali et al., "Aqueous *Azadirachta indica* (Neem) Extract Attenuates Insulin Resistance to Improve Glycemic Control and Endothelial Function in Subjects with Metabolic

Syndrome," *Journal of Medicinal Food* 24, no. 11 (November 2021): 1135–1144, doi: 10.1089/jmf.2020.4838.

26. Beena Khillare and Tulsidas G. Shrivastav, "Spermicidal Activity of Azadirachta Indica (Neem) Leaf Extract," *Contraception* 68, no. 3 (September 2003): 225–229, doi: 10.1016/s0010-7824(03)00165-3.

27. Soheil Zorofchian Moghadamtousi et al., "A Review on Antibacterial, Antiviral, and Antifungal Activity of Curcumin," *BioMed Research International* 2014 (April 29, 2014): 186864, doi: 10.1155/2014/186864.

28. Vilai Kuptniratsaikul et al., "Efficacy and Safety of Curcuma Domestica Extracts Compared with Ibuprofen in Patients with Knee Osteoarthritis: A Multicenter Study," *Clinical Interventions in Aging* 9 (March 20, 2014): 451–458, doi: 10.2147/CIA.S58535.

29. Binu Chandran and Ajay Goel, "A Randomized, Pilot Study to Assess the Efficacy and Safety of Curcumin in Patients with Active Rheumatoid Arthritis," *Phytotherapy Research* 26, no. 11) (November 2012): 1719–1725, doi: 10.1002/ptr.4639.

30. B. Lal et al., "Efficacy of Curcumin in the Management of Chronic Anterior Uveitis," *Phytotherapy Research* 13, no. 4 (June 1999): 318–322, doi: 10.1002/(SICI)1099-1573(199906)13:4<318::AID-PTR445>3.0.CO;2-7.

31. Rakhi Agarwal et al., "Detoxification and Antioxidant Effects of Curcumin in Rats Experimentally Exposed to Mercury," *Journal of Applied Toxicology* 30, no. 5 (July 1, 2010): 457–468, doi: 10.1002/jat.1517.

32. Guido Shoba et al., "Influence of Piperine on the Pharmacokinetics of Curcumin in Animals and Human Volunteers," *Planta Medica* 64, no. 4 (May 1998): 353–356, doi: 10.1055/s-2006-957450.

33. Atsushi Imaizumi, "Highly Bioavailable Curcumin (Theracurmin): Its Development and Clinical Application," *PharmaNutrition* 4, no. 1 (January 2016): 1–8, doi: 10.1016/j.phanu.2015.11.001.

34. Rohitash Jamwal, "Bioavailable Curcumin Formulations: A Review of Pharmacokinetic Studies in Healthy Volunteers," *Journal of Integrative Medicine* 16, no. 6 (November 2018): 367–374, doi: 10.1016/j.joim.2018.07.001.

35. Jamwal, "Bioavailable Curcumin Formulations," 367–374.

36. Shrikant Mishra and Kalpana Palanivelu, "The Effect of Curcumin (Turmeric) on Alzheimer's Disease: An Overview," *Annals of Indian Academy of Neurology* 11, no. 1 (January 2008): 13–19, doi: 10.4103/0972-2327.40220.

37. Mishra, "The Effect of Curcumin," 13–19.

Chapter 9

1. Bradley Leech et al., "Risk Factors Associated with Intestinal Permeability in an Adult Population: A Systematic Review," *International Journal of Clinical Practice* 73, no. 10 (October 2019): e13385, doi: 10.1111/ijcp.13385.

2. Jonathan Gan et al., "A Case for Improved Assessment of Gut Permeability: A Meta-Analysis Quantifying the Lactulose: Mannitol Ratio in Coeliac and Crohn's Disease," *BMC Gastroenterology* 22 (January 10, 2022): 16, doi: 10.1186/s12876-021-02082-z.

3. Benjamin Seethaler et al., "Biomarkers for Assessment of Intestinal Permeability in Clinical Practice," *American Journal of Physiology—Gastrointestinal and Liver Physiology* 321, no. 1 (May 19, 2021): G11–G17, doi: 10.1152/ajpgi.00113.2021.

4. Yusuke Kinashi and Koji Hase, "Partners in Leaky Gut Syndrome: Intestinal Dysbiosis and Autoimmunity," *Frontiers in Immunology* 12 (April 22, 2021): 673708, doi: 10.3389/fimmu.2021.673708.

5. Jerry M. Wells et al., "Homeostasis of the Gut Barrier and Potential Biomarkers," *American Journal of Physiology—Gastrointestinal and Liver Physiology* 312, no. 3 (March 1, 2017): G171–G193, doi: 10.1152/ajpgi.00048.2015.

6. Nicholas J. Mantis et al., "Secretory IgA's Complex Roles in Immunity and Mucosal Homeostasis in the Gut," *Mucosal Immunology* 4, no. 6 (November 2011): 603–611, doi: 10.1038/mi.2011.41.

7. Per Brandtzaeg, "Update on Mucosal Immunoglobulin A in Gastrointestinal Disease," *Current Opinion in Gastroenterology* 26, no. 6 (November 2010): 554–563, doi: 10.1097/MOG.0b013e32833dccf8.

8. Marcin Krawczyk, "Gut Permeability Might be Improved by Dietary Fiber in Individuals with Nonalcoholic Fatty Liver Disease (NAFLD) Undergoing Weight Reduction," *Nutrients* 10, no. 11 (November 18, 2018): 1793, doi: 10.3390/nu10111793.

9. Dagfinn Aune et al., "Fruit and Vegetable Intake and the Risk of Cardiovascular Disease, Total Cancer and All-cause Mortality: A Systematic Review and Dose-Response Meta-Analysis of Prospective Studies," *International Journal of Epidemiology* 46, no. 3 (June 2017): 1029–1056, doi: 10.1093/ije/dyw319.

10. Francesco Russo et al., "Inulin-Enriched Pasta Improves Intestinal Permeability and Modifies the Circulating Levels of Zonulin and Glucagon-Like Peptide 2 in Healthy Young Volunteers," *Nutrition Research* 32, no. 12 (December 2012): 940–946, doi: 10.1016/j.nutres.2012.09.010.

11. Laura M. Mar-Solis et al., "Analysis of the Anti-Inflammatory Capacity of Bone Broth in a Murine Model of Ulcerative Colitis," *Medicina (Kaunas)* 57, no. 11 (October 20, 2021): 1138, doi: 10.3390/medicina57111138.

12. Jordan L. Hawkins and Paul L. Durham, "Enriched Chicken Bone Broth as a Dietary Supplement Reduces Nociception and Sensitization Associated with Prolonged Jaw Opening," *Journal of Oral & Facial Pain and Headache* 32, no. 2 (March 6, 2018): 208–215, doi: 10.11607/ofph.1971.

13. Qianru Chen et al., "Collagen Peptides Ameliorate Intestinal Epithelial Barrier Dysfunction in Immunostimulatory Caco-2 Cell Monolayers via Enhancing Tight Junctions," *Food & Function* 3 (2017), doi: 10.1039/C6FO01347C.

14. Rebekah D. Alcock, Gregory C. Shaw, and Louise M. Burke, "Bone Broth Unlikely to Provide Reliable Concentrations of Collagen Precursors Compared with Supplemental Sources of Collagen Used in Collagen Research," *International Journal of Sport Nutrition and Exercise Metabolism* 29, no. 3 (May 1, 2019): 265–272, doi: 10.1123/ijsnem.2018-0139.

15. Satiesh Kumar Ramadass et al., "Type I Collagen and Its Daughter Peptides for Targeting Mucosal Healing in Ulcerative Colitis: A New Treatment Strategy," *European Journal of Pharmaceutical Sciences* 91 (August 25, 2016): 216–224, doi: 10.1016/j.ejps.2016.05.015.

16. Kristine L. Clark et al., "24-Week Study on the Use of Collagen Hydrolysate as a Dietary Supplement in Athletes with Activity-related Joint Pain," *Current Medical Research and Opinion* 24, no. 5 (May 2008): 1485–1496, doi: 10.1185/030079908x291967.

17. Lara Costantini et al., "Impact of Omega-3 Fatty Acids on the Gut Microbiota," *International Journal of Molecular Sciences* 18, no. 12 (December 7, 2017): 2645, doi: 10.3390/ijms18122645.

18. M. Takic et al., "Effects of Dietary α-Linolenic Acid Treatment and the Efficiency of Its Conversion to Eicosapentaenoic and Docosahexaenoic Acids in Obesity and Related Diseases," *Molecules* 27 no. 14 (2022): 4471, doi: 10.3390/molecules27144471.

19. Cuong D. Tran et al., "Zinc-fortified Oral Rehydration Solution Improved Intestinal Permeability and Small Intestinal Mucosal Recovery," *Clinical Pediatrics (Philadelphia)* 54, no. 7 (June 2015): 676–682, doi: 10.1177/0009922814562665.

20. Juana F. Willumsen, "Dietary Management of Acute Diarrhea in Children: Effect of Fermented and Amylase-Digested Weaning Foods on Intestinal Permeability," *Journal of Pediatric Gastroenterology and Nutrition* 24, no. 3 (March 1997): 235–241, doi: 10.1097/00005176-199703000-00001.

21. Eirini Dimidi et al., "Fermented Foods: Definitions and Characteristics, Impact on the Gut Microbiota and Effects on Gastrointestinal Health and Disease," *Nutrients* 11, no. 8 (August 2019): 1806, doi: 10.3390/nu11081806.

22. Matthew R. Hilimire et al., "Fermented Foods, Neuroticism, and Social Anxiety: An Interaction Model," *Psychiatry Research* 228, no. 2 (April 28, 2015): 203–208, doi: 10.1016/j.psychres.2015.04.023.

23. Hannah C. Wastyk et al., "Gut-microbiota-targeted Diets Modulate Human Immune Status," *Cell* 184, no. 16 (July 12, 2021): 4137–4153, doi: 10.1016/j.cell.2021.06.019.

24. Matthew T. Sorbara, "Inhibiting Antibiotic-resistant Enterobacteriaceae by Microbiota-mediated Intracellular Acidification," *Journal of Experimental Medicine* 216, no. 1 (January 7, 2019): 84–98, doi: 10.1084/jem.20181639.

25. Alison C. Bested et al., "Intestinal Microbiota, Probiotics and Mental Health: From Metchnikoff to Modern Advances: Part II—Contemporary Contextual Research," *Gut Pathogens* 5, no. 1 (March 14, 2013): 3, https://doi.org/10.1186/1757-4749-5-3.

26. Fabienne Laugerette et al., "Emulsified Lipids Increase Endotoxemia: Possible Role in Early Postprandial Low-grade Inflammation," *The Journal of Nutritional Biochemistry* 22, no. 1 (January 2011): 53–59, doi: 10.1016/j.jnutbio.2009.11.011.

27. Marlene Remely et al., "Increased Gut Microbiota Diversity and Abundance of *Faecalibacterium Prausnitzii* and *Akkermansia* After Fasting: A Pilot Study," *Wiener Klinische Wochenschrift* 127, no. 9–10 (March 13, 2015): 394–398, doi: 10.1007/s00508-015-0755-1.

28. Falak Zeb et al., "Effect of Time-Restricted Feeding on Metabolic Risk and Circadian Rhythm Associated with Gut Microbiome in Healthy Males," *British Journal of Nutrition* 123, no. 11 (January 6, 2020): 1216–1226, doi: 10.1017/S0007114519003428.

29. Ceren Özkul, Meltem Yalinay, and Tarkan Karakan, "Islamic Fasting Leads to an Increased Abundance of Akkermansia Muciniphila and Bacteroides Fragilis Group: A Preliminary Study on Intermittent Fasting," *Turkish Journal of Gastroenterology* 30, no. 12 (December 2019): 1030–1035, doi: 10.5152/tjg.2019.19185.

30. András Maifeld et al., "Fasting Alters the Gut Microbiome Reducing Blood Pressure and Body Weight in Metabolic Syndrome Patients," *Nature Communications* 12 (March 30, 2021): 1970, doi: 10.1038/s41467-021-22097-0.

31. Nielson T. Baxter et al., "Dynamics of Human Gut Microbiota and Short-Chain Fatty Acids in Response to Dietary Interventions with Three Fermentable Fibers," *mBio* 10, no. 1 (January–February 2019): e02566-18, doi: 10.1128/mBio.02566-18.

32. Nielson, "Dynamics of Human Gut Microbiota," e02566-18.

33. Mandy C. Szymanski et al., "Short-term Dietary Curcumin Supplementation Reduces Gastrointestinal Barrier Damage and Physiological Strain Responses during Exertional Heat Stress," *Journal of Applied Physiology* 124, no. 2 (February 1, 2018): 330–340, doi: 10.1152/japplphysiol.00515.2017.

34. QiQi Zhou et al., "Randomised Placebo-controlled Trial of Dietary Glutamine Supplements for Postinfectious Irritable Bowel Syndrome," *Gut* 68, no. 6 (June 2019): 996–1002, doi: 10.1136/gutjnl-2017-315136.

35. Jaya Benjamin et al., "Glutamine and Whey Protein Improve Intestinal Permeability and Morphology in Patients with Crohn's Disease: A Randomized Controlled Trial," *Digestive Diseases and Sciences* 57, no. 4 (April 2012): 1000–1012, doi: 10.1007/s10620-011-1947-9.

36. Zahra Vahdat Shariatpanahi et al., "Effects of Early Enteral Glutamine Supplementation on Intestinal Permeability in Critically Ill Patients," *Indian Journal of Critical Care Medicine* 23, no. 8 (August 2019): 356–362, doi: 10.5005/jp-journals-10071-23218.

37. Xi Peng et al., "Effects of Enteral Supplementation with Glutamine Granules on Intestinal Mucosal Barrier Function in Severe Burned Patients," *Burns* 30, no. 2 (March 2004): 135–139, doi: 10.1016/j.burns.2003.09.032.

38. Raymond John Playford and Michael James Weiser, "Bovine Colostrum: Its Constituents and Uses," *Nutrients* 13, no. 1 (January 2021): 265, doi: 10.3390/nu13010265.

39. Maciej Halasa et al., "Oral Supplementation with Bovine Colostrum Decreases Intestinal Permeability and Stool Concentrations of Zonulin in Athletes," *Nutrients* 9, no. 4 (April 2017): 370, doi: 10.3390/nu9040370.

40. Grégoire Wieërs et al., "How Probiotics Affect the Microbiota," *Frontiers in Cellular and Infection Microbiology* 9 (January 15, 2020): 454, doi: 10.3389/fcimb.2019.00454.

41. Jing Cheng, Arja Laitila, and Arthur C. Ouwehand, "*Bifidobacterium animalis* subsp. *lactis* HN019 Effects on Gut Health: A Review," *Frontiers in Nutrition* 8 (December 14, 2021): 790561, doi: 10.3389/fnut.2021.790561.

42. Jason C. Sniffen et al., "Choosing an Appropriate Probiotic Product for Your Patient: An Evidence-based Practical Guide," *PLoS One* 13, no. 12 (December 26, 2018): doi: 10.1371/journal.pone.0209205.

43. Antonella Orlando et al., "*Lactobacillus rhamnosus* GG Protects the Epithelial Barrier of Wistar Rats from the Pepsin-Trypsin-Digested Gliadin (PTG)-Induced Enteropathy," *Nutrients* 10, no. 11 (November 7, 2018): 1698, doi: 10.3390/nu10111698.

44. Kulandaipalayam N.C. Sindhu et al., "Immune Response and Intestinal Permeability in Children with Acute Gastroenteritis Treated with Lactobacillus Rhamnosus GG: A Randomized, Double-blind, Placebo-controlled Trial," *Clinical Infectious Diseases* 58, no. 8 (April 2014): 1107–1115, doi: 10.1093/cid/ciu065.

45. Lucio Capurso, "Thirty Years of *Lactobacillus rhamnosus* GG: A Review," *Journal of Clinical Gastroenterology* 53, suppl. 1 (March 2019): S1–S41, doi: 10.1097/MCG.0000000000001170.

46. Vibeke Rosenfeldt et al., "Effect of Probiotics on Gastrointestinal Symptoms and Small Intestinal Permeability in Children with Atopic Dermatitis," *The Journal of Pediatrics* 145, no. 5 (November 2004): 612–616, doi: 10.1016/j.jpeds.2004.06.068.

47. *Beneficial Probiotics,* accessed on February 27, 2022, http://www.floraactive.com/.

48. Cheng, "*Bifidobacterium animalis*," 790561.

49. David Groeger et al., "*Bifidobacterium infantis* 35624 Modulates Host Inflammatory Processes Beyond the Gut," *Gut Microbes* 4, no. 4 (July 1, 2013): 325–339, doi: 10.4161/gmic.25487.

50. Peter J. Whorwell et al., "Efficacy of an Encapsulated Probiotic *Bifidobacterium infantis* 35624 in Women with Irritable Bowel Syndrome," *The American Journal of Gastroenterology* 101, no. 7 (July 2006): 1581–1590, doi: 10.1111/j.1572-0241.2006.00734.x.

51. Marcin Lukaszewicz, "*Saccharomyces cerevisiae var. boulardii*—Probiotic Yeast," *Probiotics,* Everlon Rigobelo, ed. (London: IntechOpen Limited, October 3, 2012): 385–398, doi: 10.5772/50105.

52. Ener Cagri Dinleyici et al., "*Saccharomyces boulardii* CNCM I-745 in Different Clinical Conditions," *Expert Opinion on Biological Therapy* 14, no. 11 (November 2014): 1592–1609, doi: 10.1517/14712598.2014.937419.

53. Eduardo Garcia Vilela et al., "Influence of *Saccharomyces boulardii* on the Intestinal Permeability of Patients with Crohn's Disease in Remission," *Scandinavian Journal of Gastroenterology* 43, no. 7 (2008): 842–848, doi: 10.1080/00365520801943354.

54. Pedro Pais et al., "*Saccharomyces boulardii*: What Makes it Tick as Successful Probiotic?", *Journal of Fungi* 6, no. 2 (June 2020): 78, doi: 10.3390/jof6020078.

55. Shahin Ayazi et al., "Measurement of Gastric pH in Ambulatory Esophageal pH Monitoring," *Surgical Endoscopy* 23, no. 9 (September 2009): 1968–1973, doi: 10.1007/s00464-008-0218-0.

56. Hrair P. Simonian et al., "Regional Postprandial Differences in pH within the Stomach and Gastroesophageal Junction," *Digestive Diseases and Sciences* 50, no. 12 (December 2005): 2276–2285, doi: 10.1007/s10620-005-3048-0.

57. T.A. Tompkins, I. Mainville, and Y. Arcand, "The Impact of Meals on a Probiotic During Transit through a Model of the Human Upper Gastrointestinal Tract," *Beneficial Microbes* 2, no. 4 (December 2011): 295–303, doi: 10.3920/BM2011.0022.

58. M. Kilian et al., "The Oral Microbiome—An Update for Oral Healthcare Professionals," *British Dental Journal* 221 (November 18, 2016): 657–666, doi: 10.1038/sj.bdj.2016.865.

59. Priya Nimish Deo and Revati Deshmukh, "Oral Microbiome: Unveiling the Fundamentals," *Journal of Oral and Maxillofacial Pathology* 23, no. 1 (January–April 2019): 122–128, doi: 10.4103/jomfp.JOMFP_304_18.

60. Elijah O. Oyetola et al., "Salivary Bacterial Count and Its Implications on the Prevalence of Oral Conditions," *The Journal of Contemporary Dental Practice* 20, no. 2 (February 1, 2019): 184–189, https://pubmed.ncbi.nlm.nih.gov/31058633/.

61. Carol Perricone et al., "*Porphyromonas gingivalis* and Rheumatoid Arthritis," *Current Opinion in Rheumatology* 31, no. 5 (September 2019): 517–524, doi: 10.1097/BOR.0000000000000638.

62. Eduardo Gómez-Bañuelos et al., "Rheumatoid Arthritis-Associated Mechanisms of *Porphyromonas gingivalis* and *Aggregatibacter actinomycetemcomitans*," *Journal of Clinical Medicine* 8, no. 9 (September 2019): 1309, doi: 10.3390/jcm8091309.

63. Zebunnissa Memon et al., "An Orthodontic Retainer Preventing Remission in Celiac Disease," *Clinical Pediatrics (Philadelphia)* 52, no. 11 (November 2013): 1034–1037, doi: 10.1177/0009922813506254.

64. Kazumichi Abe et al., "Gut and Oral Microbiota in Autoimmune Liver Disease," *Fukushima Journal of Medical Science* 65, no. 3 (January 9, 2020): 71–75, doi: 10.5387/fms.2019-21.

65. Nikolaos G. Nikitakis, "The Autoimmunity-oral Microbiome Connection," *Oral Diseases* 23, no. 7 (October 2017): 828–839, doi: 10.1111/odi.12589.

66. Ashutosh K. Mangalam, Meeta Yadav, and Rjwardhan Yadav, "The Emerging World of Microbiome in Autoimmune Disorders: Opportunities and Challenges," *Indian Journal of Rheumatology* 16, no. 1 (March 23, 2021): 57–72, doi: 10.4103/injr.injr_210_20.

67. Kilian, "The Oral Microbiome," 657–666.

68. Shinichi Kuriyama, "The Relation between Green Tea Consumption and Cardiovascular Disease as Evidenced by Epidemiological Studies," *The Journal of Nutrition* 138, no. 8 (August 1, 2008): 1548S–1553S, doi: 10.1093/jn/138.8.1548S.

69. Sabu M. Chacko et al., "Beneficial Effects of Green Tea: A Literature Review," *Chinese Medicine* 5 (April 6, 2010): 13, doi: 10.1186/1749-8546-5-13.

70. Xiaojie Yuan et al., "Green Tea Liquid Consumption Alters the Human Intestinal and Oral Microbiome," *Molecular Nutrition & Food Research* 62, no. 12 (June 2018): 1800178, doi: 10.1002/mnfr.201800178.

71. David J. Weiss and Christopher R. Anderton, "Determination of Catechins in Matcha Green Tea by Micellar Electrokinetic Chromatography," *Journal of Chromatography A* 1011, no. 1–2 (September 5, 2003): 173–180, doi: 10.1016/s0021-9673(03)01133-6.

72. J. Steinmann et al., "Anti-infective Properties of Epigallocatechin-3-Gallate (EGCG), a Component of Green Tea," *British Journal of Pharmacology* 168, no. 5 (March 2013): 1059–1073, doi: 10.1111/bph.12009.

73. Parth Lodhia et al., "Effect of Green Tea on Volatile Sulfur Compounds in Mouth Air," *Journal of Nutritional Science and Vitaminology (Tokyo)* 54, no. 1 (February 2008): 89–94, doi: 10.3177/jnsv.54.89.

74. Oghenekome Gbinigie et al., "Effect of Oil Pulling in Promoting Oro Dental Hygiene: A Systematic Review of Randomized Clinical Trials," *Complementary Therapies in Medicine* 26 (June 2016): 47–54, doi: 10.1016/j.ctim.2016.02.011.

75. Buket Acar et al., "Effects of Oral Prophylaxis Including Tongue Cleaning on Halitosis and Gingival Inflammation in Gingivitis Patients: A Randomized Controlled Clinical Trial," *Clinical Oral Investigations* 23, no. 4 (April 2019): 1829–1836, doi: 10.1007/s00784-018-2617-5.

Chapter 10

1. Ana M. Andrade, Geoffrey W. Greene, and Kathleen J. Melanson, "Eating Slowly Led to Decreases in Energy Intake within Meals in Healthy Women," *Journal of the Academy of Nutrition and Dietetics* 108, no. 7 (July 1, 2008): 1186–1191, doi: 10.1016/j.jada.2008.04.026.

2. Hongbin Guo et al., "Associations of Whole Grain and Refined Grain Consumption with Metabolic Syndrome: A Meta-Analysis of Observational Studies," *Frontiers in Nutrition* 8 (July 1, 2021): 695620, doi: 10.3389/fnut.2021.695620.

3. Md. Ashraful Islam et al., "Trans Fatty Acids and Lipid Profile: A Serious Risk Factor to Cardiovascular Disease, Cancer and Diabetes," *Diabetes & Metabolic Syndrome* 13, no. 2 (March-April 2019): 1643–1647, doi: 10.1016/j.dsx.2019.03.033.

4. María Correa-Rodríguez et al., "Dietary Intake of Free Sugars is Associated with Disease Activity and Dyslipidemia in Systemic Lupus Erythematosus Patients," *Nutrients* 12, no. 4 (April 15, 2020): 1094, doi: 10.3390/nu12041094.

5. Sanjay Basu et al., "The Relationship of Sugar to Population-Level Diabetes Prevalence: An Econometric Analysis of Repeated Cross-Sectional Data," *PLoS One* 8, no. 2 (February 27, 2013): e57873, doi: 10.1371/journal.pone.0057873.

6. Laura O'Connor et al., "Intakes and Sources of Dietary Sugars and Their Association with Metabolic and Inflammatory Markers," *Clinical Nutrition* 37, no. 4 (August 2018): 1313–1322, doi: 10.1016/j.clnu.2017.05.030.

7. George A. Bray and Barry M. Popkin, "Dietary Sugar and Body Weight: Have We Reached a Crisis in the Epidemic of Obesity And Diabetes?: Health be Damned! Pour on the Sugar," *Diabetes Care* 37, no. 4 (April 2014): 950–956, doi: 10.2337/dc13-2085.

8. Quanhe Yang et al., "Added Sugar Intake and Cardiovascular Diseases Mortality among US Adults," *JAMA Internal Medicine* 174, no. 4 (April 2014): 516–524, doi: 10.1001/jamainternmed.2013.13563.

9. Tugba Ozdal et al., "The Reciprocal Interactions between Polyphenols and Gut Microbiota and Effects on Bioaccessibility," *Nutrients* 8, no. 2 (February 6, 2016): 78, doi: 10.3390/nu8020078.

10. Laura Lavefve, Luke R. Howard, and Franck Carbonero, "Berry Polyphenols Metabolism and Impact on Human Gut Microbiota and Health," *Food & Function* 11, no. 1 (January 29, 2020): 45–65, doi: 10.1039/c9fo01634a.

11. Sanne Ahles, Peter J. Joris, and Jogchum Plat, "Effects of Berry Anthocyanins on Cognitive Performance, Vascular Function and Cardiometabolic Risk Markers: A Systematic Review of Randomized Placebo-Controlled Intervention Studies in Humans," *International Journal of Molecular Sciences* 22, no. 12 (June 17, 2021): 6482, doi: 10.3390/ijms22126482.

12. J. Pérez-Jiménez et al., "Identification of the 100 Richest Dietary Sources of Polyphenols: An Application of the Phenol-Explorer Database," *European Journal of Clinical Nutrition* 64, S112–S120 (2010), doi: 10.1038/ejcn.2010.221.

13. Xenofon Tzounis et al., "Prebiotic Evaluation of Cocoa-Derived Flavanols in Healthy Humans by Using a Randomized, Controlled, Double-blind, Crossover Intervention Study," *The American Journal of Clinical Nutrition* 93, no. 1 (January 2011): 62–72, doi: 10.3945/ajcn.110.000075.

14. Yuji Naito, Kazuhiko Uchiyama, and Tomohisa Tagaki, "A Next-generation Beneficial Microbe: *Akkermansia muciniphila*," *Journal of Clinical Biochemistry and Nutrition* 63, no. 1 (July 2018): 33–35, doi: 10.3164/jcbn.18-57.

15. Sherif Abed et al., "Inulin as Prebiotics and Its Applications in Food Industry and Human Health; A Review," *International Journal of Agriculture Innovations and Research* 5, no. 1 (September 8, 2016): 88–97, https://www.researchgate.net/publication/318900116_Inulin_as_Prebiotics_and_its_Applications_in_Food_Industry_and_Human_Health_A_Review.

16. Abed, "Inulin as Prebiotics," 88–97.

17. Maryem Ben Salem et al., "Pharmacological Studies of Artichoke Leaf Extract and Their Health Benefits," *Plant Foods for Human Nutrition* 70, no. 4 (December 2015): 441–453, doi: 10.1007/s11130-015-0503-8.

18. Jane G. Muir et al., "Fructan and Free Fructose Content of Common Australian Vegetables and Fruit," *Journal of Agricultural and Food Chemistry* 55, no. 16 (July 11, 2007): 6619–6627, doi: 10.1021/jf070623x.

19. Solange Saxby et al., "Assessing the Prebiotic Potential of Taro (Colocasia esculenta) with Probiotic Lactobacillus Species in an In Vitro Human Digestion System (P20-022-19)," *Current Developments in Nutrition* 3, suppl. 1 (June 2019): 1784, doi: 10.1093/cdn/nzz040.P20-022-19.

20. K.L. Johnston et al., "Resistant Starch Improves Insulin Sensitivity in Metabolic Syndrome," *Diabetic Medicine* 27, no. 4 (April 2010): 391–397, doi: 10.1111/j.1464-5491.2010.02923.x.

21. Damien P. Belobrajdic et al., "Dietary Resistant Starch Dose-dependently Reduces Adiposity in Obesity-Prone and Obesity-Resistant Male Rats," *Nutrition & Metabolism* 9 (October 25, 2012): 93, doi: 10.1186/1743-7075-9-93.

22. Diane F. Birt et al., "Resistant Starch: Promise for Improving Human Health," *Advances in Nutrition* 4, no. 6 (November 2013): 587–601, doi: 10.3945/an.113.004325.

23. Birt, "Resistant Starch," 587–601.

24. Aprianita Aprianita et al., "Physicochemical Properties of Flours and Starches Derived from Traditional Indonesian Tubers and Roots," *Journal of Food Science and Technology* 51, no. 12 (December 2014): 3669–3679, doi: 10.1007/s13197-012-0915-5.

25. Irene Darmadi-Blackberry et al., "Legumes: The Most Important Dietary Predictor of Survival in Older People of Different Ethnicities," *Asia Pacific Journal of Clinical Nutrition* 13, no. 2 (2004): 217–220, https://pubmed.ncbi.nlm.nih.gov/15228991/.

26. Newswise, "New Low-Calorie Rice Could Help Cut Rising Obesity Rates," *American Chemical Society*, accessed on January 29, 2022, http://www.newswise.com/articles/new-low-calorie-rice-could-help-cut-rising-obesity-rates.

27. Jagan Mohan Rao Tingirikari, "Microbiota-accessible Pectic Poly- and Oligosaccharides in Gut Health," *Food & Function* 9, no. 10 (October 17, 2018): 5059–5073, doi: 10.1039/c8fo01296b.

28. Linda Riede, Barbara Grube, and Joerg Gruenwald, "Larch Arabinogalactan Effects on Reducing Incidence of Upper Respiratory Infections," *Current Medical Research and Opinion* 29, no. 3 (March 2013): 251–258, doi: 10.1185/03007995.2013.765837.

29. Li-Chan Yang, Ching-Yi Lai, and Wen-Chuan Lin, "Natural Killer Cell-mediated Cytotoxicity Is Increased by a Type II Arabinogalactan from *Anoectochilus formosanus*," *Carbohydrate Polymers* 155 (January 2, 2017): 466–474, doi: 10.1016/j.carbpol.2016.08.086.

30. Jay K. Udani et al., "Proprietary Arabinogalactan Extract Increases Antibody Response to the Pneumonia Vaccine: A Randomized, Double-blind, Placebo-controlled Pilot Study in Healthy Volunteers," *Nutrition Journal* 9 (August 26, 2010): 32, doi: 10.1186/1475-2891-9-32.

31. Carine Dion, Eric Chappuis, and Christopher Ripoll, "Does Larch Arabinogalactan Enhance Immune Function? A Review of Mechanistic and Clinical Trials," *Nutrition and Metabolism* 13, no. 28 (2016): doi: 10.1186/s12986-016-0086-x.

32. Buck Hanson et al. "Sulfoquinovose Is a Select Nutrient of Prominent Bacteria and a Source of Hydrogen Sulfide in the Human Gut," *The ISME journal* 15, no. 9 (2021): 2779–2791, doi: 10.1038/s41396-021-00968-0.

33. Emanuel Vamanu et al., "Therapeutic Properties of Edible Mushrooms and Herbal Teas in Gut Microbiota Modulation," *Microorganisms* 9, no. 6 (June 2021): 1262, doi: 10.3390/microorganisms9061262.

34. Jyotika Varshney et al., "White Button Mushrooms Increase Microbial Diversity and Accelerate the Resolution of Citrobacter Rodentium Infection in Mice," *The Journal of Nutrition* 143, no. 4 (April 2013): 526–532, doi: 10.3945/jn.112.171355.

35. Janina A. Krumbeck et al., "Probiotic *Bifidobacterium* Strains and Galactooligosaccharides Improve Intestinal Barrier Function in Obese Adults but Show No Synergism When Used Together as Synbiotics," *Microbiome* 6 (June 28, 2018): 121, doi: 10.1186/s40168-018-0494-4.

36. Sophia E. Agapova et al., "Additional Common Bean in the Diet of Malawian Children Does Not Affect Linear Growth, but Reduces Intestinal Permeability," *The Journal of Nutrition* 148, no. 2 (February 1, 2018): 267–274, doi: 10.1093/jn/nxx013.

37. R. Satish Kumar et al., "Traditional Indian Fermented Foods: A Rich Source of Lactic Acid Bacteria," *International Journal of Food Sciences and Nutrition* 64, no. 4 (2013): 415–428, doi: 10.3109/09637486.2012.746288.

38. Aune, "Fruit and Vegetable Intake," 1029–1056.

39. Afka Deen et al., "Chemical Composition and Health Benefits of Coconut Oil: An Overview," *Journal of the Science of Food and Agriculture* 101, no. 6 (April 2021): 2182–2193, doi: 10.1002 /jsfa.10870.

40. Aune, "Fruit and Vegetable Intake," 1029–1056.

41. Lisa Lucas, Aaron Russell, and Russell Keast, "Molecular Mechanisms of Inflammation. Anti-Inflammatory Benefits of Virgin Olive Oil and the Phenolic Compound Oleocanthal," *Current Pharmaceutical Design* 17, no. 8 (2011): 754–768, doi: 10.2174/138161211795428911.

42. Satoko Yoneyama et al., "Dietary Intake of Fatty Acids and Serum C-reactive Protein in Japanese," *Journal of Epidemiology* 17, no. 3 (May 2007): 86–92, doi: 10.2188/jea.17.86.

43. Alair Alfredo Berbert et al., "Supplementation of Fish Oil and Olive Oil in Patients with Rheumatoid Arthritis," *Nutrition* 21, no. 2 (February 2005): 131–136, doi: 10.1016/j.nut .2004.03.023.

44. Marina Aparicio-Soto et al., "The Phenolic Fraction of Extra Virgin Olive Oil Modulates the Activation and the Inflammatory Response of T Cells from Patients with Systemic Lupus Erythematosus and Healthy Donors," *Molecular Nutrition & Food Research* 61, no. 8 (August 2017): doi: 10.1002/mnfr.201601080.

45. Marta Guasch-Ferré et al., "Olive Oil Intake and Risk of Cardiovascular Disease and Mortality in the PREDIMED Study," *BMC Medicine* 12 (May 13, 2014): 78, doi: 10.1186/1741-7015-12-78.

46. Marta Guasch-Ferré et al., "Consumption of Olive Oil and Risk of Total and Cause-Specific Mortality Among US Adults," *Journal of the American College of Cardiology* 79, no. 2 (January 2022): 101–112, doi: 10.1016/j.jacc.2021.10.041.

47. H. Ramachandra Prabhu, "Lipid Peroxidation in Culinary Oils Subjected to Thermal Stress," *Indian Journal of Clinical Biochemistry* 15 (2000): 1–5, doi: 10.1007/BF02873539.

48. Y.H. Qu et al., "Genotoxicity of Heated Cooking Oil Vapors," *Mutation Research/Genetic Toxicology* 298, no. 2 (December 1992), 105–111, doi: 10.1016/0165-1218(92)90035-X.

49. Yosra Allouche et al., "How Heating Affects Extra Virgin Olive Oil Quality Indexes and Chemical Composition," *Journal of Agricultural and Food Chemistry* 55, no. 23 (November 14, 2007): 9646–9654, doi: 10.1021/jf070628u.

50. Deen, "Chemical Composition," 2182–2193.

51. Kay-Tee Khaw et al., "Randomized Trial of Coconut Oil, Olive Oil or Butter on Blood Lipids and Other Cardiovascular Risk Factors in Healthy Men and Women," *BMJ Open* 8, no. 3 (March 6, 2018): e020167, doi: 10.1136/bmjopen-2017-020167.

52. Andrew A. Meharg et al., "Speciation and Localization of Arsenic in White and Brown Rice Grains," *Environmental Science & Technology* 42, no. 4 (February 15, 2008): 1051–1057, doi: 10.1021/es702212p.

53. Y Huang et al., "Red and Processed Meat Consumption and Cancer Outcomes: Umbrella Review," *Food Chem* 356 (2021): 129697, doi: 10.1016/j.foodchem.2021.129697.

54. Romaina Iqbal et al., "Associations of Unprocessed and Processed Meat Intake with Mortality and Cardiovascular Disease in 21 Countries: Prospective Urban Rural Epidemiology (PURE) Study," *Am J Clin Nutr* 114 (2021): 1049–1058, doi: 10.1093/ajcn/nqaa448.

55. M. Karwowska et al., "Nitrates/Nitrites in Food-Risk for Nitrosative Stress and Benefits," *Antioxidants* 9 (2020): 241, doi: 10.3390/antiox9030241.

Chapter 11

1. Kasem Sharif et al., "The Role of Stress in the Mosaic of Autoimmunity: An Overlooked Association," *Autoimmunity Reviews* 17, no. 10 (October 2018): 967–983, doi: 10.1016/j .autrev.2018.04.005.

2. Savita Srivastava and James L. Boyer, "Psychological Stress is Associated with Relapse in Type 1 Autoimmune Hepatitis," *Liver International* 30, no. 10 (November 2010): 1439–1447, https:// doi.org/10.1111/j.1478-3231.2010.02333.x.

3. Qi Jiang et al., "Role of Th22 Cells in the Pathogenesis of Autoimmune Diseases," *Frontiers in Immunology* 12 (July 6, 2021): 688066, doi: 10.3389/fimmu.2021.688066.

4. Sharif, "The Role of Stress," 967–983.

5. Elizabeth K. Pradhan et al., "Effect of Mindfulness-Based Stress Reduction in Rheumatoid Arthritis Patients," *Arthritis & Rheumatology* 57, no. 7 (October 2007): 1134–1142, doi: 10.1002/art.23010.

6. Srivastava, "Psychological Stress," 1439–1447.

7. Maya C. Mizrahi et al., "Effects of Guided Imagery with Relaxation Training on Anxiety and Quality of Life Among Patients with Inflammatory Bowel Disease," *Psychology and Health* 27, no. 12 (May 10, 2012): 1463–1479, doi: 10.1080/08870446.2012.691169.

8. Braden Kuo et al., "Genomic and Clinical Effects Associated with a Relaxation Response Mind-Body Intervention in Patients with Irritable Bowel Syndrome and Inflammatory Bowel Disease," *PLoS One* 12, no. 2 (April 30, 2015): e0172872, doi: 10.1371/journal.pone.0123861.

9. Felicia A. Huppert and Daniel M. Johnson, "A Controlled Trial of Mindfulness Training in Schools: The Importance of Practice for an Impact on Well-Being," *The Journal of Positive Psychology* 5, no. 4 (August 3, 2010): 264–274, doi: 10.1080/17439761003794148.

10. Ravi Prakash et al., "Long-Term Vihangam Yoga Meditation and Scores on Tests of Attention," *Perceptual and Motor Skills* 110, no. 3 (June 1, 2010): 1139–1148, doi: 10.2466/pms.110.C.1139-1148.

11. Kimberly Carrière et al., "Mindfulness-based Interventions for Weight Loss: A Systematic Review and Meta-analysis," *Obesity Reviews* 19, no. 2 (October 27, 2017): 164–177, doi: 10.1111/obr.12623.

12. Ayman Mukerji Househam et al., "The Effects of Stress and Meditation on the Immune System, Human Microbiota, and Epigenetics," *Advances in Mind-Body Medicine* 31, no. 4 (Fall 2017): 10–25, https://pubmed.ncbi.nlm.nih.gov/29306937/.

13. Michaela C. Paskoe et al., "Mindfulness Mediates the Physiological Markers of Stress: Systematic Review and Meta-analysis," *Journal of Psychiatric Research* 95 (December 2017): 156-178, doi: 10.1016/j.jpsychires.2017.08.004.

14. Mizrahi, "Effects of Guided Imagery," 1463–1479.

15. Richard J. Davidson et al., "Alterations in Brain and Immune Function Produced by Mindfulness Meditation," *Psychosomatic Medicine* 65, no. 4 (July-August 2003): 564–570, doi: 10.1097/01.psy.0000077505.67574.e3.

16. Thaddeus W.W. Pace et al., "Effect of Compassion Meditation on Neuroendocrine, Innate Immune and Behavioral Responses to Psychosocial Stress," *Psychoneuroendocrinology* 34, no. 1 (January 2009): 87–98, doi: 10.1016/j.psyneuen.2008.08.011.

17. "Meditation's Impact on Neurochemicals: Evidence of Meditation's Impact on Neurotransmitters and Neurohormones," Sahaja Online, accessed July 11, 2022, https://sahajaonline.com/science-health/mental-health-well-being/neurochemicals/evidence-of-meditations-impact-on-neurotransmitters-neurohormones/.

18. M. Veehof et al., "Acceptance- and Mindfulness-based Interventions for the Treatment of Chronic Pain: A Meta-analytic Review," *Cogn Behav Ther* 45 no. 1 (2016): 5–31, doi: 10.1080/16506073.2015.1098724.

19. Britta K. Hölzel, "Mindfulness Practice Leads to Increases in Regional Brain Gray Matter Density," *Psychiatry Research: Neuroimaging* 191, no. 1 (January 30, 2011): 36–43, doi: 10.1016/j.pscychresns.2010.08.006.

20. Sara W. Lazar et al., "Meditation Experience is Associated with Increased Cortical Thickness," *NeuroReport* 16, no. 17 (November 28, 2005): 1893–1897, doi: 10.1097/01.wnr.0000186598.66243.19.

21. Adrienne A. Taren, J. David Creswell, and Peter J. Gianaros, "Dispositional Mindfulness Co-Varies with Smaller Amygdala and Caudate Volumes in Community Adults," *PLoS One* 8, no. 5 (May 22, 2013): e64574, doi: 10.1371/journal.pone.0064574.

22. Nicole Last, Emily Tufts, and Leslie E. Auger, "The Effects of Meditation on Grey Matter Atrophy and Neurodegeneration: A Systematic Review," *Journal of Alzheimer's Disease* 56, no. 1 (2017): 275–286, doi: 10.3233/JAD-160899.

23. Yi-Yuan Tang et al., "Short-term Meditation Induces White Matter Changes in the Anterior Cingulate," *Proceedings of the National Academy of Sciences of the United States of America* 107, no. 35 (August 31, 2010): 15649–15652, doi: 10.1073/pnas.1011043107.

24. Antoine Lutz et al., "Long-term Meditators Self-induce High-amplitude Gamma Synchrony During Mental Practice," *Proceedings of the National Academy of Sciences of the United States of America* 101, no. 46 (November 8, 2004): 16369–16373, doi: 10.1073/pnas.0407401101.

25. Yu-Rim Lee and Robert D. Enright, "A Meta-analysis of the Association Between Forgiveness of Others and Physical Health," *Psychology & Health* 34, no. 5 (May 2019): 626–643, doi: 10.1080/08870446.2018.1554185.

26. Julian F. Thayer, Shelby S. Yamamoto, and Joseph F. Brosschot, "The Relationship of Autonomic Imbalance, Heart Rate Variability and Cardiovascular Disease Risk Factors," *International Journal of Cardiology* 141, no. 2 (May 28, 2010): 122–131, doi: 10.1016/j.ijcard.2009.09.543.

27. Marjolein H. Kamphuis et al., "Autonomic Dysfunction: A Link Between Depression and Cardiovascular Mortality? The FINE Study," *The European Journal of Cardiovascular Prevention & Rehabilitation* 14, no. 6 (December 2007): 796–802, doi: 10.1097/HJR.0b013e32829c7d0c.

28. Lourdes Díaz-Rodríguez et al., "Effects of Meditation on Mental Health and Cardiovascular Balance in Caregivers," *International Journal of Environmental Research and Public Health* 18 (2021): 617, doi: 10.3390/ijerph18020617.

29. Rhonda Patrick et al., "Sauna Use as a Lifestyle Practice to Extend Healthspan," *Experimental Gerontology* 154 (2021): 111509, doi: 10.1016/j.exger.2021.111509.

30. Jay C. Fournier et al., "Antidepressant Drug Effects and Depression Severity: A Patient-Level Meta-analysis," *JAMA: Journal of the American Medical Association* 303, no. 1 (January 6, 2010): 47–53, doi: 10.1001/jama.2009.1943.

31. Tor D. Wager et al., "Placebo-induced Changes in FMRI in the Anticipation and Experience of Pain," *Science* 303, no. 5661 (February 20, 2004): 1162–1167, doi: 10.1126/science.1093065.

32. Tor D. Wager, David J. Scott, and Jon-Kar Zubieta, "Placebo Effects on Human μ-opioid Activity During Pain," *Proceedings of the National Academy of Sciences of the United States of America* 104, no. 26 (June 26, 2007): 11056–11061, doi: 10.1073/pnas.0702413104.

33. Guy Montgomery and Irving Kirsch, "Mechanisms of Placebo Pain Reduction: An Empirical Investigation," *Psychological Science* 7, no. 3 (May 1, 1996): 174–176, doi: 10.1111/j.1467-9280.1996.tb00352.x.

34. Alberto J. Espay et al., "Placebo Effect of Medication Cost in Parkinson Disease: A Randomized Double-Blind Study," *Neurology* 84, no. 8 (February 24, 2015): 794–802, doi: 10.1212/WNL.0000000000001282.

35. J. Bruce Moseley et al., "A Controlled Trial of Arthroscopic Surgery for Osteoarthritis of the Knee," *New England Journal of Medicine* 347, no. 2 (July 11, 2002): 81–88, doi: 10.1056/NEJMoa013259.

36. Laura Vagnoli et al., "Relaxation-guided Imagery Reduces Perioperative Anxiety and Pain in Children: A Randomized Study," *European Journal of Pediatrics* 178, no. 6 (June 2019): 913–921, doi: 10.1007/s00431-019-03376-x.

37. Ursula Debarnot et al., "Motor Imagery Practice Benefits During Arm Immobilization," *Scientific Reports* 11 (2021): 8928, doi: 10.1038/s41598-021-88142-6.

38. Norman Doidge, *The Brain's Way of Healing* (New York: Penguin Books, 2015): 10–15.

39. Doidge, *The Brain's Way of Healing*, 19–20.

40. "Neuroplastic Transformation," Neuroplastix, accessed January 29, 2022, http://www.neuroplastix.com/styled-2/styled-6/instructions.html.

41. Catherine Preston and Roger Newport, "Analgesic Effects of Multisensory Illusions in Osteoarthritis," *Rheumatology* 50, no. 12 (March 29, 2011): 2314–2315, doi: 10.1093/rheumatology/ker104.

42. G. Lorimer Moseley, Timothy J. Parsons, and Charles Spence, "Visual Distortion of a Limb Modulates the Pain and Swelling Evoked by Movement," *Current Biology* 18, no. 22 (November 25, 2008): PR1047–R1048, doi: 10.1016/j.cub.2008.09.031.

43. Guang Yue and Kelly J. Cole, "Strength Increases from the Motor Program: Comparison of Training with Maximal Voluntary and Imagined Muscle Contractions," *Journal of Neurophysiology* 67, no. 5 (May 1992): 1114–1123, doi: 10.1152/jn.1992.67.5.1114.

44. Vinoth K. Ranganathan et al., "From Mental Power to Muscle Power—Gaining Strength by Using the Mind," *Neuropsychologia* 42, no. 7 (2004): 944–956, doi: 10.1016/j.neuropsychologia .2003.11.018.

45. Roderik Gerritsen and Guido Band, "Breath of Life: The Respiratory Vagal Stimulation Model of Contemplative Activity," *Frontiers in Human Neuroscience* 12 (Oct. 9, 2018): 397, doi: 10.3389/fnhum.2018.00397.

46. P.Q. Yuan et al., "Acute Cold Exposure Induces Vagally Mediated Fos Expression in Gastric Myenteric Neurons in Conscious Rats," *American Journal of Physiology-Gastrointestinal and Liver Physiology* 281, no. 2 (August 2001): G560–G568, doi: 10.1152/ajpgi.2001.281.2.G560.

47. Logan J. Niehues and Victoria Klovenski, "Vagal Maneuver," in *StatPearls* (Treasure Island, Fla.: StatPearls Publishing, 2022).

48. Mark C. Genovese et al., "First-in-human Study of Novel Implanted Vagus Nerve Stimulation Device to Treat Rheumatoid Arthritis," *Annals of the Rheumatic Diseases* 78, suppl. 2 (June 2019): 264.1–264, https://doi.org/10.1136/annrheumdis-2019-eular.8716.

49. Sophie C. Payne et al., "Anti-inflammatory Effects of Abdominal Vagus Nerve Stimulation on Experimental Intestinal Inflammation," *Frontiers in Neuroscience* 13 (May 8, 2019): 418, doi: 10.3389/fnins.2019.00418.

50. Juliana M. Bottomley et al., "Vagus Nerve Stimulation (VNS) Therapy in Patients with Treatment Resistant Depression: A Systematic Review and Meta-analysis," *Comprehensive Psychiatry* 98 (December 12, 2019): 152156, doi: 10.1016/j.comppsych.2019.152156.

51. Gabriel Leonard et al., "Noninvasive Tongue Stimulation Combined with Intensive Cognitive and Physical Rehabilitation Induces Neuroplastic Changes in Patients with Multiple Sclerosis: A Multimodal Neuroimaging Study," *Multiple Sclerosis Journal—Experimental, Translational and Clinical* 3, no. 1 (February 1, 2017): 2055217317690561, doi: 10.1177/2055217317690561.

52. "FDA Authorizes Marketing of Device to Improve Gait in Multiple Sclerosis Patients," U.S. Food & Drug Administration, accessed January 29, 2022, https://www.fda.gov/news-events/press -announcements/fda-authorizes-marketing-device-improve-gait-multiple-sclerosis-patients.

53. Dion Diep, Andrew C.L. Lam, and Gordon Ko, "A Review of the Evidence and Current Applications of Portable Translingual Neurostimulation Technology," *Neuromodulation* 24, no. 8 (December 2021): 1377–1387, doi: 10.1111/ner.13260.

54. Ryan C.N. D'Arcy et al., "Portable Neuromodulation Induces Neuroplasticity to Reactivate Motor Function Recovery from Brain Injury: A High-density MEG Case Study," *Journal of NeuroEngineering and Rehabilitation* 17, no. 1 (December 1, 2020): 158, doi: 10.1186 /s12984-020-00772-5.

55. Zimmerman, Rachel, "Trauma Update: On the 'Tipping Point for Tapping' Therapy," *WBUR* (July 23, 2013), https://www.wbur.org/news/2013/07/23/trauma-update-on-the-tipping-point -for-tapping-therapy.

56. Dawson Church et al., "Psychological Trauma Symptom Improvement in Veterans Using Emotional Freedom Techniques: A Randomized Controlled Trial," *The Journal of Nervous and Mental Disease* 201, no. 2 (February 2013): 153–160, doi: 10.1097/NMD.0b013e31827f6351.

57. Alicia Valiente-Gómez et al., "EMDR Beyond PTSD: A Systematic Literature Review," *Frontiers in Psychology* 8 (September 26, 2017): 1668, doi: 10.3389/fpsyg.2017.01668.

58. Susana Roque-Lopez et al., "Mental Health Benefits of a 1-Week Intensive Multimodal Group Program for Adolescents with Multiple Adverse Childhood Experiences," *Child Abuse & Neglect* 122 (December 2021): 105349, doi: 10.1016/j.chiabu.2021.105349.

59. Valiente-Gómez, "EMDR Beyond PTSD," 1668.

60. Paramahansa Yogananda, *The Divine Romance: Collected Talks and Essays on Realizing God in Daily Life* (Los Angeles: Self-Realization Fellowship, 1986): 134.

61. "Quote of the Day: 'We are what we think. All that we are arises with our thought. With our thoughts, we make our world.'—Gautama Buddha," Good News Network, accessed June 28, 2022, https://www.goodnewsnetwork.org/gautama-buddha-quote-on-thought/.

62. Ken Keyes, Jr., *Handbook to Higher Consciousness* (Marina del Rey, Calif.: DeVorss and Company, 1975): 171.

63. Esther and Jerry Hicks, *The Astonishing Power of Emotions* (Carlsbad, Calif.: Hay House, 2007): 144–146.

64. Hicks, *The Astonishing Power of Emotions*, 52–56.

65. Julianne Holt-Lunstad, Timothy B. Smith, and J. Bradley Layton, "Social Relationships and Mortality Risk: A Meta-analytic Review," *PLoS Medicine* 7, no. 7 (July 27, 2010): e1000316, doi: 10.1371/journal.pmed.1000316.

66. Steven W. Cole, "Social Regulation of Human Gene Expression: Mechanisms and Implications for Public Health," *American Journal of Public Health* 103, suppl. 1 (October 2013): S84–S92, doi: 10.2105/AJPH.2012.301183.

67. Anna L. Boggiss et al., "A Systematic Review of Gratitude Interventions: Effects on Physical Health and Health Behaviors," *Journal of Psychosomatic Research* 135 (August 2020): 110165, doi: 10.1016/j.jpsychores.2020.110165.

68. Mikaela B. von Bonsdorff and Taina Rantanen, "Benefits of Formal Voluntary Work Among Older People: A Review," *Aging Clinical and Experimental Research* 23, no. 3 (June 2011): 162–169, doi: 10.1007/BF03337746.

69. Hein M. Tun et al., "Exposure to Household Furry Pets Influences the Gut Microbiota of Infant at 3–4 Months Following Various Birth Scenarios," *Microbiome* 5, no. 1 (April 6, 2017): 40, doi: 10.1186/s40168-017-0254-x.

Chapter 12

1. Greer McGuinness and Yeonsoo Kim, "Sulforaphane Treatment for Autism Spectrum Disorder: A Systematic Review," *EXCLI Journal* 19 (June 26, 2020): 892–903, doi: 10.17179/excli2020-2487.

2. Alena Vanduchova, Pavel Anzenbacher, and Eva Anzenbacherova, "Isothiocyanate from Broccoli, Sulforaphane, and Its Properties," *Journal of Medicinal Food* 22, no. 2 (February 2019): 121–126, doi: 10.1089/jmf.2018.0024.

3. Jun Akaogi et al., "Role of Non-protein Amino Acid L-canavanine in Autoimmunity," *Autoimmunity Reviews* 5, no. 6 (July 2006): doi: 10.1016/j.autrev.2005.12.004.

4. Martin Vermeulen et al., "Bioavailability and Kinetics of Sulforaphane in Humans After Consumption of Cooked Versus Raw Broccoli," *Journal of Agricultural and Food Chemistry* 56, no. 22 (November 26, 2008): 10505–10509, doi: 10.1021/jf801989e.

5. Olukayode Okunade et al., "Supplementation of the Diet by Exogenous Myrosinase via Mustard Seeds to Increase the Bioavailability of Sulforaphane in Healthy Human Subjects after the Consumption of Cooked Broccoli," *Molecular Nutrition & Food Research* 62, no. 18 (September 2018): e1700980, doi: 10.1002/mnfr.201700980.

6. Sarah C. Ray et al., "Oral $NaHCO_3$ Activates a Splenic Anti-Inflammatory Pathway; Evidence Cholinergic Signals are Transmitted via Mesothelial Cells," *Journal of Immunology* 200, no. 10 (May 15, 2018): 3568–3586, doi: 10.4049/jimmunol.1701605.

7. Lars R. McNaughton et al., "Recent Developments in the Use of Sodium Bicarbonate as an Ergogenic Aid," *Current Sports Medicine Reports* 15, no. 4 (July-August 2016): 233–244, doi: 10.1249/JSR.0000000000000283.

8. Jozo Grgic et al., "Effects of Sodium Bicarbonate Supplementation on Muscular Strength and Endurance: A Systematic Review and Meta-analysis," *Sports Medicine* 50, no. 7 (July 2020): 1361–1375, doi: 10.1007/s40279-020-01275-y.

9. Igor Loniewski and Donald E. Wesson, "Bicarbonate Therapy for Prevention of Chronic Kidney Disease Progression," *Kidney International* 85, no. 3 (March 2014): 529–535, doi: 10.1038/ki.2013.401.

10. Ching-Mao Chang et al., "Integrative Therapy Decreases the Risk of Lupus Nephritis in Patients with Systemic Lupus Erythematosus: A Population-based Retrospective Cohort Study," *Journal of Ethnopharmacology* 196 (January 20, 2017): 201–212, doi: 10.1016/j.jep.2016.12.016.

11. Yuxi Di et al., "Catalpol Inhibits Tregs-to-Th17 Cell Transdifferentiation by Up-Regulating Let-7g-5p to Reduce STAT3 Protein Levels," *Yonsei Medical Journal* 63, no. 1 (January 2022): 56–65, doi: 10.3349/ymj.2022.63.1.56.

12. Kyungsun Han et al., "Rehmannia Glutinosa Reduced Waist Circumferences of Korean Obese Women Possibly Through Modulation of Gut Microbiota," *Food & Function* 6, no. 8 (August 2015): 2684–2692, doi: 10.1039/c5fo00232j.

13. Mahdieh Abbasalizad Farhangi et al., "The Effects of Nigella Sativa on Thyroid Function, Serum Vascular Endothelial Growth Factor (VEGF)—1, Nesfatin-1 and Anthropometric Features in Patients with Hashimoto's Thyroiditis: A Randomized Controlled Trial," *BMC Complementary and Alternative Medicine* 16 (November 16, 2016): 471, doi: 10.1186/s12906-016-1432-2.

14. Tamer A. Gheita and Sanaa A. Kenawy, "Effectiveness of Nigella Sativa Oil in the Management of Rheumatoid Arthritis Patients: A Placebo Controlled Study," *Phytotherapy Research* 26, no. 8 (August 2012): 1246–1248, doi: 10.1002/ptr.3679.

15. Geert A. Buijze et al., "The Effect of Cold Showering on Health and Work: A Randomized Controlled Trial," *PLoS One* 11, no. 9 (September 15, 2016): e0161749, doi: 10.1371/journal.pone.0161749.

16. Nikolai A. Shevchuk, "Adapted Cold Shower as a Potential Treatment for Depression," *Medical Hypotheses* 70, no. 5 (2008): 995–1001, doi: 10.1016/j.mehy.2007.04.052.

17. A. Mooventhan and L. Nivethitha, "Scientific Evidence-based Effects of Hydrotherapy on Various Systems of the Body," *North American Journal of Medicine and Science* 6, no. 5 (May 2014): 199–209, doi: 10.4103/1947-2714.132935.

18. Travor R. Higgins, David A. Greene, and Michael K. Baker, "Effects of Cold Water Immersion and Contrast Water Therapy for Recovery From Team Sport: A Systematic Review and Meta-analysis," *Journal of Strength and Conditioning Research* 31, no. 5 (May 2017): 1443–1460, doi: 10.1519/JSC.0000000000001559.

19. Sheng Hui and Joshua D. Rabinowitz, "An Unexpected Trigger for Calorie Burning in Brown Fat," *Nature* 560, no. 7716 (August 2018): 38–39, doi: 10.1038/d41586-018-05619-7.

20. Maria Chondronikola et al., "Brown Adipose Tissue Improves Whole-Body Glucose Homeostasis and Insulin Sensitivity in Humans," *Diabetes* 63, no. 12 (December 1, 2014): 4089–4099, doi: 10.2337/db14-0746.

21. D.A. Fraser et al., "Serum Levels of Interleukin-6 and Dehydroepiandrosterone Sulphate in Response to Either Fasting or a Ketogenic Diet in Rheumatoid Arthritis Patients," *Clinical and Experimental Rheumatology* 18, no. 3 (May–June 2000): 357–362, https://pubmed.ncbi.nlm.nih.gov/10895373/.

22. András Maifeld et al., "Fasting Alters the Gut Microbiome Reducing Blood Pressure and Body Weight in Metabolic Syndrome Patients," *Nature Communications* 12 (March 30, 2021): 1970, doi: 10.1038/s41467-021-22097-0.

23. Mo'ez Al-Islam E. Faris et al., "Intermittent Fasting During Ramadan Attenuates Proinflammatory Cytokines and Immune Cells in Healthy Subjects," *Nutrition Research* 32, no. 12 (December 2012): 947–955, doi: 10.1016/j.nutres.2012.06.021.

24. Rittika Chunder et al., "Antibody Cross-Reactivity Between Casein and Myelin-Associated Glycoprotein Results in Central Nervous System Demyelination," *Proceedings of the National Academy of Sciences of the United States of America* 119, no. 10 (March 2, 2022): e2117034119, doi: 10.1073/pnas.2117034119.

25. Horst Müller, Françoise Wilhelmi de Toledo, and Karl Ludwig Resch, "Fasting Followed by Vegetarian Diet in Patients with Rheumatoid Arthritis: A Systematic Review," *Scandinavian Journal of Rheumatology* 30, no. 1 (2001): 1–10, doi: 10.1080/030097401750065256.

26. Giovanni Damiani et al., "The Impact of Ramadan Fasting on the Reduction of PASI Score, in Moderate-to-Severe Psoriatic Patients: A Real-Life Multicenter Study," *Nutrients* 11, no. 2 (2019): 277, doi: 10.3390/nu11020277.

27. Francesca Cignarella et al., "Intermittent Fasting Confers Protection in CNS Autoimmunity by Altering the Gut Microbiota," *Cell Metabolism* 27, no. 6 (June 5, 2018): 1222–1235, doi: 10.1016/j.cmet.2018.05.006.

28. In Young Choi et al., "Diet Mimicking Fasting Promotes Regeneration and Reduces Autoimmunity and Multiple Sclerosis Symptoms," *Cell Reports* 15, no. 10 (June 7, 2016): 2136–2146, doi: 10.1016/j.celrep.2016.05.009.

29. Krista A. Varady et al., "Cardiometabolic Benefits of Intermittent Fasting," *Annual Review of Nutrition* 41 (October 11, 2021): 333–361, doi: 10.1146/annurev-nutr-052020-041327.

30. Hamed Varkaneh Kord et al., "The Influence of Fasting and Energy-restricted Diets on Leptin and Adiponectin Levels in Humans: A Systematic Review and Meta-analysis," *Clinical Nutrition* 40, no. 4 (April 2021): 1811–1821, doi: 10.1016/j.clnu.2020.10.034.

31. Astrid Hjelholt et al., "Growth Hormone and Obesity," *Endocrinology and Metabolism Clinics of North America* 49, no. 2 (June 2020): 239–250, doi: 10.1016/j.ecl.2020.02.009.

32. Sebastian Brandhorst et al., "A Periodic Diet that Mimics Fasting Promotes Multi-System Regeneration, Enhanced Cognitive Performance, and Healthspan," *Cell Metabolism* 22, no. 1 (July 7, 2015): 86–99, doi: 10.1016/j.cmet.2015.05.012.

33. In Young Choi, "Diet Mimicking Fasting," 2136–2146.

34. "Reset & Rejuvenate: The Fasting Plan That Lets You Eat," Prolon, accessed May 14, 2022, https://prolonfmd.com/.

35. Chanthawat Patikorn et al., "Intermittent Fasting and Obesity-Related Health Outcomes: An Umbrella Review of Meta-analyses of Randomized Clinical Trials," *JAMA Network Open* 4, no. 12 (December 1, 2021): e2139558, doi: 10.1001/jamanetworkopen.2021.39558.

36. Tiina Karu, "Is It Time to Consider Photobiomodulation as a Drug Equivalent?", *Photomedicine and Laser Surgery* 31, no. 5 (May 2013): 189–191, doi: 10.1089/pho.2013.3510.

37. Victoria A. Wickenheisser et al., "Laser Light Therapy in Inflammatory, Musculoskeletal, and Autoimmune Disease," *Current Allergy and Asthma Reports* 19, no. 8 (July 2, 2019): 37, doi: 10.1007/s11882-019-0869-z.

38. Joseph Tafur and Paul J. Mills, "Low-intensity Light Therapy: Exploring the Role of Redox Mechanisms," *Photomedicine and Laser Surgery* 26, no. 4 (August 2008): 323–328, doi: 10.1089/pho.2007.2184.

39. Doidge, *The Brain's Way of Healing*, 126–127.

40. Patricia Pereira Alfredo et al., "Efficacy of Low-level Laser Therapy Associated with Exercises in Knee Osteoarthritis: A Randomized Double-blind Study," *Clinical Rehabilitation* 26, no. 6 (June 2012): 523–533, doi: 10.1177/0269215511425962.

41. Ali Gur et al., "Efficacy of Different Therapy Regimes of Low-Power Laser in Painful Osteoarthritis of the Knee: A Double-blind and Randomized-controlled Trial," *Lasers in Surgery and Medicine* 33, no. 5 (2003): 330–338, doi: 10.1002/lsm.10236.

42. Ron Clijsen et al., "Effects of Low-level Laser Therapy on Pain in Patients with Musculoskeletal Disorders: A Systematic Review and Meta-analysis," *European Journal of Physical and Rehabilitation Medicine* 53, no. 4 (August 2017): 603–610, doi: 10.23736/S1973-9087.17.04432-X.

43. Wei Wang et al., "Clinical Efficacy of Low-level Laser Therapy in Plantar Fasciitis: A Systematic Review and Meta-analysis," *Medicine (Baltimore)* 98, no. 3 (January 2019): e14088, doi: 10.1097/MD.0000000000014088.

44. Margaret A. Naesar and Michael R. Hamblin, "Potential for Transcranial Laser or LED Therapy to Treat Stroke, Traumatic Brain Injury, and Neurodegenerative Disease," *Photomedicine and Laser Surgery* 29, no. 7 (July 2011): 443–446, doi: 10.1089/pho.2011.9908.

45. Wickenheisser, "Laser Light Therapy," 37.

46. Xu-Sheng Qiu, Xu-Gang Li, and Yi-Xin Chen, "Pulsed Electromagnetic Field (PEMF): A Potential Adjuvant Treatment for Infected Nonunion," *Medical Hypotheses* 136 (March 2020): 109506, doi: 10.1016/j.mehy.2019.109506.

47. Davide Cappon et al., "Transcranial Magnetic Stimulation (TMS) for Geriatric Depression," *Ageing Research Reviews* 74 (February 2022): 101531, doi: 10.1016/j.arr.2021.101531.

48. Jie Tong, "The Efficacy of Pulsed Electromagnetic Fields on Pain, Stiffness, and Physical Function in Osteoarthritis: A Systematic Review and Meta-analysis," *Pain Research & Management* 2022 (May 9, 2022): 9939891, doi: 10.1155/2022/9939891.

49. Xin Sun et al., "Efficacy of Pulsed Electromagnetic Field on Pain and Physical Function in Patients with Low Back Pain: A Systematic Review and Meta-analysis," *Clinical Rehabilitation* 36, no. 5 (May 2022), doi: 10.1177/02692155221074052.

50. Jared Younger, Luke Parkitny, and David McLain, "The Use of Low-Dose Naltrexone (LDN) as a Novel Anti-Inflammatory Treatment for Chronic Pain," *Clinical Rheumatology* 33, no. 4 (April 2014): 451–459, doi: 10.1007/s10067-014-2517-2.

51. Guttorm Raknes and Lars Småbrekke, "Low Dose Naltrexone: Effects on Medication in Rheumatoid and Seropositive Arthritis. A Nationwide Register-based Controlled Quasi-experimental Before-After Study," *PLoS One* 14, no. 10 (February 14, 2019): doi: 10.1371/journal.pone.0212460.

52. Jarred Younger et al., "Low-dose Naltrexone for the Treatment of Fibromyalgia: Findings of a Small, Randomized, Double-blind, Placebo-controlled, Counterbalanced, Crossover Trial Assessing Daily Pain Levels," *Arthritis & Rheumatology* 65, no. 2 (February 2013): 529–538, doi: 10.1002/art.37734.

53. Ryan C. Keefe et al., "BCG Therapy Is Associated with Long-term, Durable Induction of Treg Signature Genes by Epigenetic Modulation," *Scientific Reports* 11, no. 14933 (July 22, 2021), doi: 10.1038/s41598-021-94529-2.

54. Alok K. Singh, Mihai G. Netea, and William R. Bishai, "BCG Turns 100: Its Nontraditional Uses Against Viruses, Cancer, and Immunologic Diseases," *The Journal of Clinical Investigation* 131, no. 11 (June 1, 2020): e148291, doi: 10.1172/JCI148291.

55. William M. Kühtreiber et al., "Long-term Reduction in Hyperglycemia in Advanced Type 1 Diabetes: The Value of Induced Aerobic Glycolysis with BCG Vaccinations," *NPJ Vaccines* 3, no. 23 (June 21, 2018), doi: 10.1038/s41541-018-0062-8.

56. Cindy Orvain et al., "Is There a Place for Chimeric Antigen Receptor-T Cells in the Treatment of Chronic Autoimmune Rheumatic Diseases?", *Arthritis & Rheumatology* 73, no. 11 (November 2021): 1954–1965, doi: 10.1002/art.41812.

57. Dimitrios Mougiakakos et al., "CD19-Targeted CAR T Cells in Refractory Systemic Lupus Erythematosus," *New England Journal of Medicine* 385, no. 6 (August 5, 2021): 567–569, doi: 10.1056/NEJMc2107725.

58. Györgyi Müzes and Ferenc Sipos, "Issues and Opportunities of Stem Cell Therapy in Autoimmune Diseases," *World Journal of Stem Cells* 11, no. 4 (April 26, 2019): 212–221, doi: 10.4252/wjsc.v11.i4.212/.

59. "Biologic Refractory Rheumatoid Arthritis," Mesoblast, accessed May 8, 2022, https://www.mesoblast.com/product-candidates/immune-mediated-inflammatory-conditions/rheumatoid-arthritis.

60. Luciane de Fátima Caldeira et al., "Fecal Microbiota Transplantation in Inflammatory Bowel Disease Patients: A Systematic Review and Meta-Analysis," *PLoS One* 15, no. 9 (September 18, 2020): e0238910, doi: 10.1371/journal.pone.0238910.

61. Karuna E.W. Vendrik et al., "Fecal Microbiota Transplantation in Neurological Disorders," *Frontiers in Cellular and Infection Microbiology* 10 (March 24, 2020): 98, doi: 10.3389/fcimb .2020.00098.

62. Arthi Chinna Meyyappan et al., "Effect of Fecal Microbiota Transplant on Symptoms of Psychiatric Disorders: A Systematic Review," *BMC Psychiatry* 20, no. 1 (June 15, 2020): 299, doi: 10.1186/s12888-020-02654-5.

Chapter 13

1. Gebriela Leite et al., "The Duodenal Microbiome Is Altered in Small Intestinal Bacterial Overgrowth," *PLoS One* 15, no. 7 (July 9, 2020): e0234906, doi: 10.1371/journal.pone.0234906.

2. Will Takakura and Mark Pimentel, "Small Intestinal Bacterial Overgrowth and Irritable Bowel Syndrome—An Update," *Frontiers in Psychiatry* 11 (July 10, 2020): 664, doi: 10.3389 /fpsyt.2020.00664.

3. Xin Feng and Xiao-Qing Li, "The Prevalence of Small Intestinal Bacterial Overgrowth in Diabetes Mellitus: A Systematic Review and Meta-analysis," *Aging (Albany, NY)* 14, no. 2 (January 27, 2022): 975–998, doi: 10.18632/aging.203854.

4. Erika Ruback Bertges and Júlio Maria Fonseca, "Prevalence and Factors Associated with Small Intestinal Bacterial Overgrowth in Patients with Crohn's Disease: A Retrospective Study at a Referral Center," *Arq Gastrenterol* 57, no. 3 (July–September 2020): 283–288, doi: 10.1590 /S0004-2803.202000000-64.

5. Yongbo Zhang et al., "Prevalence of Small Intestinal Bacterial Overgrowth in Multiple Sclerosis: A Case-Control Study from China," *Journal of Neuroimmunology* 301 (December 15, 2016): 83–87, doi: 10.1016/j.jneuroim.2016.11.004.

6. Jeremy Liu Chen Kiow et al., "High Occurrence of Small Intestinal Bacterial Overgrowth in Primary Biliary Cholangitis," *Journal of Neurogastroenterology and Motility* 31, no. 11 (November 2019): e13691, doi: 10.1111/nmo.13691.

7. Beata Polkowska-Pruszynska et al., "Small Intestinal Bacterial Overgrowth in Systemic Sclerosis: A Review of the Literature," *Archives of Dermatological Research* 311, no. 1 (January 2019): 1–8, doi: 10.1007/s00403-018-1874-0.

8. Melissa A. Nickles et al., "Alternative Treatment Approaches to Small Intestinal Bacterial Overgrowth: A Systematic Review," *Journal of Alternative and Complementary Medicine* 27, no. 2 (February 2021): 108–119, doi: 10.1089/acm.2020.0275.

9. Mahnaz Sandoughi et al., "Effects of Dehydroepiandrosterone on Quality of Life in Premenopausal Women with Rheumatoid Arthritis: A Preliminary Randomized Clinical Trial," *International Journal of Rheumatic Diseases* 23, no. 12 (December 2020): 1692–1697, doi: 10.1111/1756-185X.13975.

10. Jason R. Bobe et al., "Recent Progress in Lyme Disease and Remaining Challenges," *Frontiers in Medicine* 8 (August 18, 2021): 666554, doi: 10.3389/fmed.2021.666554.

11. Paul M. Lantos et al., "Clinical Practice Guidelines by the Infectious Diseases Society of America (IDSA), American Academy of Neurology (AAN), and American College of Rheumatology (ACR): 2020 Guidelines for the Prevention, Diagnosis, and Treatment of Lyme Disease," *Arthritis Care & Research* (Hoboken, NJ) 73, no. 1 (January 2021): 1–9, doi: 10.1002/acr.24495.

12. Daniel J. Cameron et al., "Evidence Assessments and Guideline Recommendations in Lyme Disease: The Clinical Management of Known Tick Bites, *Erythema Migrans* Rashes and Persistent Disease," ILADS, accessed May 8, 2022, https://www.ilads.org/patient-care/ilads-treatment-guidelines/.

13. Michael T. Melia and Paul G. Auwaerter, "Time for a Different Approach to Lyme Disease and Long-Term Symptoms," *The New England Journal of Medicine* 374 (March 31, 2016): 1277–1278, doi: 10.1056/NEJMe1502350.

14. Leena Meriläinen et al., "Morphological and Biochemical Features of *Borrelia Burgdorferi* Pleomorphic Forms," *Microbiology* 161, pt. 3 (March 2015): 516–527, doi: 10.1099/mic.0.000027.

15. Peter Kraiczy, "Hide and Seek: How Lyme Disease Spirochetes Overcome Complement Attack," *Frontiers in Immunology* 7 (September 26, 2016): 385, doi: 10.3389/fimmu.2016.00385.

16. Felipe C. Cabello et al., "*Borreliella Burgdorferi* Antimicrobial-Tolerant Persistence in Lyme Disease and Posttreatment Lyme Disease Syndromes," *mBio* 13, no. 3 (June 28, 2022): e0344021, doi:10.1128/mbio.03440-21.

17. Giuseppe Conte et al., "Mycotoxins in Feed and Food and the Role of Ozone in Their Detoxification and Degradation: An Update," *Toxins (Basel)* 12, no. 8 (July 30, 2020): 486, doi: 10.3390/toxins12080486.

18. Maciej Zelechowski et al., "Patterns of Diversity of *Fusarium* Fungi Contaminating Soybean Grains," *Toxins (Basel)* 13, no. 12 (December 10, 2021): 884, doi: 10.3390/toxins13120884.

19. Michael R. Gray et al., "Mixed Mold Mycotoxicosis: Immunological Changes in Humans Following Exposure in Water-Damaged Buildings," *Archives of Environmental Health* 58, no. 7 (July 1, 2003): 410–420, doi: 10.1080/00039896.2003.11879142.

20. Tamara Tuuminen and Kyösti Sakari Rinne, "Severe Sequelae to Mold-Related Illness as Demonstrated in Two Finnish Cohorts," *Frontiers in Immunology* 8 (April 3, 2017): 382, doi: 10.3389/fimmu.2017.00382.

21. Mohamed Bahie Abou-Donia, Allan Lieberman, and Luke Curtis, "Neural Autoantibodies in Patients with Neurological Symptoms and Histories of Chemical/Mold Exposures," *Toxicology and Industrial Health* 34, no. 1 (January 2018): 44–53, doi: 10.1177/0748233717733852.

22. Andrew W. Campbell et al., "Neural Autoantibodies and Neurophysiologic Abnormalities in Patients Exposed to Molds in Water-Damaged Buildings," *Archives of Environmental Health* 58, no. 8 (August 7, 2010): doi: 10.3200/AEOH.58.8.464-474.

23. William J. Rea et al, "Effects of Toxic Exposure to Molds and Mycotoxins in Building-Related Illnesses," *Archives of Environmental Health* 58, no. 7 (December 9, 2003): 399–405, doi: 10.1080/00039896.2003.11879140.

24. "Environmental Relative Moldiness Index (ERMI)," Environmental Protection Agency, accessed May 25, 2022, https://www.epa.gov/air-research/environmental-relative-moldiness-index-ermi.

25. Robert K. Naviaux, "Metabolic Features of the Cell Danger Response," *Mitochondrion* 16 (May 2014): 7–17, doi: 10.1016/j.mito.2013.08.006.

26. "Acupuncture: In Depth," National Center for Complementary and Integrative Health, accessed May 8, 2022, https://www.nccih.nih.gov/health/acupuncture-in-depth.

27. Jing Wang et al., "Therapeutic Effect and Mechanism of Acupuncture in Autoimmune Diseases," *The American Journal of Chinese Medicine* 50, no. 3 (March 10, 2022): 639–652, doi: 10.1142/S0192415X22500252.

28. Daniel E. Furst et al., "Double-blind, Randomized, Controlled Pilot Study Comparing Classic Ayurvedic Medicine, Methotrexate, and Their Combination in Rheumatoid Arthritis," *Journal of Clinical Rheumatology* 17, no. 4 (June 2011): 185–192, doi: 10.1097/RHU .0b013e31821c0310.

29. Jie Kie Phang et al., "Complementary and Alternative Medicine for Rheumatic Diseases: A Systematic Review of Randomized Controlled Trials," *Complementary Therapies in Medicine* 37 (April 2018): 143–157, doi: 10.1016/j.ctim.2018.03.003.

30. Rajkala P. Patil, Panchakshari D. Patil, Anup B. Thakar, "*Panchakarma* in Autoimmune Pancreatitis: A Single-case Study," *AYU* 40, no. 4 (October–December 2019): 242–246, doi: 10.4103 /ayu.AYU_15_20; Rahul K. Shingadiya et al., "Autoimmune Bullous Skin Disease Managed with Ayurvedic Treatment: A Case Report," *Ancient Science of Life* 36, no. 4 (April–June 2017): 229–233, doi: 10.4103/asl.ASL_91_16.

Chapter 14

1. J. Michael Gaziano et al., "Multivitamins in the Prevention of Cancer in Men: The Physicians' Health Study II Randomized Controlled Trial," *Journal of the American Medical Association* 308, no. 18 (November 14, 2012): 1871–1880, doi: 10.1001/jama.2012.14641.

2. Muhammad Shahzeb Khan et al., "Dietary Interventions and Nutritional Supplements for Heart Failure: A Systematic Appraisal and Evidence Map," *European Journal of Heart Failure* 23, no. 9 (September 2021): 1468–1476, doi: 10.1002/ejhf.2278.

3. Haseeb Ahsan et al., "Pharmacological Potential of Tocotrienols: A Review," *Nutrition & Metabolism (London)* 11, no. 1 (November 12, 2014): 52, doi: 10.1186/1743-7075-11-52.

4. Donald R. Davis, Melvin D. Epp, and Hugh D. Riordan, "Changes in USDA Food Composition Data for 43 Garden Crops, 1950 to 1999," *Journal of the American College of Nutrition* 23, no. 6 (December 23, 2004): 669–682, doi: 10.1080/07315724.2004.10719409.

5. Jayme L. Workinger, Robert P. Doyle, and Jonathan Bortz, "Challenges in the Diagnosis of Magnesium Status," *Nutrients* 10, no. 9 (September 1, 2018): 1202, doi: 10.3390/nu10091202.

6. Alessandro Sanna et al., "Zinc Status and Autoimmunity: A Systematic Review and Meta-Analysis," *Nutrients* 10, no. 1 (January 11, 2018): 68, doi: 10.3390/nu10010068.

7. "Micronutrient Inadequacies in the US Population: An Overview," Oregon State University, accessed November 5, 2021, https://lpi.oregonstate.edu/mic/micronutrient-inadequacies /overview.

8. Workinger, "Challenges in the Diagnosis of Magnesium Status," 1202.

9. Clementina Sitzia et al., "Intra-erythrocytes Magnesium Deficiency Could Reflect Cognitive Impairment Status Due to Vascular Disease: A Pilot Study," *Journal of Translational Medicine* 18 (December 3, 2020): 458, doi: 10.1186/s12967-020-02645-w.

10. Tomoka Ao, Junichi Kikuta, and Masaru Ishii, "The Effects of Vitamin D on Immune System and Inflammatory Diseases," *Biomolecules* 11, no. 11 (November 3, 2021): 1624, doi: 10.3390 /biom11111624.

11. Nipith Charoenngam et al., "Vitamin D and Rheumatic Diseases: A Review of Clinical Evidence," *International Journal of Molecular Sciences* 22, no. 19 (October 1, 2021): 10659, doi: 10.3390/ijms221910659.

12. Jill Hahn et al., "Vitamin D and Marine n-3 Fatty Acid Supplementation and Prevention of Autoimmune Disease in the VITAL Randomized Controlled Trial," *Arthritis & Rheumatology* 73, suppl. 10 (2021), https://acrabstracts.org/abstract/vitamin-d-and-marine-n-3-fatty-acid -supplementation-and-prevention-of-autoimmune-disease-in-the-vital-randomized-controlled -trial/.

13. Nipith Charoenngam, "Vitamin D and Rheumatic Diseases: A Review of Clinical Evidence," *International Journal of Molecular Sciences* 22, no. 19 (October 1, 2021): 10659, doi: /10.3390 /ijms221910659.

14. Workinger, "Challenges in the Diagnosis of Magnesium Status," 1202.

15. Marta Pelczynska, Malgorzata Moszak, and Pawel Bogdanski, "The Role of Magnesium in the Pathogenesis of Metabolic Disorders," *Nutrients* 14, no. 9 (May 2022): 1714, doi: 10.3390 /nu14091714.

16. Jeroen J.F. de Baaij, Joose G.J. Hoenderop, and René J.M. Bindels, "Magnesium in Man: Implications for Health and Disease," *Physiological Reviews* 95, no. 1 (January 2015): 1–46, doi: 10.1152/physrev.00012.2014.

17. Paulina Ihnatowicz et al., "The Importance of Nutritional Factors and Dietary Management of Hashimoto's Thyroiditis," *Annals of Agricultural and Environmental Medicine* 27, no. 2 (June 19, 2020): 184–193, doi: 10.26444/aaem/112331.

18. Ana Kelen Rodrigues, Ana Elisa Melo, and Caroline Pereira Domingueti, "Association Between Reduced Serum Levels of Magnesium and the Presence of Poor Glycemic Control and Complications in Type 1 Diabetes Mellitus: A Systematic Review and Meta-analysis," *Diabetes & Metabolic Syndrome* 14, no. 2 (March–April 2020): 127–134, doi: 10.1016/j.dsx.2020.01.015.

19. May M. Cheung et al., "The Effect of Combined Magnesium and Vitamin D Supplementation on Vitamin D Status, Systemic Inflammation, and Blood Pressure: A Randomized Double-Blinded Controlled Trial," *Nutrition* 99-100 (July–August 2022): 111674, doi: 10.1016/j .nut.2022.111674.

20. "Magnesium: Fact Sheet for Health Professionals," National Institutes of Health, Office of Dietary Supplements, accessed May 17, 2022, https://ods.od.nih.gov/factsheets/Magnesium -HealthProfessional/.

21. Marta R. Pardo et al., "Bioavailability of Magnesium Food Supplements: A Systematic Review," *Nutrition* 89 (September 2021): 111294, doi: 10.1016/j.nut.2021.111294.

22. Alessandro Sanna et al., "Zinc Status and Autoimmunity: A Systematic Review and Meta-Analysis," *Nutrients* 10, no. 1 (January 11, 2018): 68, doi: 10.3390/nu10010068.

23. Jennifer Kaltenberg et al., "Zinc Signals Promote IL-2-Dependent Proliferation of T Cells," *European Journal of Immunology* 40, no. 5 (May 2010): 1496–1503, doi: 10.1002/eji.200939574.

24. Elahe Nirooei et al., "Blood Trace Element Status in Multiple Sclerosis: A Systematic Review and Meta-analysis," *Biological Trace Element Research* 200, no. 1 (January 2022): 13–26, doi: 10.1007/s12011-021-02621-5.

25. Paulina Ihnatowicz et al., "The Importance of Nutritional Factors and Dietary Management of Hashimoto's Thyroiditis," *Annals of Agricultural and Environmental Medicine* 27, no. 2 (June 19, 2020): 184–193, doi: 10.26444/aaem/112331.

26. Sanna, "Zinc Status and Autoimmunity," 68.

27. Sanna, "Zinc Status and Autoimmunity," 68.

28. Cuong D. Tran et al., "Zinc-fortified Oral Rehydration Solution Improved Intestinal Permeability and Small Intestinal Mucosal Recovery," *Clinical Pediatrics (Philadelphia)* 54, no. 7 (June 2015): 676–682, doi: 10.1177/0009922814562665.

29. "Zinc: Fact Sheet for Health Professionals," National Institutes of Health, Office of Dietary Supplements, accessed July 12, 2022, https://ods.od.nih.gov/factsheets/Zinc-HealthProfessional/.

30. Dina C. Simes et al., "Vitamin K as a Diet Supplement with Impact in Human Health: Current Evidence in Age-Related Diseases," *Nutrients* 12, no. 1 (January 2020): 138, doi: 10.3390/nu12010138.

31. Katarzyna Maresz, "Growing Evidence of a Proven Mechanism Shows Vitamin K2 Can Impact Health Conditions Beyond Bone and Cardiovascular," *Integrative Medicine: A Clinician's Journal* 20, no. 4 (August 2021): 34–38, https://www.ncbi.nlm.nih.gov/pmc/articles /PMC8483258/.

32. Meiyu Zhang, "Vitamin K2 Suppresses Proliferation and Inflammatory Cytokine Production in Mitogen-Activated Lymphocytes of Atopic Dermatitis Patients through the Inhibition of Mitogen-Activated Protein Kinases," *Biological and Pharmaceutical Bulletin* 44, no. 1 (2021): 7–17, doi: 10.1248/bpb.b20-00079.

33. Leon J. Schurgers and Cees Vermeer, "Determination of Phylloquinone and Menaquinones in Food. Effect of Food Matrix on Circulating Vitamin K Concentrations," *Haemostasis* 30, no. 6 (November–December 2000): 298–307, doi:10.1159/000054147.

34. Xueyan Fu et al., "Measurement of Multiple Vitamin K Forms in Processed and Fresh-Cut Pork Products in the U.S. Food Supply," *Journal of Agricultural and Food Chemistry* 64, no. 22 (June 8, 2016), doi: 10.1021/acs.jafc.6b00938.

35. Sonya J. Elder et al., "Vitamin K Contents of Meat, Dairy, and Fast Food in the U.S. Diet," *Journal of Agricultural and Food Chemistry* 54, no. 2 (December 27, 2005): 463–467, doi: 10.1021/jf052400h.

36. Kazumasa Hirauchi et al., "Measurement of K Vitamins in Animal Tissues by High-Performance Liquid Chromatography with Fluorimetric Detection," *Journal of Chromotography* 497 (December 29, 1989): 131–137, doi: 10.1016/0378-4347(89)80012-x.

37. K. Hojo et al., "Quantitative Measurement of Tetrahydromenaquinone-9 in Cheese Fermented by Propionibacteria," *Journal of Dairy Science* 90, no. 9 (September 2007): 4078–4083, doi: 10.3168/jds.2006-892.

38. Xiaoxi Li et al., "Therapeutic Potential of ω-3 Polyunsaturated Fatty Acids in Human Autoimmune Diseases," *Frontiers in Immunology* 10 (September 27, 2019): 2241, doi: 10.3389 /fimmu.2019.02241.

39. William S. Harris and Clemens Von Schacky, "The Omega-3 Index: A New Risk Factor for Death from Coronary Heart Disease?", *Preventive Medicine* 39, no. 1 (July 2004): 212–220, doi: 10.1016/j.ypmed.2004.02.030.

40. Aleix Sala-Vila et al., "Red Blood Cell DHA Is Inversely Associated with Risk of Incident Alzheimer's Disease and All-Cause Dementia: Framingham Offspring Study," *Nutrients* 14, no 12 (2022): 2408, doi: 10.3390/nu14122408.

41. Michael I. McBurney et al., "Using an Erythrocyte Fatty Acid Fingerprint to Predict Risk of All-cause Mortality: The Framingham Offspring Cohort," *The American Journal of Clinical Nutrition* 114, no. 4 (October 2021): 1447–1454, doi: 10.1093/ajcn/nqab195.

42. Xiaoxi Li, "Therapeutic Potential of ω-3 Polyunsaturated Fatty Acids," 2241.

43. "Physical Activity for Different Groups," Centers for Disease Control and Prevention, accessed June 21, 2022, https://www.cdc.gov/physicalactivity/basics/age-chart.html.

44. Jinbing Bai, Yi-Juan Hu, and Deborah Watkins Bruner, "Composition of Gut Microbiota and Its Association with Body Mass Index and Lifestyle Factors in a Cohort of 7–18 Years Old Children from the American Gut Project," *Pediatric Obesity* 14, no. 4 (November 11, 2018), doi: 10.1111/ijpo.12480.

45. Siobhan F. Clarke et al., "Exercise and Associated Dietary Extremes Impact on Gut Microbial Diversity," *Gut* 63, no. 12 (December 2014): 1913–1920, doi: 10.1136/gutjnl-2013-306541.

46. Hassane Zouhal et al., "Effects of Exercise Training on Anabolic and Catabolic Hormones with Advanced Age: A Systematic Review," *Sports Medicine* 52, no. 6 (June 2022): 1353–1368, doi: 10.1007/s40279-021-01612-9.

47. Pedro Lopez et al., "Benefits of Resistance Training in Physically Frail Elderly: A Systematic Review," *Aging Clinical and Experimental Research* 30, no. 8 (August 2018): 889–899, doi: 10.1007/s40520-017-0863-z.

48. Ana Kovacevic et al., "The Effect of Resistance Exercise on Sleep: A Systematic Review of Randomized Controlled Trials," *Sleep Medicine Reviews* 39 (June 2018): 52–68, doi: 10.1016/j.smrv.2017.07.002.

49. Hidde P. van der Ploeg et al., "Sitting Time and All-Cause Mortality Risk in 222497 Australian Adults," *Archives of Internal Medicine* 172, no. 6 (March 26, 2012): 494–500, doi: 10.1001/archinternmed.2011.2174.

50. Alpa V. Patel et al., "Leisure Time Spent Sitting in Relation to Total Mortality in a Prospective Cohort of US Adults," *American Journal of Epidemiology* 172, no. 4 (August 15, 2010): 419–429, doi: 10.1093/aje/kwq155.

51. Bethany J. Howard et al., "Associations of Overall Sitting Time and TV Viewing Time with Fibrinogen and C Reactive Protein: The Ausdiab Study," *British Journal of Sports Medicine* 49, no. 4 (February 2015): 255–258, doi: 10.1136/bjsports-2013-093014.

52. Genevieve N. Healy et al., "Sedentary Time and Cardio-Metabolic Biomarkers in US Adults: NHANES 2003–06," *European Heart Journal* 32, no. 5 (March 2011): 590–597, doi: 10.1093/eurheartj/ehq451.

53. Elin Ekblom-Bak, Mai-Lis Hellénius, and Björn Ekblom, "Are We Facing a New Paradigm of Inactivity Physiology?", *British Journal of Sports Medicine* 44, no. 12 (n.d.), doi: 10.1136/bjsm.2009.067702.

54. John D. Akins et al., "Inactivity Induces Resistance to the Metabolic Benefits Following Acute Exercise," *Journal of Applied Physiology* 126, no. 4 (April 1, 2019): 1088–1094, doi: 10.1152/japplphysiol.00968.2018.

55. Joan Vernikos, *Sitting Kills, Moving Heals* (Fresno: Linden Publishing, 2011).

Index

About the Author

Akil Palanisamy, MD, is a Harvard-trained physician who practices integrative medicine, blending his conventional medical expertise with holistic approaches including functional medicine and Ayurveda. "Dr. Akil" attended Harvard University and graduated magna cum laude with a Bachelor of Arts in biochemical sciences. He earned an MD from the University of California, San Francisco (UCSF) and completed family medicine residency training at Stanford University. He then graduated from a fellowship in integrative medicine with Dr. Andrew Weil at the University of Arizona, and received certification in mind-body medicine from the Georgetown University Center.

Dr. Akil is the Department Chair for Integrative Medicine at the Sutter Health Institute for Health and Healing (IHH). He also serves as IHH Physician Director for Community Education and leads their educational initiatives and programs. Dr. Akil has been a consultant with the Medical Board of California for many years.

A widely known speaker and educator, he is the author of *The Paleovedic Diet: A Complete Program to Burn Fat, Increase Energy, and Reverse Disease*. As he has done for over two decades, Dr. Akil sees patients and conducts clinical research studies in the San Francisco Bay Area. In his free time, he enjoys playing tennis, traveling, and spending time with his wife and daughter.

3